THE
TESTOSTERONE
OPTIMIZATION
THERAPY
BIBLE

THE ULTIMATE GUIDE
TO LIVING A FULLY
OPTIMIZED LIFE

JAY CAMPBELL & JIM BROWN

Published by Best Seller Publishing®, Pasadena, CA
Best Seller Publishing® is a registered trademark
Printed in the United States of America.
ISBN 978-1-946978-53-0

This publication is designed to provide accurate and authoritative information with regard to the subject matter covered. It is sold with the understanding that the publisher is not engaged in rendering legal, accounting, or other professional advice. If legal advice or other expert assistance is required, the services of a competent professional should be sought. The opinions expressed by the authors in this book are not endorsed by Best Seller Publishing® and are the sole responsibility of the author rendering the opinion.

Most Best Seller Publishing® titles are available at special quantity discounts for bulk purchases for sales promotions, premiums, fundraising, and educational use. Special versions or book excerpts can also be created to fit specific needs.

For more information, please write:
Best Seller Publishing®
1346 Walnut Street, #205
Pasadena, CA 91106
or call 1(626) 765 9750
Toll Free: 1(844) 850-3500
Visit us online at: www.BestSellerPublishing.org

Praise for The TOT Bible

I doubt there is a single disease, disorder, or deficiency that doctors haven't managed to confuse, complicate, and coerce into conforming to their belief that "their way is the best way." Nowhere is this hubris more apparent and problematic than in hormone optimization therapy. With Jay and Jim's *The TOT Bible*, order has been brought to the chaos and clarity to the confusion. Based on years of experience, tens of thousands of hours of research, and hundreds of interviews with the top thought leaders in TOT, Jay and Jim have successfully synthesized the true best practices into a clear and concise resource that should occupy every man's (patient and physician's) library.

Jim Meehan, MD
Chief Medical Officer, BodMD, PC

Every now and then a book is published that literally can and will change the trajectory of your life. The *TOT Bible: The Ultimate Guide to Living a Fully Optimized Life* is a must read for the physician and the patient. The field of interventional endocrinology has advanced dramatically in the past decade, exposing the numerous subtleties required for expert hormone replacement therapy. Jay and Jim have interviewed and assembled powerful insights into this field of endeavor, giving you, the reader, their years of expertise and authoritarian information that brings you to the pinnacle of TOT. Insights from numerous thought leaders with decades of clinical experience will educate, inform and enlighten. Welcome to the "Tip of the Spear"!

Rob Kominiarek, D.O., FACOFP
Founder ReNue Health

Jay Campbell's *The TOT Bible* serves as both a primer and a DEEP DIVE that supersedes much of the academic writing out there. Our practitioners have mirrored many of the ideas from the book with tremendous and life-changing effects to our clients.

Aaron Grossman, MD
Founder and President of CHEKD.com,
Leading Expert in Health Optimization.

With *The TOT Bible*, Jay Campbell has created an avenue for all men to begin to enjoy a more healthy and fulfilling life. Medicine today is literally incapable of producing a reference text with the information Jay has compiled. He seeks the truth through science and real life clinical data/experience. Traditional medicine is a victim of its own system, and it takes true compassionate practitioners like Jay to convey the message of testosterone's crucial role in optimizing men's health. Anyone interested in maximizing his healthspan needs to read this book. His message is strong and clear. The real world guidance he provides is precisely what is needed to begin to "right your own ship" of health and wellness.

H. Merrill Matschke, MD
Board Certified Urologist and Fellowship trained expert in Andrology/
Men's Sexual Health & Wellness. BetterHealthCarolinas.com

What I REALLY like about my good friend Jay Campbell's book is it covers ALL areas of men's health; not just the Interventional Endocrinology, but also diet, supplementation, exercise, and the "anti's": anti-inflammation, anti-cancer and anti-heart disease. It's truly a one stop shopping manual for the man who wants to optimize his health and happiness....from a guy who is the best living example of his own great advice!

John Crisler, D.O., Age Management Medicine
Founder of AllThingsMale.com

The Testosterone Optimization Therapy Bible by Jay Campbell and Jim Brown is the most comprehensive, up to date, and insightful book on this exciting and very important topic. For men interested in health and longevity, combined with the willingness to take control of their destiny, this book is an absolute must read. The information herein is well written, easy to read, scientifically informative, and can be appreciated by non-physicians and physicians alike.

Christopher Foucher, MD
Clinical Associate Professor at MSU-COM's
Anesthesiology Residency Program

Jay Campbell's knowledge in testosterone optimization therapy is simply stunning. His books gave me such great and practical advice to use with my patients. The wisdom he shares is profound, offering a much better quality of life and increased longevity. I have recommended his book to every single Age Management Practicing Doctor I know in South America.

Vicente Coutinho, MD, VPC
Integrative Medicine Clinic, São Paulo Brazil

The Testosterone Optimization Therapy Bible, written by Jay Campbell and Jim Brown, should be read by any man who seeks to achieve optimal health. He brilliantly explains the benefits and risks of testosterone replacement therapy (TOT) in a way that is easy to understand, yet it has depth. I have noticed in my practice that the men who have read this book are extremely knowledgeable about TOT, and it actually makes my interaction much easier as they are already educated patients. I decided to read the book as a result of my patients raving about it. Though I am very experienced with prescribing TOT, I actually picked up many pearls from reading it. This book is a must read for patients as well as physicians!

Lynese Lawson, D.O.
Founder of Pro-Active Wellness Centers Vienna Virginia

The Testosterone Optimization Therapy Bible is the real deal. It gives the reader years of medical research, experience from the gym and a real world, yet scientific understanding of TOT, delivered in a format which will help anyone wanting to help themselves. Jay and Jim's book is THE resource manual for professionals, strength trainers, athletes and anyone else wanting to utilize testosterone safely and in the context of long term health.

Leonard A. Farber, MD
Clinical Director of Radiation Oncology of Lower Manhattan
The Farber Center for Radiation Oncology

Jay Campbell, in *The Testosterone Optimization Therapy Bible,* has synthesized a vast body of evidence, as well as the extensive experience of countless doctors and other professionals, into a concise, understandable, and immediately applicable manual. Whether you are a man in need of direction in the much misaligned and misinformed arena of TOT, or a physician interested in doing a better job for your patients, this book is written precisely for you. Read it, reference it and put it into practice.

James D. Dickie, MD
Leader in Age Management Medicine and Hormone
Replacement. Founder of UnstoppableLife.net

Jay Campbell has been a visionary in men's health for nearly two decades. His passion and commitment to help people navigate the broken medical system comes shining through in his new must read book *The TOT Bible: The Ultimate Guide to Living a Fully Optimized Life.*

Russ Scala
Founder, The Institute of Nutritional Medicine
and Cardiovascular Research

If you're looking to obtain, and maintain, youth, strength and sexual vitality as you age, Jay Campbell is the man you need to listen to. *The TOT Bible* provides a clear cut blueprint on how to optimize hormone levels for health, performance and freedom from the ills of aging. Don't succumb to old age gracefully — fight it tooth and nail! This book will show you how.

Nelson Montana
Author-The Bodybuilding Truth, Writer for Muscle & Fitness, Muscular Development, Iron Man and Testosterone Nation

The concept of "health" has become compartmentalized by the modern fitness and medical fields to be narrow definitions of exercises, diets, and normal range lab tests. Regarding hormonal health and the role of testosterone, there has been a dearth of quality information available, and millions of men operate today in total ignorance of how their own hormones are affecting their daily well being. What Jay has done with *The Testosterone Optimization Therapy Bible* is create an unparalleled, holistic resource that synthesizes the science, data, and real world evidence into a practical guide for all men everywhere to understand and take control of their health on all fronts. Any man with this guide is no longer in the dark about what optimal health means. *The TOT Bible* provides the tools to create that for himself.

Alexander Juan Antonio Cortes
Writer, Author, Top 10 Most Influential Fitness Writer

Inspiring is Jay's knowledge of hormone replacement and human physiology, which surpasses that of many of my medical colleagues. This he brings to you, the reader, in the pages of his much-needed and timely opus. Open your eyes, read and digest Jay's words. This book is the chapter that I was scared to write.

Brett Osborn, MD

Diplomate, American Board of Neurological Surgery Diplomate, American Academy of Anti-Aging Medicine CSCS, National Strength and Conditioning Association, Author of *Get Serious, A Neurosurgeon's Guide To Optimal Health and Fitness*

The Testosterone Optimization Therapy Bible presents practical information about the best ways to maximize benefits and minimize side effects of testosterone replacement therapy. It accomplishes this goal in the most visually appealing way I have ever seen in this field. This book is an enjoyable and highly empowering read for any man who wants to take charge of his health and quality of life.

Nelson Vergel, CEO

ExcelMale.com and DiscountedLabs.com, Author of *Testosterone: A Man's Guide: Practical Tips For Boosting Physical, Mental and Sexual Vitality*

If there's one thing the health care debate has made clear, it's that everyone is ultimately responsible for their own health and wellness. And for men today, that includes educating themselves on the growing epidemic of low testosterone. In *The TOT Bible*, Jay Campbell and Jim Brown break down the causes, symptoms, and available treatment modalities for low testosterone, and how to work with your physician to obtain the safest, most effective care available. This book is a must-read for every man who wants to live up to his full potential.

Bryan Krahn CSCS

National Strength and Conditioning Association, Writer for Men's Health, Bodybuilding.com and AskMen.com.

The TOT Bible by Jay Campbell and Jim Brown is an excellent source of information regarding the basics of hormonal optimization. The text is written in a very engaging yet simple form, allowing the beginner to understand the hormonal aspects of hypogonadism. I highly recommend it for any man who wishes to change his quality of life especially moving into middle age. I have to admit that my supervisor, who is a general pathologist, found it really informative.

George Touliatos, MD

Biopathology Specialist, expert on medical prevention regarding PEDs use in sports. Medical Contributor for Anabolics 11th edition (2017), Writer for Anabolic.org, Musclemag & Muscular Development magazines.

Jay Campbell and Jim Brown's *The TOT Bible: The Ultimate Guide to Living a Fully Optimized Life,* delivers a punch to the face of hormonophobia governing modern societies around the globe. Critical aspects of male interventional endocrinology are broken down and explained in a simple, clear, enjoyable and highly educative manner. Jay Campbell's commitment, accompanied by his vast knowledge in the testosterone optimization therapy field, resulted in the creation of a helpful and applicable hormonal optimization tool for both patients and physicians. Every single man dreaming of an ultimate optimized everyday life should get their hands on this manual as quickly as possible. Aging has finally met its match.

Nick Sakkas, DVM, MD, PhD

Candidate in Molecular Endocrinology, School of Medicine, University of Ioannina, Greece.

Jay Campbell's *The TOT Bible: The Ultimate Guide to Living a Fully Optimized Life,* is a must read for all physicians interested in optimizing the health of their male patients and for any patients looking to live a life full of vitality. This book serves as a guide for all men who desire to take responsibility for their own health, acquire the right knowledge to help them make the right decisions, and want to be cutting edge. Our modernized environment is sabotaging our hormone balances. A proactive approach to living an optimized life as outlined in the pages of this book serves as the ultimate resource for men.

Bob Harding, D.O.
Men's Integrative and Functional Medicine Physician, Austin, Texas

I have nothing but praise for Jay Campbell's book, *The Testosterone Optimization Therapy Bible*. As an Age Management Physician, I was quite impressed with the context, format and well referenced chapters. Without reservation, I feel this book is a must have for any physician or male patient interested in OPTIMAL healthy aging for lifespan quality as well as quantity in years.

Stephen M. Ellestad, D.O.

Table of Contents

Disclaimer

(1) Introduction

This disclaimer governs the use of this book. [By using this book, you accept this disclaimer in full. / We will ask you to agree to this disclaimer before you can access the book.] No part of this book may be reproduced in any written, electronic, recording, or photocopying without written permission of the publisher or authors. All trademarks are the exclusive property of TRTRevolution.com

(2) Credit

This disclaimer was created using an SEQ Legal template.

(3) No advice

The book contains information about Testosterone Optimization Therapy. The information is not advice, and should not be treated as such. You must not rely on the information in the book as an alternative to medical advice from an appropriately qualified professional. If you have any specific questions about any matter you should consult an appropriately qualified medical professional. If you think you may be suffering from any medical condition you should seek immediate medical attention. You should never delay seeking medical advice, disregard medical advice, or discontinue medical treatment because of information in this book

(4) No representations or warranties

To the maximum extent permitted by applicable law and subject to section 6 below, we exclude all representations, warranties, undertakings and guarantees relating to the book. Without prejudice to the generality of the foregoing paragraph, we do not represent, warrant, undertake or guarantee:

- that the information in the book is correct, accurate, complete or non-misleading;

- that the use of the guidance in the book will lead to any particular outcome or result;

(5) Limitations and exclusions of liability

The limitations and exclusions of liability set out in this section and elsewhere in this disclaimer: are subject to section 6 below; and govern all liabilities arising under the disclaimer or in relation to the book, including liabilities arising in contract, in tort (including negligence) and for breach of statutory duty. We will not be liable to you in respect of any losses arising out of any event or events beyond our reasonable control. We will not be liable to you in respect of any business losses, including without limitation loss of or damage to profits, income, revenue, use, production, anticipated savings, business, contracts, commercial opportunities or goodwill. We will not be liable to you in respect of any loss or corruption of any data, database or software. We will not be liable to you in respect of any special, indirect or consequential loss or damage.

(6) Exceptions
Nothing in this disclaimer shall: limit or exclude our liability for death or personal injury resulting from negligence; limit or exclude our liability for fraud or fraudulent misrepresentation; limit any of our liabilities in any way that is not permitted under applicable law; or exclude any of our liabilities that may not be excluded under applicable law.

(7) Severability
If a section of this disclaimer is determined by any court or other competent authority to be unlawful and/or unenforceable, the other sections of this disclaimer continue in effect.

If any unlawful and/or unenforceable section would be lawful or enforceable if part of it were deleted, that part will be deemed to be deleted, and the rest of the section will continue in effect.

(8) Law and jurisdiction
This disclaimer will be governed by and construed in accordance with law in the United States of America, and any disputes relating to this disclaimer will be subject to the exclusive jurisdiction of the courts of the United States of America. Testosterone is classified as a controlled substance under the Anabolic Steroids Control Act of 1990 and has been assigned to Schedule III. It is regulated by the Drug Enforcement Agency (DEA).The use of testosterone is illegal in the United States for those without a valid medical diagnosis and prescription justifying their use.

(9) Our details
In this disclaimer, "we" means (and "us" and "our" refer to) Jay Campbell (Southern California, USA) and Jim Brown (South Florida, USA) and or any future addresses, temporary or permanent.

Acknowledgments

This is the most challenging aspect of writing a book. Because there are so many people who have profoundly influenced our lives, it would be impossible to acknowledge and thank them all. But we have to start somewhere.

First, we could not have attempted to write this book, let alone finish it, without the help of the greatest things that ever happened to us—our wives—Monica Campbell and Rosie Brown. Their enormous self-sacrifice and encouragement compelled us to do and be more in every aspect of our lives, this book included. Through their example, we've both learned the greatest form of acceptance—unyielding and unwavering love and gratitude.

Second, heartfelt praise and gratitude to Joshua Smith, our business partner and mentor whose internet marketing mastery is allowing us to change the face of the sports supplement and hormonal optimization industries.

To doctors Jim Meehan, John Crisler, Merrill Matschke, Rob Kominiarek, Aaron Grossman, Brett Osborn and Joseph Cruise, whose visions are creating a personalized health care revolution. To Nelson Vergel for being the original torchbearer and passionate men's health advocate. To Natalie Minh for her uncanny wisdom and creative insights into the Fitness space. To Binais Begovic for providing us the global platform to extend our knowledge. To Matt Lawrence for his design skill and website architecture expertise. To Humbert Glaffo for his amazing cover artwork.

To all our families, friends and social media and forum brothers, ex-wives, girlfriends, clients, and fitness industry peers, thank you for the assistance and intel you provided in our times together while researching this material for more than 25 years.

Last but not least, thanks to our editing team and dear friends Tom Zakharov, Alexander Cortes, Daniel Kelly, Michael Kocsis and Austin Gunter for their editorial oversight and help turning this book into the bible of total life optimization.

This book is dedicated to Lee Myer, the amazing and devoted husband and father who also founded PeakTestosterone.com.

Lee was killed in a tragic car accident while picking up his children from school in January of 2018. He was a man who toiled in the shadows for years when Therapeutic Testosterone was not accepted in the public eye. His website was responsible for educating millions of of men unable to get proper care and treatment from the Medical profession. Much of his research and work guided me in writing both of my books.

I only wish I could have met him in person. Both Jim and I are humbly indebted to him for his sharp wit and excellent evidence based research. May he rest in peace.

Foreword

I'm incredibly honored to have the opportunity to write the foreword for this amazing book! My good friends Jay Campbell and Jim Brown, along with the content inside this book, have completely changed my life. I would like to share my story about how all of it happened.

In my early 20s, I lost my health. As a teenager, I was in good shape and working out was a large part of my life. Then, in my early 20s, I became seriously depressed and stopped taking care of my health. Before I knew it, I had gained over 100 pounds of pure fat and was morbidly obese. After a couple years of going down this path, I decided that it wasn't for me. I made a firm commitment to my health and lost the weight through hard work and patience.

Despite successfully losing 118 pounds, I wasn't doing any physical activity. At that point, I was what Jay refers to as "skinny fat." I was skinny with very little muscle and moderately high levels of body fat. That's not the outcome I wanted, so I decided to turn that around by working out with weights and eating an extremely clean diet. During this process, I started realizing how much internal damage I had done to my body from being morbidly obese and consuming so much junk food.

Fast forward to 2015, where I am now 33 years old. I am working out with weights 5 times per week, doing cardio at least 4 times per week and I am eating extremely clean. When I say that I was eating extremely clean, I am talking about eating nothing but "organic" foods, juicing greens and taking all the right supplements. According to my family doctor, I was in absolutely amazing health. All's well that ends well, right?

Not quite, because there was still one major issue: My energy levels were HORRIBLE. How could someone at 33 years old be in 'absolutely amazing health' but still feel awful at the same time? For the life of me, I could not figure out why I had low energy, low sex drive and high levels of brain fog. I thought it was because I was an entrepreneur who ran several busy companies at once, while taking care of 3 young kids at home. As much as I tried to accept this condition, there was still a burning feeling inside of me that said "This is not right, I should have more energy and feel better."

I refused to accept that my low energy levels were due to old age, or my current stage of life. Luckily, that's when I was first introduced to Jay Campbell. We were initially introduced by a mutual friend and had scheduled a 15-minute call to talk. That 15-minute call quickly turned into a 3-hour conversation that ultimately changed the course of my life.

Jay told me that all the symptoms I was experiencing were because of low testosterone levels. To be completely honest, I didn't want to believe him. Being a grown adult man, I immediately correlated low testosterone levels with poor performance in the bedroom. Of course, like most men, I thought "Nope, I'm good in that department." And having adopted such an "organic lifestyle," I refused to put "chemicals" into my body.

Fortunately, Jay and I quickly developed a close friendship, probably because we are both entrepreneurs and have a lot in common. Every day, I thank God that he did not give up on convincing me to get my blood work done and my testosterone levels checked.

Several months later, I finally got to that level of frustration that most of us get to when we're ready to make a change in our lives. I called up Jay, asked him where I should go to get my testosterone levels checked, and followed his instructions. One week later, I got my blood work back and I was SHOCKED! My testosterone levels weren't just low: At the ripe age of 33, I had the testosterone levels of a healthy 80-year-old man!

I couldn't believe it! Getting those test results back was a harsh yet eye-opening experience for me. With this realization in hand, I was finally ready to listen and apply everything Jay had been telling me for months.

I began working with a progressive physician and was prescribed something called "Testosterone Optimization Therapy." Within 2 weeks, I felt like an entirely new man. I had massive amounts of energy, insane amounts of mental clarity, and zero brain fog. My sex drive was back, and I found myself sexually desiring my wife again! Not only that, but my performance in the gym also skyrocketed and I was CRUSHING all of my workouts!

Before following the protocols described in this book, I was only having sex a couple of times a month. I just chalked it up to being an extremely busy entrepreneur, having 3 young kids at home. I would never have imagined it was due to low testosterone levels.

Looking back on all this, it makes me wonder how many marriages are needlessly wrecked due to men having low testosterone levels. They still find their wives to be attractive, but they just don't "want" her in the way that they used to. Sadly, the wives end up finding the attention they desire somewhere else. I was extremely fortunate to discover this issue and fix it before it became a real deal-breaking problem inside my own marriage. If you are reading this book now, you owe it to yourself and your wife to avoid becoming yet another broken marriage statistic.

Fast-forward a few months from this discovery, and Jay introduces me to his mentor Jim Brown. Hands down, Jim is one of the most brilliant individuals I have ever met! I have never met anyone that has his insane amount of knowledge about the human body, how it works and how to live a truly optimized lifestyle. In addition to everything I had learned and adopted from Jay, I started adopting the workout protocols, nutrition plans and supplementation protocols that Jim was teaching me. So far, the results have been nothing short of life-changing!

By following the protocols that Jay and Jim discuss in this book, along with the "Metabolic Blowtorch Diet" (their Amazon bestseller on optimizing intermittent fasting, get your FREE COPY at MetabolicBlowTorchDiet.com), I can honestly say that every aspect of my life has improved. I am a much better husband, father and entrepreneur than I ever thought was possible. My energy, my focus, the way I feel and the way I look - all of these things continue to improve on a daily basis.

At the end of the day, it is entirely up to each and every one of us to become proactive and take our health into our own hands. The government isn't going to do it for you, and neither will your family doctor. The simple fact is this: NOBODY is going to do it for you. It is up to you to take full ownership of your health and live what Jay and Jim refer to as a "fully optimized life."

Personally, I don't want to go through my life with 'good' health. I want to have EXCEPTIONAL health and have the energy and stamina to do the things I want to do, regardless of my age.

When you read this amazing book, I truly hope that you take the time to learn the information and apply it. I want you to understand it at a personal level so that you can take the MASSIVE action needed to transform your own life, ultimately giving you the life you truly want and deserve!

A personal note to the authors: Jay Campbell and Jim Brown, you have both had such a profound impact on my life that I can never personally thank you enough. Not just for changing my life, but for the amazing impact you have on so many others!

I truly appreciate and love you both!

Joshua Smith, CEO
Perfect Storm, Revisto Real Estate, GSDMode.com
and Co-Owner of TRT Revolution LLC and
Optimized Life Nutrition

INTRODUCTION
The Unapologetic Truth About Testosterone

We live in some interesting times for men. Our bodies are fragile and aging prematurely from the constant assault of urban environments, poor nutrition, and sedentary lifestyles, and this is causing many men to question their own masculinity. Is it any wonder our role in Western society is being questioned as well? These are not disconnected phenomena. Male health is faltering and too many men are living lives of quiet desperation, wishing for their weak bodies to become fit, wondering where their zest for life went, and abandoning any thought of ever getting it back.

But there is hope. The research has never been clearer, not only about how how male bodies are being destroyed by our modern environments and lifestyles, but ALSO how proven medical therapies can reverse the trend and return men to lives of vitality and contribution. In this book, we provide you with the scientifically proven method for optimizing the most important hormone in your body: Testosterone. And by the time you're done reading, you'll understand why optimizing your testosterone will transform your body, mind, and spirit.

Make no mistake, this book is about much more than undergoing testosterone therapy for purely physical or cosmetic reasons. We're going to show you how to optimize your testosterone, *and your entire life*. Throughout this book, we will emphasize that testosterone therapy is a complete lifestyle, and is much more than simply taking a therapeutic dose of testosterone under your doctor's care. Rather than simply viewing it as Testosterone *Replacement* Therapy, we invite you to make the shift and begin to see it as Testosterone *Optimization* Therapy **(TOT)**.

Why?

Observant readers will note that much of the literature around testosterone therapy to date uses the term "Testosterone Replacement Therapy (TRT)." In this book, we put an end to that acronym for good. The idea of *replacing* "normal" testosterone levels in a world where the average man has suboptimal and consistently declining natural levels of testosterone makes no sense. This book goes far beyond merely replacing anything. This book is about optimizing testosterone levels in order for men to reach peak levels of health.

As a result, we will exclusively use the term **Testosterone Optimization Therapy** (TOT) throughout the book, and say with absolute confidence that if you use our book as a guide while working closely with the right physician, you will reach levels of health beyond anything you believed could be possible for you.

And whether you're already convinced of the merits of **TOT**, or just starting to learn about the foundational role testosterone plays in your life, there is a single fact that bears repeating:

Testosterone is what makes men, MEN.

If you are one of the seekers who has already experienced the indisputable benefits of therapeutic testosterone, this book will educate you on the latest and most cutting-edge science behind TOT. We analyze and dissect the best testosterone optimization protocols so that you can make the most informed decision possible when working with a progressive physician and/or when designing your own customized testosterone therapy protocol.

Alternatively, you may be one of the millions of men whose natural testosterone levels have declined so dramatically that your zest for life no longer exists. Whether you're in your 20s, your 30s, or even approaching "middle age," you wonder if you are destined to spend the rest of your life feeling lousy, tired, and lethargic. Deep down, you know you don't have to, and that's why you've picked up this book.

As you read the book, you'll see how TOT is the paradigm-changing solution you need for living an exciting and purposeful life. And we should know: We have been living the pursuit of optimization for close to 30 years. We have tinkered, experimented, played human guinea pig, and bio-hacked our way to the physical and spiritual manifestation of OPTIMIZED MEN. Doing the work on ourselves has afforded us the opportunity to give back and help countless men around the world radically optimize and ultimately transform their lives.

In writing this book, we have 3 goals in mind to help men achieve this testosterone-fueled vision for themselves:

First, we want to stop men from being deceived by false claims from supplement companies selling ineffective testosterone booster supplements. We will demonstrate that there is no scientifically proven way to meaningfully raise your testosterone levels, other than through TOT.

Second, we want to offer the world THE definitive resource guide for all men seeking knowledge of legitimate testosterone products, testosterone optimization therapy, and everything that it entails. This book is your bible for truly living a testosterone-optimized lifestyle.

Finally, we want men to fully understand the greater sociopolitical climate and the controversy manufactured by the media to frame "testosterone" as taboo and polarizing. When men fully understand the false social narratives, it will become easier to fight the good fight and seize their natural potential.

Chapter Summaries

Here's what we'll cover, chapter-by-chapter, in this book.

Chapter 1 - Why Men are Losing Their Masculinity in the 21st Century shows you why so many men around the world have become emasculated, along with the importance of taking accountability for your health by working with a progressive physician.

Chapter 2 - Why Optimizing Your Blood Testosterone Levels Will Transform Your Physique is a deep dive into the physical benefits of optimizing your blood testosterone levels. You will discover how therapeutic testosterone serves to improve health in every system of the body.

Chapter 3 - The Power of Testosterone to Transform Your Life takes the previous chapter one step further by providing the intimate details on how optimal blood testosterone levels can literally transform every aspect of your life beyond the physical, from your personal affairs to growing your business.

Chapter 4 - The Natural Testosterone Boosting Myth shows you how to avoid falling for false promises of "all-natural" testosterone boosters, and clearly demonstrates how most supplements that claim to boost your testosterone levels are ineffective and a waste of money.

Chapter 5 - Testosterone 101: Understanding the Biological Role of Testosterone provides you a quick, concise and easy-to-understand breakdown of the biological role that testosterone plays in your body. Think of it as your "Endocrinology for Dummies" Cliff Notes guide.

Chapter 6 - Choosing When to Optimize Your Testosterone Levels is a pivotal chapter that teaches you how to recognize whether you may be suffering from suboptimal levels of testosterone. You will learn about the symptoms of low testosterone, the specific tests you must take to determine your symptoms, what really defines normal testosterone levels, and how to get tested properly.

Chapter 7 - Testosterone Optimization Therapy: Non Injectable Options will introduce you to the various non-injectable delivery systems for testosterone: creams, gels, nasal sprays, pellets, troches and patches. We cover them all and show you which ones are worthy solutions for lifelong TOT.

Chapter 8 - The Optimal TOT Protocol: Injectable Testosterone will teach you what has taken us nearly 20 years to learn: *The OPTIMAL Testosterone Optimization Protocol.* We go in-depth and analyze all the various injectable formulations of testosterone (Undecanoate, Propionate, Cypionate, Enanthate) and we also mention Sustanon for our European friends. We also discuss the importance of choosing the right doctor and the costs involved.

Chapter 9 - How to Properly and Safely Inject Yourself for Life covers everything you need to know about properly (and safely) injecting yourself with testosterone for life. We also discuss how and where to inject testosterone, the exact syringes to use, the correct needle gauge, and the optimal withdrawing procedures. You'll quickly become a testosterone-injecting expert!

Chapter 10 - Potential Side Effects, Their Likelihood and How to Alleviate Them gets into the details of avoiding and minimizing the side effects of testosterone. This is a great chapter that teaches you EXACTLY how, when, and why you may encounter side effects. It also teaches you how to handle and effectively treat (if not eliminate altogether) side effects when administering testosterone.

Chapter 11 - Eliminating Gynecomastia Permanently offers much-needed help for the millions of men who suffer from gynecomastia and don't know where to turn for an effective solution (If you think you might have 'bitch tits', this chapter is for you!).

Chapter 12 - Monitoring TOT for Optimum Health is not only for you, the patient, but for your doctor as well. We cut to the chase about monitoring your health, and taking regular labs and biomarker measurements as you age. This chapter is packed with research, studies, and citations that back up our recommendations on how to optimize your health for lifelong TOT administration.

Chapter 13 - The Critical Role of Nutrition in TOT examines the role nutrition plays in helping you get the most out of TOT. We break down the three major macronutrients (Protein, Carbs, and Fats) and discuss how supplements and specific vitamins & nutrients affect TOT. Additionally, you'll hear our very strong opinions on alcohol, soy proteins, and sugar/High Fructose Corn Syrup.

Chapter 14 - What is Insulin Controlled Living and Why Is it Essential? is a layered and supremely important analysis of Insulin Controlled Living (ICL), and why you must embrace it to maximize TOT. There are very few books written in existence that discuss this complex topic in an easy-to-understand way, and/or offer actionable advice you can apply immediately. We do both.

Chapter 15 - Agents of Change is a chapter many of you will want to read right away. It contains the synthesis of Jim and

Jay's 30 years of biohacking efforts and being their own guinea pigs to discover the substances that optimize performance and alter the human physique. This chapter contains our very best recommendations, and gives you the foundation for biohacking yourself into a fully optimized life.

Chapter 16 - TOT and Fitness is a deep dive into the optimal ways to build muscle and lose fat through highly specific resistance and cardiovascular training protocols. You'll also find out more about the often underestimated and undervalued role of sleep. And in maybe the most unique section of the entire book, you'll learn why embracing the power of the now (i.e. spiritual fitness) might be the key to unlocking an entirely new and upgraded you.

Chapter 17 - The State of the Science in Male Hormonal Optimization: An Exclusive Interview with Dr. Rob Kominiarek is a groundbreaking and highly revealing interview with Dr. Rob Kominiarek, who offers profound insights regarding hormonal optimization in males. Dr. Rob has been prescribing testosterone for 22 years in his thousands of patients while also using it on himself. There are very few physicians with his experiential knowledge and insights on TOT.

BONUS: Chapter 18 - Hormonal Optimization for Women: Doing It the Right Way is an eye opening yet practical summary from Dr. Jim Meehan and co-author Monica Campbell on hormonal optimization for women. It's a perfect lead-in for their book coming out in 2018 titled *Cracking the Fountain of Youth Code - The Complete Women's Guide to Becoming Leaner, Sexier, and Empowered for Life*. Women will definitely want to read this chapter!

BONUS: Chapter 19 - The Stone Cold Truth About Anabolic Steroids is an excellent, high-level summary from Alexander

Juan Antonio Cortes about Anabolic Steroids and how they differ from the usage of therapeutic testosterone. This chapter gives the average reader a very good understanding of how these two things are fundamentally different, despite what we have been led to believe.

BONUS: Chapter 20 - TOT and US Military Veterans: The Problem and Solution is a concise, yet powerful summary of the terrible situation that U.S. military veterans find themselves in when coming back from active duty, and trying to get properly evaluated by the VA. You will hear about veteran and ex special forces soldier Andrew DeMar, along with Dr. Mark Gordon, both of whom founded the Warrior Angel Foundation to help members of the U.S. military diagnosed with TBI (Traumatic Brain Injury) and PTSD (Post Traumatic Stress Disorder).

Chapter 21 - Conclusion reminds you that TOT is always based on a clinical need. Above all else, it is the conscious choice of a man who wants a better way to combat the modern day societal assault on his endocrine system and ultimately his long-term health.

THE GOLDEN RULES OF TOT contains 20 of the most important insights revealed inside the pages of the book. Each provides the reader with life-changing concepts they will now be able to apply to their own optimization quest.

FAQ's are the best questions Jim and Jay have collected from the last 3 years regarding the use of TOT for lifelong health and happiness. These questions cover both hormonal and life optimization from every conceivable angle and aspect.

TOT Resources contain the best of the best in podcasts, websites, and articles that we believe will further inform you as you seek to optimize your life.

Private Coaching/Success Stories let you hear from (and see) some of the men who've completely transformed their lives while working with Jim and Jay utilizing the strategies found inside this book.

About the Authors shows you how to find Jay and Jim online and understand their missions.

The Science Team provides the profiles of the amazing progressive physicians who contributed to the research and insights found inside the book. It also allows you to directly interface with each so that you may consider them as an option in your decision to optimize your health.

The Editing Team provides the profiles of the amazing men who have taken Jay and Jim's clinical research and made it understandable by all men and women in an easy-to-read and engaging way.

A Sincere Request is a friendly reminder to share this book with family and friends who may desperately need it. More importantly, we ask you to leave us an honest review (preferably 5 stars) on Amazon so that we positively impact millions of lives.

Each chapter will end with **Key Takeaways** designed to summarize the information, and restate the important bullet points to remember. There's a lot of research condensed into each chapter, so you can review the Key Takeaways to reinforce the most important information found within.

NOTE We'll use the word *optimize* a lot in this book. Before we go any further, let's take a brief moment to define what optimize and optimization means in the context of health. Optimization means improving *all* your health markers from every conceivable and measurable angle. It also means optimizing your mind and your spirit as well. The health of your body, mind, and spirit all go hand in hand, and this book will touch on each of them.

CHAPTER 1
Why are Men Losing Their Masculinity In The 21st Century?

The truth about the connection between testosterone and optimal health is hard to find. Despite living in an era of scientific inquiry and skepticism, there is an incredible amount of confusion and misinformation about the most important hormone in the male body.

But the truth is simple. Without testosterone, you are not a man. It is the hormone responsible for normal growth and development of male sex characteristics. If you doubt the power contained within this hormone, take a look at transgender women who inject this drug to transition into men and become champion athletes.

Testosterone formulations first came into existence when steroid chemist Adolf Butenandt of Schering partially synthesized them from a cholesterol base in 1935[1]. This work was done in collaboration with fellow chemist Leopold Ruzicka and the pair were awarded the Nobel Prize in Chemistry in 1939[2].

Testosterone and its derivatives quickly became the target of invention and application to both humans and animals, and 'testosterone esters' were finally developed during what can be

---

[1]   Szöllösi-Janze, Margit (2001). *Science in the Third Reich (German Historical Perspectives)*. Oxford, UK: Berg Publishers. ISBN 1-85973-421-9.

[2]   Karl Grandin, ed. (1939). "Leopold Ružička Biography." *Les Prix Nobel*. The Nobel Foundation. Retrieved 2008-10-21.

called the "golden age" of testosterone chemistry (from 1950 to the mid-1960s)[3]. These newly developed chemical compounds were specifically designed to reduce the speed at which testosterone breaks down in the human body. Using testosterone esters allowed physicians to better study and effectively treat a variety of medical conditions, including hypogonadism, anemia, wasting diseases, burns, recovery from surgery and trauma, age-related frailty, and many others.

As you can see, testosterone does a lot more for your body than increase the size of your biceps. It's essential for every part of what makes you happy, healthy, and wise.

Most professional bodybuilders, fitness competitors, pro athletes, celebrity actors, and political leaders who use testosterone are forced to conceal their use of it. They must pretend to be 100% natural in order maintain their squeaky-clean image, and because the U.S. government classifies non-prescription testosterone use as a felony crime.

The modern-day reality is this: Testosterone levels in men are dramatically decreasing, and have been for more than 20 years across the USA[4]. Lower concentrations of testosterone increase a man's risk for age-related diseases, depression and infertility[5]. Look at the accompanying data proving the population wide decline in testosterone over the 80's, 90's and 2000's. Extrapolating this trend into the current day position, this is

---

[3] Schwarz S, Onken D, Schubert A (July 1999). "The steroid story of Jenapharm: from the late 1940s to the early 1970s." Steroids 64 (7): 439–45.

[4] A population-level decline in serum testosterone levels in American men. J Clin Endocrinol Metab. 2007 Jan;92(1):196-202. Epub 2006 Oct 24.

[5] Testosterone, sex hormone-binding globulin, and the development of type 2 diabetes in middle-aged men: prospective results from the Massachusetts male aging study. Stellato RK, Feldman HA, Hamdy O, Horton ES, McKinlay JB. Diabetes Care. 2000 Apr; 23(4):490-4.

clearly a burgeoning crisis that the current medical community is either ignoring or completely unaware of.

FIG. 1.

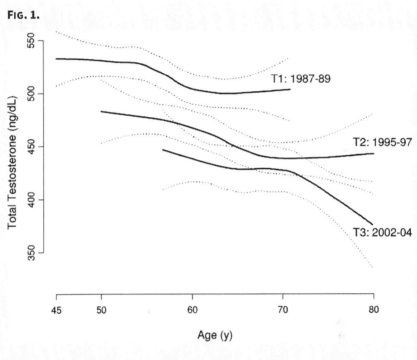

Crude mean TT concentrations, by MMAS study wave (T1, T2, T3) with confidence bands (*dotted lines*). Estimates are obtained from a generalized additive model with a lowess smoothing term.

6

---

6   A population-level decline in serum testosterone levels in American men. J Clin Endocrinol Metab. 2007 Jan;92(1):196-202. Epub 2006 Oct 24.

TABLE 2.

Total and calculated bioavailable T concentrations, by study wave and corresponding age range

Study wave	Observation years	Age range (yr)	n	TT (ng/dl) [a]		Bioavailable T (ng/dl) [a]	
				Median	Interquartile range	Median	Interquartile range
T1	1987–89	45–71	1383	501	392–614	237	179–294
T2	1995–97	50–80	955	435	350–537	188	150–234
T3	2002–04	57–80	568	391	310–507	130	101–163

[a] May be converted to nmol/liter via multiplication by 0.03467.

7

NOTE We want to be clear on something: This book is not meant as a backhanded slight to the established medical community who otherwise attempt to offer help by prescribing a wide range of therapeutic testosterone protocols to their patients. Many are doing the best they can with the limited information and long-term studies available to them. One of the primary purposes of this book is to be a resource guide for both the patient and the doctor to maximize TOT.

It's also of significant concern and worry that there is no standard 'patient of care' model for optimizing hormone levels for men or women. The medical schools in the USA are sadly

---

7   A population-level decline in serum testosterone levels in American men. J Clin Endocrinol Metab. 2007 Jan;92(1):196-202. Epub 2006 Oct 24.

lacking when it comes to teaching TOT as a practice. Many of the Urology and Endocrinology physicians are only familiar with the "theories" and "textbook science[8]" of managing male endocrine systems. Unfortunately, they don't have real first-hand knowledge gained from experiential learning (and managing thousands of patients). This privilege is only attained and shared by a select few. As with most things in medicine, practice-based experience is essential to provide the most up to date and advanced understanding of TOT.

If you want to safely and effectively optimize your blood testosterone levels, it is extremely important to consult with a prescribing doctor with considerable practice-based experience. Unfortunately, while this eliminates a huge percentage of physicians[9], the purpose of this book is to guide you to a physician who is successful in prescribing therapeutic testosterone, thereby allowing you to achieve optimal health.

What this Book Is

This book is the first of its kind to create a better resource guide for **Testosterone-Optimizing Therapy (TOT)** physicians and their patients. You heard that correctly! This book displaces the tired and worn-out acronym **"T-R-T" (Testosterone Replacement Therapy)**, and replaces it with something more instructive and positively inspirational for any man seeking to level up in his life. It also offers the hard-earned wisdom and calculated advice

---

[8]   Nieschlag, Eberhard, Nieschlag, Susan M., Behre, Hermann M. Testosterone: Action, Deficiency, Substitution. Hardcover, Cambridge Univ Pr, 2012, ISBN13 9781107012905.

[9]   Are We Testing Appropriately for Low Testosterone?: Characterization of Tested Men and Compliance with Current Guidelines. Malik RD1, Lapin B, Wang CE, Lakeman JC, Helfand BT. J Sex Med. 2014 Nov 10.

of men who have optimized their testosterone for nearly two decades under the supervision of experienced and forward-thinking doctors. This advice is backed by scientific research, citations, and data to clearly separate the truths from widely held myths and misbeliefs.

This book also relies heavily on molecular biology, bio-chemistry, and endocrinology to explain how TOT works while demonstrating its proven benefits. At the same time, it is written for all men to easily understand. All the TOT misnomers and conventional beliefs held by so many men for decades will be debunked and dispelled. In short, this book offers scientific and practical information on TOT that no aging man should be without.

As the authors of the book, we are not owned by any corporation or person. We can, and WILL tell you the whole truth about testosterone. We hold nothing back and give you everything that you need to know in order to make an informed decision about your health and well-being.

What this Book is Not

This is not a book about how to use Anabolic Steroids. There have been plenty of authoritative books written by superb researchers and scientists about using anabolics[10,11]. This book is a resource written for men on how to use testosterone productively and holistically for life. There is a difference between testosterone use and testosterone abuse.

---

[10] Roberts Anthony, Clapp Brian-*Anabolic Steroids Ultimate Research Guide Volume 1*. 2005 Anabolic Information LLC. www.anabolicbooks.com

[11] William Llewellyn, Anabolics 10th Edition. 2010 Molecular Nutrition.

This book provides crystal-clear strategies designed to optimize physical and mental performance, while enjoying the life-changing benefits of TOT. This allows you to become happier, more driven, improve your relationships, and live an incredible life.

A WORD OF CAUTION:

If you follow the advice and guidance in this book, and do so under the supervision of a medical doctor who understands Testosterone Optimization Therapy, you will see every area of your health improve. And your life will be transformed as well.

So, with that out of the way...

Are you ready to learn how Testosterone Optimization Therapy can improve your life in every way possible?

CHAPTER 1 KEY TAKEAWAYS

- Testosterone is essential for every conceivable aspect of a man's physical and mental health.

- Testosterone levels in men are dramatically decreasing, and have been for more than 20 years across the world. Lower concentrations of testosterone increase your risk for age-related diseases, depression and infertility.

- If you want to safely and effectively optimize your blood testosterone levels, it is essential to consult with a prescribing doctor with practice based experience.

- The authors of this book offer scientific and practical information on TOT that no aging man should be without. We WILL tell you the whole truth about testosterone.

- This book is NOT about how to use Anabolic Steroids, as other books have been written on that subject. It is specifically about the life enhancing USE (not ABUSE) of therapeutic testosterone.

CHAPTER 2
Why Optimizing Your Blood Testosterone Levels Will Transform Your Physique

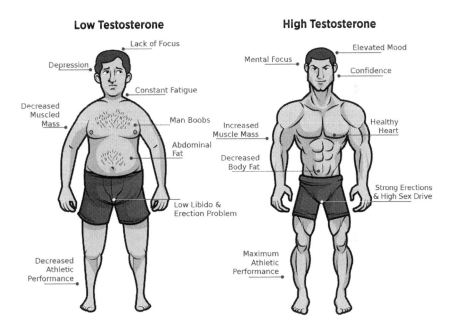

Why men need more testosterone

People often ask why they should consider having their testosterone levels measured at all. The ONLY answer worthy of the question is this:

TO UNDERSTAND IF YOU ARE FUNCTIONING OPTIMALLY AS A MAN.

There is some controversy regarding the key signs which indicate that a man would benefit from (or even require) testosterone supplementation. This is due to a lack of large-scale, long-term studies assessing the benefits and risks of TOT.

Despite few sanctioned studies, reports from hundreds of thousands of men and their doctors prescribing TOT indicate that it often produces a wide range of benefits. Testosterone usage is not yet widespread, but the number of patients with a testosterone prescription rose from 1.3 million people in 2010 to 2.3 million in 2013[12]. More than 50% of testosterone prescriptions are written by primary care physicians[13] for middle-aged and older men with age-related declines in testosterone[14]. And these numbers are not even reflective of the global male population using TOT without a doctor's prescription! The best estimates of this population grouping suggests that roughly 6 million people[15] (without a prescription) are using anabolic and/or androgenic steroids (including testosterone) every year.

According to the U.S. Census Bureau, approximately 15 million men suffer from testosterone deficiency, a condition in which significant decreases in testosterone levels take place[16]. Shockingly, very few of these men will seek treatment. 'Male hypogonadism', a recognized medical condition in which the human

---

[12]   http://www.hcplive.com/medical-news/will-the-fda-tighten-the-use-of-testosterone-replacement-therapy

[13]   http://www.aafp.org/afp/2017/1001/p441.html#afp20171001p441-b2

[14]   http://www.aafp.org/afp/2017/1001/p441.html#afp20171001p441-b1

[15]   http://www.criminaldefenselawyer.com/resources/illegal-steroids-and-human-growth-hormone-hgh.htm

[16]   Andropause: Current concepts .Indian J Endocrinol Metab. 2013 Dec;17(Suppl 3):S621-9. doi: 10.4103/2230-8210.123552

body does not produce enough testosterone, remains danger-ously underdiagnosed by many doctors.

Hypogonadism is often underdiagnosed for the following reasons:

1. Men don't report it to their doctors because they are embarrassed to report symptoms that are sexual in nature. Additionally, they are conditioned to accept that these symptoms are typical of 'old age' and are therefore unfixable.

2. Men will often present nonspecific symptoms such as lack of motivation, depression, listlessness, and so on. Rarely is low testosterone investigated as the potential source for these symptoms.

3. There isn't a definitive biochemical test for hypogonadism, nor is there a standard 'patient of care model' for physicians to follow.

4. There is a distinct lack of physician awareness regarding the condition. Many doctors do not understand what blood tests to order, as well as how to effectively and correctly identify the symptoms of a testosterone deficiency.

5. The U.S. Food and Drug Administration clarified in 2015 that prescribing testosterone due to aging constitutes off-label use. This institutes fear and disinterest in inexperienced primary care doctors (which are the majority of prescribers).

6. Many newer primary care physicians abide by the Endocrine Society's recommendation: male hypogonadism should only be diagnosed if total serum testosterone levels are low on at least two early morning blood draws. This prevents many men who are suffering from symptoms from getting accurately diagnosed.

A very recent study shows that up to 40% of all tested men are dealing with suboptimal levels of testosterone[17], and are suffering from the effects. Anecdotally, many progressive physicians report a much higher number of patients suffering from suboptimal levels of testosterone. Dr. Merrill Matschke[18], a board certified urologist in a large suburban practice in Chicago (interviewed in Chapter 12), observes that 90% of his patients show up with subclinical levels of testosterone. He specifically states he rarely sees men with total testosterone levels higher than 400 ng/dL in his office.

That's all the bad news, so here's the good news: There are an endless amount of benefits to optimizing your testosterone levels, many of which you have never heard of or even thought were possible. And when you head down the life-altering testosterone optimization pathway, you'll experience those benefits far sooner than you think!

---

[17] https://www.prognos.ai/abstracts/incidence-low-testosterone-40-tested-men-40-years-highest-prevalence-found-men-living-southern-states-results-nationwide-database/

[18] www.betterhealthcarolinas.com

Testosterone Decreases Body Fat

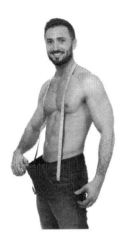

Testosterone is essential to the regulation of insulin, glucose, and fat storage[19]. Managing your body's insulin production is the key to reducing inflammation as one ages (we will discuss the role of insulin much more in Chapters 13 and 14). As testosterone levels plummet, so does your body's ability to process insulin, glucose, and fat. Simply put, a decrease in testosterone levels is directly correlated with an increase in fat storage[20].

To make matters worse for obese men (25% body fat or higher), an increase in fat also lowers testosterone levels. The fatter you become, the lower your testosterone levels go. This vicious cycle is a huge contributor to the obesity pandemic sweeping the world. As of October 2017, the CDC in the United States is reporting that 4 out of 10 adults are obese[21].

In obese males, there is increased aromatase activity (aromatase is the enzyme directly responsible for converting testosterone into estrogen), which results in decreased testosterone levels and elevated estrogen levels. However, obese and high body fat men alike can break this cycle by undergoing TOT due to

---

[19]   The interactions between hypothalamic-pituitary-adrenal axis activity, testosterone, insulin-like growth factor I and abdominal obesity with metabolism and blood pressure in men. Int J Obes Relat Metab Disord. 1998 Dec;22(12):1184-96.

[20]   Obesity in men: The hypogonadal–estrogen receptor relationship and its effect on glucose homeostasis Cohen, Paul G.Medical Hypotheses, Volume 70, Issue 2, 358 - 360.

[21]   https://www.cdc.gov/obesity/data/adult.html

testosterone being lipolytic[22] (i.e. fat burning). Studies have also shown that one of the positive benefits of testosterone treatment is a decrease in abdominal adiposity (also known as fat storage)[23]. The relationship between testosterone, aromatase, and obesity will be discussed in far greater detail in Chapter 10.

Testosterone Increases Muscle Mass

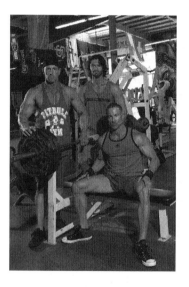

As the most essential muscle building (i.e. anabolic) hormone, testosterone improves muscle protein synthesis and therefore leads to more muscle growth[24]. The testosterone molecule is the foundation of muscle, strength, and the source of what makes men powerful.

What does that mean? It means that if you exercise with progressively heavier weights[25] while using testosterone, you'll increase your overall strength and build a more

22 Høst C, Gormsen LC, Christensen B, et al. Independent Effects of Testosterone on Lipid Oxidation and VLDL-TG Production: A Randomized, Double-Blind, Placebo-Controlled, Crossover Study. Diabetes 2013;62(5):1409-1416. doi:10.2337/db12-0440.

23 Predictors of skeletal muscle mass in elderly men and women. Mech Ageing Dev. 1999;107:123–136. [PubMed].

24 132. Verhaar HJJ, Samson MM, Aleman A, de Vries WR, de Vreede PL, Koppeschaar HPF. The relationship between indices of muscle function and circulating anabolic hormones in healthy.Aging Male. 2000;3:75–80.

25 www.advancedforgedtraining.com.

muscular physique. Remember: Muscle mass is the single greatest deterrent to the diseases of aging. The more muscle you possess, the more metabolically active you are and the more calories you burn at rest (i.e. sitting at your desk).

All of this leads to a body you'll be proud of when you look at yourself in the mirror, whether naked or clothed. Building muscle is also of critical importance to combat sarcopenia (age related muscle loss) due to its protective effects on your joints, tendons, ligaments and bones.

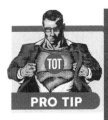

PRO TIP

It is important to understand that a clean diet[26] and a sound resistance training program[27] are absolutely necessary to maximize the potential benefits of TOT[28]. We discuss these in detail in Chapters 13 and 16, respectively.

Testosterone Improves Heart Health

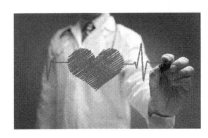

Until very recently, researchers have been divided on the topic of how testosterone affects heart health. Previously, researchers had claimed that high levels of testosterone were linked to heart disease, while more recent

---

[26]   www.metabolicblowtorchdiet.com.

[27]   www.advancedforgedtraining.com.

[28]   Effects of progressive resistance training on growth hormone and testosterone levels in young and elderly subjects. Craig BW, Brown R, Everhart J. Mech Ageing Dev. 1989 Aug; 49(2):159-69.

studies have found that low testosterone levels are responsible for an increased risk of heart ailments[29,30]. Ultimately, there is now an overwhelming amount of recently published data[31] which shows that maintaining optimal testosterone levels can help prevent cardiovascular disease[32].

"Help" is the key word here. The benefits that come with healthy testosterone levels (not testosterone alone) are what allow the heart to maintain its strength.

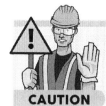

CAUTION

The hysteria created by mainstream media about therapeutic testosterone causing an increased number of CVD (cardiovascular disease) events in otherwise normal and healthy men is unsupported[33]. There is little data or proof substantiating the national TV, newsprint, and internet ads you may have seen and/or heard from legal groups and attorneys around 2014-2016 when they claimed that TOT increases the risk of heart attacks, stroke, CVD, and so on.

---

[29] http://www.pharmaceutical-journal.com/opinion/insight/why-the-evidence-for-testosterone-therapy-adds-up/20202972.article.

[30] Prevention of coronary artery disease in men: Male hormone, female hormone, or both? Yang, Changsheng et al. Medical Hypotheses, Volume 75, Issue 6, 671 - 673.

[31] https://medicalxpress.com/news/2017-02-testosterone-therapy-cardiovascular.html

[32] Testosterone as an atrial fibrillation treatment and stroke preventative in aging men: Case histories and hypothesis. Eby, George. Medical Hypotheses, Volume 75, Issue 2, 269 - 270.

[33] http://www.trtrev.com/wp-content/uploads/2015/10/Testosterone-Therapy-and-Cardiovascular-Risk.pdf

Unsurprisingly, the foundational study[34] that prompted this witch hunt for CVD risk came from a clinical trial called "Testosterone in Older Men" (**TOM**) which investigated the use of topical testosterone (a.k.a. transdermal, which is suboptimal and will be covered later in Chapter 7) in men over 65 with limited mobility. Put another way, this was a study done on men who could barely walk or move on their own[35].

I mean c'mon. How can any reasonable person assume that this study isn't completely flawed due to the physical limitations of the subjects involved? And to think it was this tragically flawed study data a recent jury (October 2017) used to award a $140 million dollar settlement to a plaintiff who sued AbbVie, the maker of Androgel[36]. A plaintiff who turned out to be morbidly obese with high blood pressure, no less. Talk about an ironically hidden agenda!

NOTE Thankfully, a U.S. Court of Appeals Judge overturned this ruling on Dec 22nd 2017 and ordered a new trial set for March 5th, 2018[37].

Even with all of that, the preponderance of evidence clearly indicates an increased risk of cardiovascular disease and death

---

[34] LeBrasseur NK, Lajevardi N, Miciek R, Mazer N, Storer TW, Bhasin S. Effects of Testosterone Therapy on Muscle Performance and Physical Function in Older Men with Mobility Limitations (The TOM Trial): Design and Methods. *Contemporary clinical trials.* 2009;30(2):133-140. doi:10.1016/j.cct.2008.10.005.

[35] Basaria S, Davda MN, Travison TG, Ulloor J, Singh R, Bhasin S. Risk Factors Associated With Cardiovascular Events During Testosterone Administration in Older Men With Mobility Limitation. *The Journals of Gerontology Series A: Biological Sciences and Medical Sciences.* 2013;68(2):153-160. doi:10.1093/gerona/gls 138.

[36] https://www.usnews.com/news/us/articles/2017-10-05/abbvie-hit-with-140-million-verdict-in-androgel-trial-lawyer

[37] https://www.reuters.com/article/us-abbvie-androgel/u-s-judge-tosses-verdict-against-abbvie-in-androgel-case-idUSKBN1EG28U

in men with low or low-normal testosterone blood levels[38]. Therapeutic testosterone, when dosed and maintained to optimal levels, offers no increased risk of CVD and in recent studies[39] offers clear protection from CVD. We offer much more information (including the latest research) about testosterone and its effect on the heart and vascular networks later in Chapter 12. Hint: it is supremely positive.

Testosterone and the Brain

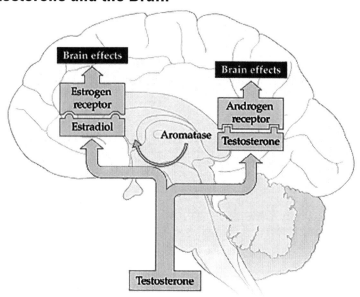

Testosterone exerts important biological effects on brain development and function throughout male life. Testosterone

---

[38]   Xu L, Freeman G, Cowling BJ, Schooling CM. Testosterone therapy and cardiovascular events among men: a systematic review and meta-analysis of placebo-controlled randomized trials. *BMC Medicine* 2013;11:108. doi:10.1186/1741-7015-11-108.

[39]   Testosterone Replacement Modulates Cardiac Metabolic Remodeling after Myocardial Infarction by Upregulating PPARα. PPAR Res. 2016;2016:4518754. doi: 10.1155/2016/4518754. Epub 2016 Jun 16.

modulates the response of the amygdala (a key brain structure for generating and processing emotions) and the prefrontal cortex (a region of the brain involved in regulating emotional responses and reactions). Studies indicate that higher testosterone levels are associated with higher risk-taking, potentially leading to greater reward in both business and life[40].

Testosterone and Dopamine

Testosterone's most noticeable effect on the brain is its ability to boost dopamine. Dopamine is a neurotransmitter (chemical messenger) that is responsible for transmitting signals between the nerve cells (neurons) of the brain. Dopamine is normally released when something good or exciting happens. According to this specific study, 'testosterone can enhance dopamine release in the mesolimbic system, which may protect against depression and the associated decrease in dopamine activity in reward-related brain pathways'[41]. The brain is heavily dependent on testosterone to boost dopamine, as it's one of the keys for a robust sex life. Many men feel the effects of increased dopamine (ridding of depression, more positive outlook, more energetic, etc.) immediately after beginning a TOT regimen.

Testosterone and Depression

One of global societies' biggest health problems is depression. This afflicts hundreds of millions of men worldwide every year. Many scientists are stuck trying to figure out a biological riddle

---

[40]   Stanton SJ, Mullette-Gillman OA, McLaurin RE, et al. Low- and High-Testosterone Individuals Exhibit Decreased Aversion to Economic Risk. Psychological science. 2011;22(4):447-453. doi:10.1177/0956797611401752.

[41]   Alderson LM, Baum MJ. Differential effects of gonadal steroids on dopamine metabolism in mesolimbic and nigro-striatal pathways of male rat brain. Brain research. 1981;218:189-206.

akin to the "chicken vs. the egg": does low testosterone cause depression, or does depression cause low testosterone?

Sadly, the standard treatment (even to this day) is to prescribe selective serotonin reuptake inhibitor (SSRI) medications in lieu of submitting for a blood testosterone test. Despite this confusion, research now demonstrates that men undergoing TOT for suboptimal levels of testosterone report improvements in mood and other issues related to depression[42]. In fact, there are many studies showing that it dramatically improves depression and mood[43].

Another study found that TOT may have an antidepressant effect in depressed patients, especially those with hypogonadism[44]. What is remarkable is that this study was willing to go on record and state that "the route by which TT [testosterone] is administered may play a role in treatment response." In other words, they actually admitted that testosterone can have a place in proper treatment of depression (in men with low testosterone levels).

Testosterone and Memory

Many studies have shown that testosterone improves working memory in men[45]. Working memory is the basis for nearly everything needed for proper brain function. Almost all

[42] Journal of Psychiatric Practice, Jul 2009, 14(4):289-305, "Testosterone and Depression: Systematic Review and Meta-Analysis."

[43] Am J Psychiatry, Jan 2003, 160:105-111, "Testosterone Gel Supplementation for Men With Refractory Depression: A Randomized, Placebo-Controlled Trial."

[44] The Journal of Clinical Endocrinology & Metabolism, Feb 1 1999, 84(2):573-577, "Bioavailable Testosterone and Depressed Mood in Older Men: The Rancho Bernardo Study."

[45] Journal of Cognitive Neuroscience, May 2000, 12(3):407-414, "Sex Steroids Modify Working Memory."

processed information goes through working memory before it is analyzed, stored or synthesized by other parts of the brain.

Further studies have shown that visual and verbal memory improve in men who are given testosterone[46]. Even your ability to think is profoundly affected by testosterone! If that's not enough, additional studies have shown that testosterone increases spatial processing power in both young and older men[47].

In fact, the brain fog exhibited by men suffering from testosterone deficiency (also known by the clinical diagnosis acronym TD, which stands for Testosterone Deficiency) is often eliminated when men start TOT. The fastest and most noticeable positive effects of TOT are clearer thinking and an improved mood. As you can see, TOT's ability to improve memory and increase cognition is quite possibly its most pronounced effect.

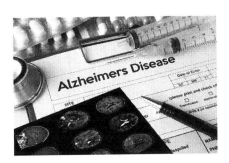

Testosterone Combats Alzheimer's Disease and Improves Cognition

Studies show that many older men with mild cognitive issues suffer from low blood levels of testosterone[48]. Many

---

46 Neurology, July 10 2001, 57(1):80-88, "Testosterone supplementation improves spatial and verbal memory in healthy older men."

47 Aging Male, 2006 Dec, 9(4):195-9, "Testosterone and the brain."

48 Gillett MJ, Martins RN, Clarnette RM, Chubb SA, Bruce DG, Yeap BB. Relationship between testosterone, sex hormone binding globulin and plasma amyloid beta peptide 40 in older men with subjective memory loss or dementia. J Alzheimers Dis. 2003;5:267-269. [PubMed]

of these men eventually develop Alzheimer's[49]. At the University of Southern California, researchers noted that increasing testosterone levels in older men stalled the development of Alzheimer's[50]. This has led scientists to speculate that maintaining healthy testosterone levels may actually prevent Alzheimer's[51]. There is also clear and substantial evidence to demonstrate TOT's ability to improve memory (both long-term and short-term) in men as they age[52].

Long story short: If you are an aging man and are interested in preserving your memory well into your golden years, make sure that your testosterone levels are optimized. It is one of the best preventative measures you will ever take for your mental and physical health.

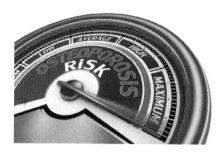

Testosterone Prevents Osteoporosis and Frailty

In multiple studies involving aging men, low testosterone levels are associated with lower skeletal muscle mass,

49   Plasma testosterone levels in Alzheimer and Parkinson diseases. Okun MS, DeLong MR, Hanfelt J, Gearing M, Levey A. Neurology. 2004 Feb 10;62(3): 411-3.

50   Gouras GK, Xu H, Gross RS, et al. Testosterone reduces neuronal secretion of Alzheimer's β-amyloid peptides. *Proceedings of the National Academy of Sciences of the United States of America.* 2000;97(3):1202-1205.

51   Cunningham RL, Singh M, O'Bryant SE, Hall JR, Barber RC. Oxidative stress, testosterone, and cognition among Caucasian and Mexican American men with and without Alzheimer's disease. Journal of Alzheimer's disease : JAD. 2014;40(3):563-573. doi:10.3233/JAD-131994.

52   Can testosterone replacement decrease the memory problem of old age? Lim, David et al. Medical Hypotheses, Volume 60, Issue 6, 893 - 896.

muscle strength, physical function, bone mineral density and higher risk of fractures and death[53]. Low testosterone levels clearly cause bone disease in men, as testosterone is indisputably linked to bone health[54].

Optimized blood testosterone levels increase bone density and impede the normal bone resorption issues that come with age (i.e. breakdown and destruction of bone tissue)[55]. Men who suffer from bone disease usually have suboptimal levels of testosterone, and this leads to frailty in old age[56]. The last thing any man wants is to end up with a deteriorated hip or spine that completely limits their range of motion later in life. No man wants to be a shadow of his former glory, stuck in a rocking chair and unable to move.

If you want ideal bone health into your later years, you owe it to yourself to optimize your testosterone levels.

Testosterone Fights Inflammation

Cellular inflammation is the core component of many aging-related diseases. It is the chief culprit of vascular disease, erectile dysfunction, autoimmune disease, and cancer[57]. Low

---

[53]   Baumgartner RN, Koehler KM, Gallagher D et al. Epidemiology of Sarcopenia among the elderly in New Mexico. AM J Epidemiol 147: 755-63.

[54]   Selective estrogen receptor modulators: A possible new treatment of osteoporosis in males. Kastelan, Darko et al. Medical Hypotheses, Volume 67, Issue 5, 1052 - 1053.

[55]   Male osteoporosis: clinical approach and management in family practice. Singapore Med J. 2014 Jul;55(7):353-7.

[56]   Fink HA, Ewing SK, Ensrud KE, et al. Association of testosterone and estradiol deficiency with osteoporosis and rapid bone loss in older men. J Clin Endocrinol Metab. 2006;91(10):3908-39015. [PubMed].

[57]   Du C, Bhatia M, Tang SCW, Zhang M, Steiner T. Mediators of Inflammation: Inflammation in Cancer, Chronic Diseases, and Wound Healing. *Mediators of Inflammation*. 2015;2015:570653. doi:10.1155/2015/570653.

levels of testosterone have been associated with a number of chronic inflammatory diseases, including an increase in cardiovascular disease markers[58], mortality[59], diabetes[60], metabolic syndrome[61], and an increased risk for bone fracture (i.e. the bone breaking). One of the primary ways testosterone improves biological systems is by decreasing inflammation.

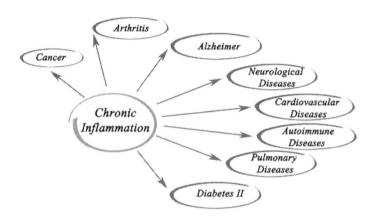

Excessive inflammation affects Leydig cell (located in the testicles) function and suppresses testosterone production. There is evidence from experimental studies that *IL-6, TNF-alpha*

---

58   Alderson LM, Baum MJ. Differential effects of gonadal steroids on dopamine metabolism in mesolimbic and nigro-striatal pathways of male rat brain. Brain research. 1981;218:189–206.

59   Laughlin GA, Barrett-Connor E, Bergstrom J. Low serum testosterone and mortality in older men. J Clin Endocrinol Metab. 2008;93:68–75.

60   Stellato RK, Feldman HA, Hamdy O, Horton ES, McKinlay JB. Testosterone, sex hormone-binding globulin, and the development of type 2 diabetes in middle-aged men: prospective results from the Massachusetts male aging study. Diabetes Care. 2000;23:490–494.

61   Laaksonen DE, Niskanen L, Punnonen K, Nyyssonen K, Tuomainen TP, Valkonen VP, Salonen R, Salonen JT. Testosterone and sex hormonebinding globulin predict the metabolic syndrome and diabetes in middle-aged men. Diabetes Care. 2004;27:1036–1041.

and *IL-1 beta* (the primary cytokines and major inflammatory markers) inhibit testosterone production by their suppressive influence on the Hypothalamus-Pituitary-Testes-Axis (HPTA)[62]. In plain English, *IL-6*, *TNF-alpha* and *IL-1 beta* control the levels of inflammation in the human body.

Studies have conclusively shown that suboptimal levels of testosterone lead to increased inflammation throughout the body. As such, we think it makes a lot of sense to briefly discuss the major inflammatory markers and how TOT has specifically been shown to improve each and every one of them.

Adiponectin is not an inflammatory cytokine per se, but it affects inflammation as it's a chief culprit of decreasing insulin sensitivity (we discuss insulin sensitivity in much greater detail in Chapter 14). As men age, usually due to poor diet, fat gain and lack of exercise, adiponectin levels drop. TOT, on the other hand, raises adiponectin levels[63].

As for the primary inflammatory cytokine *IL-1*, it is found in a number of conditions (such as rheumatoid arthritis). Researchers have proven that TOT inhibits IL-1 production[64]. *TNF alpha* is the primary cause of cardiovascular disease, and TOT has been found to lower TNF-alpha levels[65]. *IL-6* is found

---

[62] Eur J Endocrinol, 2007 May, 156(5):595-602, "The effect of testosterone replacement therapy on adipocytokines and C-reactive protein in hypogonadal men with type 2 diabetes."

[63] Obes Rev, 2005 Feb, 6(1):13-21, "Adiponectin: action, regulation and association to insulin sensitivity."

[64] Clinical and Experimental Rheumatology, 1993, 11(2):157-162, "Effect of gonadal steroids on the production of IL-1 and IL-6 by blood mononuclear cells in vitro."

[65] Cellular Physiology and Biochemistry, 2007, 20:847-852, "Effects of Testosterone on Cytokines and Left Ventricular Remodeling Following Heart Failure."

in diabetes, cancer, and Alzheimer's. Guess what? Studies show that TOT decreases IL-6 levels[66]!

CRP (C-Reactive Protein) is now a common test given by progressive doctors to measure systemic inflammation levels. High readings are extremely well correlated to increased risk for heart disease, Alzheimer's, and Fatty Liver Disease (discussed in much greater detail later in Chapter 12). Testosterone deficiency has been found to be associated with higher CRP levels from insulin resistance, Type 2 diabetes, metabolic syndrome and vascular disease[67].

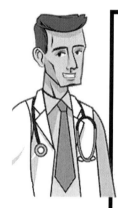

CRP values are easily affected by variable lifestyle changes such as colds, sinus infections, heavy and or intense physical training. Understanding this, it's important for physicians to take this into consideration when evaluating CRP lab measurement numbers. It is also recommended Doctors test specifically for hs-CRP (high sensitivity-C-Reactive Protein) for a more accurate analysis of cardiovascular disease risk.

Although there has not been enough research regarding the link between testosterone and inflammation, the studies listed above provide conclusive evidence that testosterone suppresses pro-inflammatory cytokines ('bad' cytokines) and stimulates

---

[66] Journal of Endocrinological Investigation, 2005, 28(11 Suppl Proceedings):116-119, "The relationship between testosterone and molecular markers of inflammation in older men."

[67] Journal of Andrology, Jan/Feb 2009, 30(1), "The Dark Side of Testosterone Deficiency: II. Type 2 Diabetes and Insulin Resistance."

anti-inflammatory cytokines[68] ('good' cytokines). Testosterone also seems to have a protective effect on beta cells (which make insulin) through its suppression and control of these inflammatory cytokines. In Chapter 20, you'll see an example of the powerful anti-inflammatory effect of testosterone and how it was used to heal a wounded Veteran.

---

[68]   Chris J. Malkin, Peter J. Pugh, Richard D. Jones, Dheeraj Kapoor, Kevin S. Channer and T. Hugh Jones. The Effect of Testosterone Replacement on Endogenous Inflammatory Cytokines and Lipid Profiles in Hypogonadal Men. J. Clin. Endocrinol. Metab. 2004 89: 3313-3318, doi: 10.1210/jc.2003-031069.

CHAPTER 2 KEY TAKEAWAYS

- Therapeutic dosages of testosterone will completely change your physique via decreasing body fat and increasing muscle mass, but ONLY when living a dialed-in lifestyle consisting of a clean diet and productive resistance and cardiovascular training.

- TOT improves heart health while simultaneously preventing cardiovascular disease. The hysteria created by mainstream media about therapeutic testosterone increasing the risk of cardiovascular disease in otherwise normal and healthy men is scientifically unsupported.

- TOT exerts powerful biological effects on brain development and brain function by increasing dopamine, alleviating depression, improving cognition/memory and ultimately combating Alzheimer's and dementia.

- TOT also prevents osteoporosis and frailty in aging men and women (which are usually the number 1 causes of death for the elderly).

- Finally, TOT has a profound effect on fighting inflammation via suppression of inflammatory cytokines and stimulation of anti-inflammatory cytokines.

CHAPTER 3

The Power of Testosterone to Transform Your Life

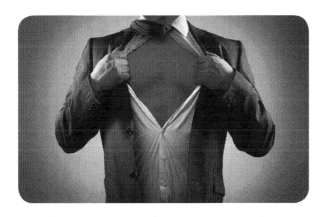

The physiological effects of optimized testosterone levels will transform men into healthier, happier, and incredibly productive human beings. However, the psychological effects will also change how you think and feel as a man. Your mindset, your will and your sense of self will change for the better as you optimize your blood testosterone levels and overall lifestyle.

Testosterone and the Manifestation of Will

Most men today do not realize the power that testosterone has to improve overall well-being, or how suboptimal levels of testosterone can prevent them from living fulfilled lives. And while we'll cover the many health benefits of optimized testosterone levels, the link between life fulfillment and testosterone usually gets ignored.

This sounds too good to be true, but men who have optimized testosterone levels report having a dramatically improved outlook on life and a supreme confidence that they can take control of their destiny in a way they didn't comprehend prior to using TOT.

Testosterone will Improve Your Sexual Confidence with Partners

In the animal world, high testosterone levels have been linked to dominance in the battle for mates[69]. The same is true for human beings[70].

Studies have shown that when two men were instructed to fight for the affection of a woman, the man's aggression, ability to direct the interaction, and chances of attracting the women were positively associated with their testosterone levels (i.e. higher testosterone levels means more aggression, greater ability & higher chances of success) before the task[71]. There is truth to the idea that boldness is a powerful key to attracting potential mates, and there is little doubt that testosterone is responsible for this boldness.

---

[69] Onyango PO, Gesquiere LR, Altmann J, Alberts SC. Testosterone positively associated with both male mating effort and paternal behavior in savanna baboons *(Papio cynocephalus). Hormones and behavior.* 2013;63(3):430-436. doi:10.1016/j.yhbeh.2012.11.014.

[70] Heany SJ, van Honk J, Stein DJ, Brooks SJ. A quantitative and qualitative review of the effects of testosterone on the function and structure of the human social-emotional brain. *Metabolic Brain Disease.* 2016;31:157-167. doi:10.1007/s11011-015-9692-y.

[71] Sex-hormone dependent perception of androstenone suggests its involvement in communicating competition and aggression. Lübke KT1, Pause BM. Physiol Behav. 2014 Jan 17;123:136-41. doi: 10.1016/j.physbeh.2013.10.016. Epub 2013 Oct 25.

Improving your testosterone levels can improve your ability to approach women and build quick rapport. From a standpoint of evolutionary biology, women can sense higher testosterone levels in men and they enjoy communication with males who give off this aura of high testosterone (in other words, they are more attracted to them)[72].

There is even research[73] indicating that women can 'smell' higher testosterone levels and seek them out during various points of their menstrual cycle. If you know this and are currently struggling with approaching women, or dating in general, why would you not want to investigate the route of TOT as a potential solution?

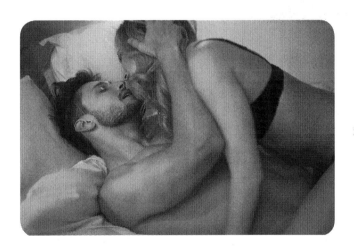

---

72 Sex-hormone dependent perception of androstenone suggests its involvement in communicating competition and aggression. Lübke KT1, Pause BM. Physiol Behav. 2014 Jan 17;123:136-41. doi: 10.1016/j.physbeh.2013.10.016. Epub 2013 Oct 25.

73 http://www.huffingtonpost.com/2013/04/18/mens-smell-testosterone-attractive-to-women-study_n_3110182.html

More Testosterone Equals Heightened Sex Drive and Libido

There's an entire industry devoted to correcting low libido and erectile dysfunction through the use of artificial chemicals. However, nothing beats out the natural and awesome power of optimized blood levels of testosterone.

Testosterone Optimization Therapy can significantly improve your sex drive while improving the quality AND quantity of erections[74]. Testosterone is undeniably the most powerful male sex hormone, and many male sexual issues can be reversed through a well-designed testosterone improvement regimen.

Unfortunately, many men who suffer from low testosterone are routinely scripted Viagra (and/or Cialis) and an anti-depressant (ex. an SSRI) when they tell a doctor about their lowered libido. These solutions are treating symptoms instead of addressing the underlying cause.

For this reason, it is critical that TOT-trained physicians learn how to decipher the difference between a patient who has a true lack of desire, and a patient who has a real-life inability to perform due to suboptimal levels of testosterone.

This will be stated numerous times throughout the book but it is worth mentioning this here:

Symptoms, and <u>then</u> blood panels - MUST be taken into account before dispensing erectile dysfunction and mood-altering medications to patients.

---

[74] Wang C, Cunningham G, Dobs A, et al. Long-term testosterone gel (AndroGel) treatment maintains beneficial effects on sexual function and mood, lean and fat mass, and bone mineral density in hypogonadal men. J Clin Endocrinol Metab. 2004;89:2085–2098. [PubMed].

The Competitive Edge Gained From Using Testosterone

Testosterone is responsible for the masculine need for victory and challenge[75]. One study even shows that a man's testosterone levels may predict whether he will persevere through defeat or give in when faced with adversity[76]. Testosterone tangibly speeds up reaction times, improves eyesight and physical endurance, and produces feelings of invulnerability[77].

Think of the times in your life when you've experienced the "thrill of victory" as your favorite sports teams won a big game, whether you were watching or participating. It's exhilarating!

The same is felt in the business world when you close a big sale or sign the paperwork on a huge deal. There is ample scientific evidence showing that testosterone levels in men increase exponentially for days after winning a game or achieving something of great significance[78].

Now, imagine incorporating those feelings into your everyday life when using therapeutic testosterone, because that's EXACTLY what it's like. Aren't you looking to get that competitive edge

---

[75] Intercollegiate soccer: saliva cortisol and testosterone are elevated during competition, and testosterone is related to status and social connectedness with teammates. Edwards DA1, Wetzel K, Wyner DR. PLoS One. 2012;7(4):e34814. doi: 10.1371/journal.pone.0034814. Epub 2012 Apr 18.

[76] Implicit power motivation predicts men's testosterone changes and implicit learning in a contest situation. Schultheiss OC1, Rohde W. Horm Behav. 2002 Mar;41(2):195-202.

[77] Serum testosterone, growth hormone, and insulin-like growth factor-1 levels, mental reaction time, and maximal aerobic exercise in sedentary and long-term physically trained elderly males. Int J Neurosci. 2004 May;114(5):623-37.

[78] Testosterone and cortisol release among Spanish soccer fans watching the 2010 World Cup final. van der Meij L1, Almela M, Hidalgo V, Villada C, Ijzerman H, van Lange PA, Salvador A.

back into your life? Of course you are, and TOT can help you become a much more productive entrepreneur and/or business person.

Testosterone Helps You Take Risks And Achieve Higher Social Status

Testosterone has been linked to risk-taking and higher status in men. Men with high testosterone have higher social status and tend to be more risk-prone (i.e. take greater risks and take them more often) than their low testosterone, lower-status brethren[79]. Many people (including the authors of this book) believe that the ability to calculate and assume risk throughout one's life is what separates the truly successful from those wishing for success.

Testosterone levels rise after every victory a person experiences[80]. This creates a positive feedback loop where a man with higher levels of testosterone may triumph over an opponent with greater skill but lower testosterone levels. Testosterone is your winning streak! A recent landmark study on testosterone in rugby players provided amazing insights on how experienced individuals with optimal testosterone levels are more tactical, rather than dominant:

---

[79] Diekhof EK, Wittmer S, Reimers L. Does Competition Really Bring Out the Worst? Testosterone, Social Distance and Inter-Male Competition Shape Parochial Altruism in Human Males. Lamm C, ed. PLoS ONE. 2014;9(7):e98977. doi:10.1371/journal.pone.0098977.

[80] Changes in testosterone mediate the effect of winning on subsequent aggressive behaviour. Carré JM1, Campbell JA, Lozoya E, Goetz SM, Welker KM. Psychoneuroendocrinology. 2013 Oct;38(10):2034-41. doi: 10.1016/j.psyneuen.2013.03.008. Epub 2013 Apr 12.

*"...Testosterone induces dominant behaviour among higher ranking individuals and obedience or submissiveness among lower ranking individuals. We found no main or interaction effects of game type on acquiescence, but did find a significant interaction between seniority and testosterone. Senior players acquiesced **less** if their testosterone was high rather than low, while junior players acquiesced **more** if their testosterone was high rather than low.*

*This interaction effect between testosterone and social status among persons embedded in hierarchical relationships is a novel finding, which suggests the interesting possibility **that testosterone is implicated in behavior that could be characterised as tactical rather than dominant**[81].*

Optimal Testosterone Levels Lead to Your Most Powerful and Enlightened Self

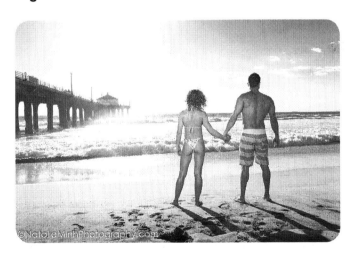

---

[81]   Inoue Y, Takahashi T, Burriss RP, Arai S, Hasegawa T, Yamagishi T, Kiyonari T. Testosterone promotes either dominance or submissiveness in the Ultimatum Game depending on players' social rank. Sci Rep. 2017;7(1):5335.

When you have higher levels of testosterone, your ability to be supremely confident in your decisions and take decisive action increases exponentially. You are assertive and purposeful in everything you do and say. Your decisions empower you to behave in ways others find attractive. You are no longer a man of words, but a man of calculated and tactical action.

TOT will help a depressed man become more assertive, giving him character traits that invoke his latent assertive spirit. And for the already assertive men out there, TOT will make you even more focused, determined and a stronger leader amongst your peers.

Being hormonally optimized gives you the mindset and focus to achieve your big goals. The connection between what you can accomplish, and the state of your physical health, is something that most men ignore. But once you realize what you can accomplish when your body is healthy, you'll never look back.

We believe that everyone has something to contribute to the world. Optimizing your testosterone levels will dump high octane fuel in your tank so you can serve and do more for your community, your friends and your loved ones. This summary quote from deceased US tennis player Arthur Ashe regarding testosterone and altruism is a perfect way to express the awe-inspiring potential of optimized testosterone levels:

> *"True heroism is remarkably sober, very undramatic. It is not the urge to surpass all at whatever cost, but the urge to serve others at whatever cost. And endogenous testosterone appears to be one important driving source of this type of prosociality in human males."*

CHAPTER 3 KEY TAKEAWAYS

- Optimizing your blood testosterone levels has the potential to radically transform your business and personal life. Specifically, the physiological effects of optimized testosterone levels make for healthier, happier, and more productive men.

- Optimal levels of testosterone will improve your outlook on life and give you absolute confidence that you can take control of your own destiny.

- TOT will improve your confidence amongst sexual partners and improve your ability to approach women and build quick rapport. It will also improve your performance in the bedroom (via enhanced libido, and better quality and quantity of erections).

- TOT will dramatically improve and strengthen your mindset, thereby allowing you to possess and maintain a competitive edge.

- TOT will provide a sense of invulnerability, which potentially leads to high rewards and a higher social status. One study even suggested that individuals with optimal testosterone levels are more tactical, rather than dominant.

- Optimized testosterone levels will allow you to become the best and strongest version of yourself. In particular, your ability to be supremely confident in your decisions and take decisive action increases exponentially. You are assertive and purposeful in everything you do and say. Your decisions empower you to behave in ways others find attractive.

CHAPTER 4
The Natural Testosterone Boosting Myth

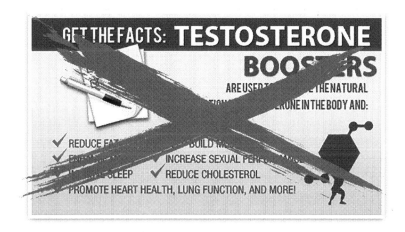

GET THE FACTS: **TESTOSTERONE BOOSTERS**

ARE USED TO ... THE NATURAL ... RONE IN THE BODY AND:

✓ REDUCE FAT   ✓ BUILD ...
... ✓ INCREASE SEXUAL PERF...
...SLEEP ✓ REDUCE CHOLESTEROL
PROMOTE HEART HEALTH, LUNG FUNCTION, AND MORE!

In the past 25 years, you've been bombarded by marketing gimmicks and 'sounds-too-good-to-be-true' ad campaigns from every conceivable form of media trying to sell you the latest and greatest "testosterone booster" supplement.

If you're reading this book, there's a very good chance you've already fallen prey to these ads and invested your hard-earned money into one of those "natural testosterone boosters." We're here to tell you unequivocally that nearly every one of those so-called boosters is a total scam[82]. These products are nothing

---

[82] Heavy Resistance Training and Supplementation With the Alleged Testosterone Booster Nmda has No Effect on Body Composition, Muscle Performance, and Serum Hormones Associated With the Hypothalamo-Pituitary-Gonadal Axis in Resistance-Trained Males. J Sports Sci Med. 2014 Jan 20;13(1):192-9. eCollection 2014.

more than unproven snake oil sold to millions of unsuspecting men who believe and buy into the hype. Men (maybe like yourself) who would do anything to look and feel better. The only thing these supplements have ever done is emptied the bank accounts of those people who swallow the "magic pills."

The companies that sell these boosters claim you can naturally raise testosterone levels through the use of their carefully selected herbal supplements. They make false promises and say that you'll notice a better sex drive, bigger muscles, or even a larger penis from taking these natural remedies. However, none of them actually deliver on their claims. These solutions are ripoffs and will not provide a meaningful increase in your testosterone levels.

So why do they stay in business despite being so ineffective? Well, there are several factors behind their popularity.

First, we live in an 'instant gratification' society that encourages people to seek immediate results without doing the actual work. Our modern culture bows at the altar of the overnight success and the quick fix. Why spend years painstakingly building a testosterone-optimized lifestyle on a foundation of diet, exercise, and sleep when you can just take an "all-natural" testosterone booster and get the same results?

Fitness gurus on YouTube will market testosterone boosters to impressionable young men who see their extreme muscularity and believe that they will achieve a similar physique in "just 60 days" by using these boosters.

Testosterone deficiency is a real, global phenomenon afflicting a massive number of men and it will only continue to grow. This means that there's a growing market of millions of men who are looking for help. But after decades of media misinformation about testosterone, while mislabelling the use of therapeutic testosterone as 'anabolic steroids' or 'juicing', many men are reluctant to undergo hormone optimization due to erroneous concerns over dangerous side effects. As a result, they look to slickly marketed natural remedies in the hopes of boosting their testosterone levels. And now, tons of fraudsters have spun up YouTube channels and portrayed themselves as experts in order to turn a profit.

So what's the cold hard truth about testosterone boosters?

The truth is that there's little to **NO SCIENTIFIC EVIDENCE** which supports the claims made by supplement companies about their testosterone boosters actually raising testosterone levels.

We'll discuss the five most popular herbal supplements typically found in testosterone boosters, and we'll show why using them to raise testosterone levels is a pointless endeavor that will fail every single time.

Tongkat Ali

Eurycoma longifolia, also known as Tongkat Ali, is a herbal supplement that has gained popularity in biohacking circles for its

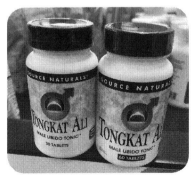

supposed ability to boost testosterone levels. However, most of the studies done on the potential of Tongkat Ali to raise testosterone levels have been done on rat populations, and the results are inconclusive. In one of the few studies done on humans, researchers tested the effects of 200 mg of water-soluble Tongkat Ali per day on men with late-onset hypogonadism[83].

After 5 weeks, the mean increase in serum testosterone levels in 76 men was the equivalent to 80 ng/dL. This increase in testosterone is insufficient to notice any significant benefits when measured using the total testosterone measurement scale provided by Labcorp. We will discuss total testosterone level measurements in depth in Chapter 6.

Tribulus Terrestris

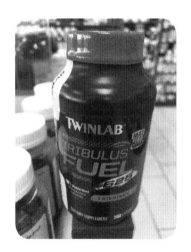

Tribulus terrestris is a plant extract that serves as a key ingredient in many testosterone boosters. However, its benefits appear to be confined solely to an ability to enhance libido. There is virtually zero scientific evidence to correlate *Tribulus terrestris* with a measurable increase in testosterone.

In a double blind study, 22 elite male rugby players took 450 mg of *Tribulus terrestris* daily versus a control group who took a placebo[84]. After 5 weeks, there were no noted differences in urinary testosterone levels and

---

[83] Rochester JR, Bisphenol A and Human Health: A review of the literature., Reproductive Toxicology (2013), http://dx.doi.org/10.1016/j.reprotox.2013.08.008.

[84] S Rogerson et al. "The effect of five weeks of Tribulus terrestris supplementation on muscle strength and body composition during preseason training in elite rugby league players." J Strength Cond Res. 2007 May;21(2):348-53.

lean body mass between the groups, both of which would be important qualitative indicators of higher testosterone levels. A further study of *Tribulus terrestris* supplementation in 21 young men showed no increase in testosterone levels after 4 weeks[85].

Zinc Magnesium Aspartate (ZMA)

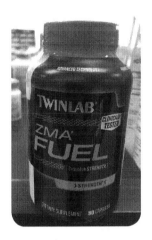

Another popular supplement purported to increase testosterone is Zinc Magnesium Aspartate (ZMA). Indeed, there is sparse evidence to demonstrate ZMA's ability to increase testosterone levels. However, both overtraining and zinc deficiency (not necessarily in conjunction) *are* associated with a reduction in testosterone. When zinc is supplemented in these scenarios, it appears to increase testosterone but only minimally (without any enhancement in training-associated performance).

In the absence of overtraining and a zinc deficiency, zinc appears to have little effect on testosterone levels[86,87]. Similarly, in one double-blind study, magnesium was shown to have

---

[85] Neychev VK,, Mitev VI. "The aphrodisiac herb Tribulus terrestris does not influence the androgen production in young men." J Ethnopharmacol. 2005 Oct 3;101(1-3):319-23.

[86] Kili M et al. "The effect of exhaustion exercise on thyroid hormones and testosterone levels of elite athletes receiving oral zinc." Neuro Endocrinol Lett. 2006 Feb-Apr;27(1-2):247-52.

[87] Netter A, Hartoma R, Nahoul K. "Effect of zinc administration on plasma testosterone, dihydrotestosterone, and sperm count." Arch Androl. 1981 Aug;7(1):69-73.

no statistically significant influence on testosterone levels[88]. And in another study, the effects of ZMA supplementation on anabolism markers (which indicate muscle growth) in 42 resistance-trained males (i.e. males who regularly lift weights) showed no increase in testosterone levels after 8 weeks[89].

Fenugreek

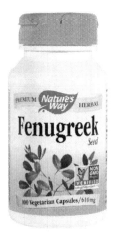

Fenugreek, a plant believed to have the ability to increase libido and testosterone, is also a mainstay in testosterone boosters.

However, the literature differs on Fenugreek's testosterone-raising capabilities. In one study of Fenugreek as an aromatase and 5 α-reductase inhibitor on hormone levels[90], average increases of 6.75% were noted in serum testosterone over an 8-week period. This means a man with serum testosterone levels of 350 ng/dL would see an increase to 374 ng/dL. This tiny increase is not enough to notice any significant benefits to health and/or well-being. Furthermore, the study is suspect because it was

---

[88]   Steels E, Rao A, Vitetta L. Effects of magnesium supplementation on testosterone levels of athletes and sedentary subjects at rest and after exhaustion. Phytother Res. 2011 Sep;25(9):1294-300. doi: 10.1002/ptr.3360. Epub 2011 Feb 10.

[89]   Wilborn C D, et al. "Effects of Zinc Magnesium Aspartate (ZMA) Supplementation on Training Adaptations and Markers of Anabolism and Catabolism." J Int Soc Sports Nutr. 2004; 1(2): 12–20. Published online 2004 Dec 31. doi: 10.1186/1550-2783-1-2-12

[90]   Wilborn C et al. "Effects of a purported aromatase and 5α-reductase inhibitor on hormone profiles in college-age men." Int J Sport Nutr Exerc Metab. 2010 Dec;20(6):457-65.

funded by a company that manufactures a Fenugreek-based workout supplement.

In a study on resistance-trained males, Fenugreek was shown to have no effect on hormonal levels, especially not testosterone[91]. And a randomized placebo study on the effects of Fenugreek on libido involved 60 healthy males taking 600 mg of Fenugreek daily[92]. After 6 weeks, positive improvements were noted in the males' libido, but there was no effect on serum (i.e. total) testosterone levels.

D-Aspartic Acid

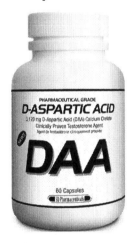

D-Aspartic acid is an amino acid that naturally occurs in the body and can be found in the adrenal gland, pituitary gland and testes[93]. Recently, D-Aspartic acid has gained popularity as a testosterone booster because of its purported involvement in the synthesis and release of testosterone in the body. Therefore, the premise is simple - supplement with D-Aspartic acid and you will be able to boost your testosterone levels!

91   Steels E, Rao A, Vitetta L. "Physiological aspects of male libido enhanced by standardized Trigonella foenum-graecum extract and mineral formulation." Phytother Res. 2011 Sep;25(9):1294-300. doi: 10.1002/ptr.3360. Epub 2011 Feb 10.

92   Bushey, Brandon; Taylor, Lem W.; Wilborn, Colin W.; Poole, Chris; Foster, Cliffa A.; Campbell, Bill; Kreider, Richard B.; and Willoughby, Darryn S. (2009) "Fenugreek Extract Supplementation Has No effect on the Hormonal Profile of Resitance-Trained Males," International Journal of Exercise Science: Conference Proceedings: Vol. 2 : Iss. 1 , Article 13.

93   The putative effects of D-Aspartic acid on blood testosterone levels: A systematic review. Int J Reprod Biomed (Yazd). 2017 January; 15(1): 1–10.

However, upon review of the literature, a familiar story emerges. There are minimal human studies on the efficacy of D-Aspartic acid and the results are inconsistent. One study was done on healthy male volunteers between the ages of 27 and 38 to determine the effect of D-Aspartic acid on fertility[94]. A total of 23 subjects consumed 3.12 grams of D-Aspartic acid for 12 consecutive days. Luteinizing Hormone (LH) levels and serum testosterone levels increased from basal levels by 33% and 42% respectively. At first glance, these results appear promising. However, on further inspection we find several holes in this study. Indeed, no inclusion or exclusion criteria of the sample population were included, and the only detail provided about the participants was their age. Therefore, we cannot truly determine if specific lifestyle factors (e.g. physical activity, supplementation, etc.) had any effect on the study.

Another randomized, double-blind study observed the effect of 3 to 6 grams of D-Aspartic acid daily in resistance trained men. Twenty healthy resistance-trained men, ages 18-36, performed weight training 4 days a week and took either a 3g placebo, 3g D-Aspartic acid or 6g D-Aspartic acid daily[95]. It's interesting to note the participants had to be able to bench press 100% of their body weight to be eligible for the study. After 28 days, no significant effect on strength, body mass or testosterone levels were seen. Furthermore, 6 daily grams of D-Aspartic acid "significantly reduced" total testosterone and free testosterone levels.

---

[94] The role and molecular mechanism of D-aspartic acid in the release and synthesis of LH and testosterone in humans and rats. J Int Soc Sports Nutr. 2015; 12: 15.

[95] Three and six grams supplementation of d-aspartic acid in resistance trained men. J Int Soc Sports Nutr. 2015; 12: 15.

THE NATURAL TESTOSTERONE BOOSTING MYTH

The Only Proven Way to Raise Testosterone

Some studies on herbal supplements do demonstrate a small increase in testosterone levels. However, these increases are both temporary and miniscule, and they cannot always be attributed to the supplement alone.

At best, you could use Tongkat Ali and MAYBE increase your total testosterone from 250 ng/dL to 330 ng/dL - a 32% increase. The problem is that you would still be suffering from suboptimal levels of testosterone, according to the total testosterone measurement scale of LabCorp (These measurement numbers of total testosterone are discussed further in Chapters 6 and 12).

There's no reason to choose that option when a clinical dose of therapeutic testosterone is scientifically proven to optimize your testosterone levels by improving both your total and free measurement lab numbers. TOT works to elevate and optimize your testosterone levels, plain and simple.

With a TOT prescription, you can take your total testosterone from 250 ng/dL to the top of the range at 1000 ng/dL **- a 233% increase**. And trust us when we say that the difference in the way you feel at those higher ranges is NIGHT AND DAY!

Regardless of what you think of the pharmaceutical industry, it is heavily regulated by the FDA, and companies must perform rigorous laboratory tests so they can back their claims with hard evidence. By comparison, the supplement industry in North America is UNREGULATED. This means the majority of supplement companies can make claims on their products without providing any proof. So not only do these boosters not raise your testosterone, you don't actually know for sure if the ingredients used are genuine (i.e. do they actually work)[96]. Another point worth mentioning is that some of these so-called boosters might actually reduce your testosterone levels (as in the aforementioned study with the D-Aspartic acid)!

Raise Libido, Raise Testosterone?

Even though we've thoroughly debunked testosterone boosters, you may still think, 'If it increases my libido, surely it increases testosterone?' That's correlation, but not causation (i.e. increasing libido does not directly cause an increase in testosterone levels). The one underlying theme uniting all these supplements IS their reputation to enhance libido, and in some cases they've been used for centuries as aphrodisiacs. But this doesn't mean that they raise testosterone levels. Your libido is comprised of more than just the amount of testosterone in your blood!

Testosterone itself is a pervasive symbol of masculinity, associated with sex drive and virility. And low testosterone is linked to a lack of sex drive in men. This is precisely where supplement companies trick unsuspecting consumers: By enhancing one's libido, testosterone boosters can make it appear as if they've also increased one's testosterone levels!

However, increased libido doesn't automatically mean you have meaningfully increased your testosterone levels. Research shows that testosterone is not always a decisive factor in libido, and indeed estrogen also plays a vital role in male sexual function. In one study, for example, men with testosterone deficiency received exogenous estradiol (i.e. estrogen delivered

---

[96] O'Connor, Anahad. Herbal Supplements Are Often Not What They Seem. The New York Times. 2013 Nov 3.

into the body from an outside source) and experienced an increase in libido[97]. So think twice about buying any alleged libido enhancers in the vain hope that they will also increase your testosterone levels.

Nonetheless, we're not here to toss out all supplements as garbage - far from it. As we'll see later in the book, there are some fantastic supplements available that can be extremely beneficial to your health. However, there is minimal to no credible scientific research that suggests any nutritional supplements can meaningfully increase and optimize your testosterone levels.

Now, there wouldn't be such a market for testosterone boosters if millions of men weren't aware that their levels were below normal. And as you've already been shown, testosterone levels have been declining for the past several decades[98] and the high market demand for testosterone supplements means that men like you are waking up to this reality.

Which leads many men to ask the following question:

"Why is my testosterone so low in the first place, and why isn't there a natural solution?"

The next few chapters will dive deeper into the science behind testosterone and why powerful environmental factors are currently overshadowing most men's efforts to naturally fix their own testosterone levels.

---

[97]   Schulster M et al. "The role of estradiol in male reproductive function." Asian Journal of Andrology (2016) 18, 1–6.

[98]   A population-level decline in serum testosterone levels in American men. J Clin Endocrinol Metab. 2007 Jan;92(1):196-202. Epub 2006 Oct 24.

If you have low testosterone, does it mean TOT is your only alternative? Not necessarily - it's not that cut and dry. As we've demonstrated in this chapter, most testosterone boosters are bunk but you will very likely get some mileage by modifying your lifestyle. There is one product, Mike Mahler's Aggressive Strength Testosterone Booster[99], that provides clinical studies asserting the effectiveness of the product's individual ingredients in boosting your testosterone levels. For an excellent article on how to maximize natural testosterone production, take a look at Alexander Juan Antonio Cortes' "50 Natural Ways To Increase Your Testosterone"[100].

If you're like most men, there's a good chance that you will benefit from the lifestyle changes Alexander recommends, including a modest increase in your testosterone levels. However, the reality is that modern-day environmental living continues to place our endocrine systems and metabolic health under siege, dramatically reducing our ability to produce testosterone naturally while also remaining lean and healthy. A pharmaceutical approach (i.e. TOT) is the only be-all, end-all solution to ensure successful hormonal optimization. So much so, in fact, that Dr. Rob Kominiarek reveals the percentage of men that can optimize their testosterone naturally in his interview in Chapter 17. The data is shocking.

---

[99]   https://mikemahler.com/nutrition-supplements/aggressive-strength-testosterone-booster

[100]   https://alexanderjuanantoniocortes.com/50-ways-to-naturally-increase-testosterone/

CHAPTER 4 KEY TAKEAWAYS

- Almost every single "testosterone boosting" supplement sold today is a scam. The cold hard truth is that there's little to NO SCIENTIFIC EVIDENCE which supports the claims made by supplement companies about their testosterone boosters actually raising testosterone levels.

- There are various reasons why supplement companies are able to get away with marketing their garbage testosterone boosters. On top of being in an industry where they are exempt from strict rules and regulations, there is a growing market consisting of millions of men who are suffering from testosterone deficiency.

- The 5 most popular testosterone boosting supplements (Tongkat Ali, Tribulus Terrestris, ZMA, Fenugreek and D-Aspartic Acid) have all been thoroughly studied, tested, and proven to be ineffective, leading to insignificant changes in testosterone levels at best. Some of these so-called boosters might actually reduce your testosterone levels!

- While you can use some of the supplements discussed in this chapter to raise libido, this does not correlate to increasing testosterone at all (i.e. increasing libido does not directly cause one's testosterone levels to go up).

- The only proven way to raise and optimize testosterone is through pharmaceutical means (i.e. utilizing TOT). This is because powerful factors in our modern-day environment are constantly placing our endocrine systems under siege. This environmental assault overshadows most men's natural ability to produce testosterone and their efforts to fix low testosterone levels.

CHAPTER 5

Testosterone 101: Understanding the Biological Role of Testosterone

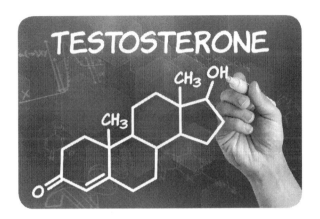

This is going to be a short chapter, because even though it's jam-packed with the science of testosterone production, it still won't come close to an exhaustive analysis of the male endocrine and reproductive system. You can and should do your own research, using this book as a starting point. Instead, what follows is a pragmatic explanation of what testosterone is and how it works in the human body.

What is Testosterone and How is It Made?

Testosterone is a hormone that males and females need in the right amount for optimal mental health and physical performance. Our focus in this chapter, therefore, is twofold.

1. We want to help men who don't want to live within what is incorrectly defined as the "normal range" of testosterone by many medical doctors (what they call normal is far below optimal), and

2. Prevent men from enduring the symptoms of what is clinically diagnosed as *Testosterone Deficiency*[101] (TD), and sometimes as *Partial Androgen Deficiency*[102], and help them experience all the life-changing potential that comes with having optimized testosterone levels.

Testosterone plays many different roles as we age. In early development it is vital for brain, sex, and bone formation. Later in life, it's important for maintaining proper brain chemistry, keeping muscle mass intact, and retaining sexual function[103].

The human body has several regulation systems in place to keep things working properly. For example, if you eat sugar, your body has chemical receptors that pick up the increase of glucose in your bloodstream, and in response it releases insulin from your pancreas to regulate your blood sugar and maintain homeostasis.

Just like how your body has a system for regulating blood glucose levels, it has a system for regulating your testosterone, which we explain below.

---

[101] The Laboratory Diagnosis of Testosterone Deficiency. Paduch, Darius A. et al. Urology, Volume 83, Issue 5, 980 - 988.

[102] Amore M, Innamorati M, Costi S, Sher L, Girardi P, Pompili M. Partial Androgen Deficiency, Depression, and Testosterone Supplementation in Aging Men. *International Journal of Endocrinology.* 2012;2012:280724. doi:10.1155/2012/280724.

[103] Mooradian AD, Morley JE, Korenman SG (February 1987). "Biological actions of androgens." Endocr. Rev. 8 (1): 1–28. doi:10.1210/edrv-8-1-1. PMID 3549275.

The Hypothalamo-pituitary Testicular Axis

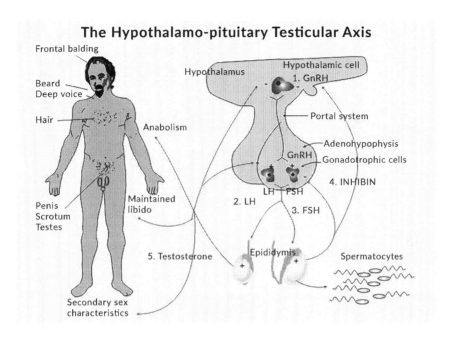

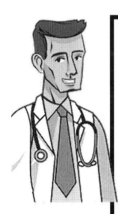

The testosterone production process begins when your brain sends a chemical signal to the hypothalamus (the part of your brain that connects the endocrine system with the nervous system) and tells it to make some testosterone. In turn, the hypothalamus releases a chemical messenger called gonadotropin (GnRH) that gets picked up by the pituitary gland (the part of your brain that controls other hormone glands in your body). This causes the pituitary gland to release two hormones: luteinizing hormone (LH) and follicle-stimulating hormone (FSH). These hormones signal the Leydig cells in the testes to produce testosterone. The testosterone is then released into the bloodstream, where it will either be bound to sex hormone-binding globulin (SHBG) and albumin, or remain in its free form and in turn find other targeted cells to bind with.

When there is enough testosterone in the human body, a negative feedback loop known as the **Hypothalamic-Pituitary-Testicular-Axis** (HPTA) [a.k.a. the hypothalamic–pituitary–gonadal axis (HPGA)] sends messages to the pituitary saying that there is enough testosterone freely circulating around. The pituitary then slows production of LH, and eventually FSH. Testosterone will be reduced (i.e. broken down) into a number of other metabolites that serve important functions, such as dihydrotestosterone (DHT) or estradiol (E2). We will discuss these metabolites in greater detail in Chapter 10.

In a perfect world, this homeostatic process works to keep men at optimal levels of testosterone. Unfortunately, homeostasis is rarely maintained in male endocrine systems in the present day (for many reasons soon to be explained).

Why Do Men Stop Producing Optimal Levels of Testosterone?

As we age, our body becomes less efficient at maintaining proper testosterone production and our testosterone levels begin to decrease. This could be in response to an injury, such as damaged testes. For example, blunt trauma[104] to

---

[104]   http://www.webmd.com/men/guide/testicle-injuries

your testicles accounts for 75% of testicular injuries. But most men don't have testicular injuries, and yet they still have low testosterone levels. Why is that?

Endocrine Disruption from Modern Day Societal Living

The truth, which not enough people are acknowledging, is that the modern environments we live in are catastrophic to our endocrine systems. Living in cities, working all day under fluorescent lights, and eating manufactured GMO foods is slowly but surely destroying our bodies. The increase in environmental pollutants, contaminants, and particulates in the air[105] produced by industrial factories, smog, emissions from cars, and more are bombarding our systems[106] and lowering testosterone levels on a global scale[107]. Men are also under siege from hormone-suppressing phytoestrogens[108] (such as soy protein by-products[109]) and a host of other toxins that our bodies were not designed to handle, yet are commonplace today.

Exposure to *phthalates* (chemicals found in plastics and personal care products) is "feminizing" males by blocking normal

---

[105] Lao XQ, Zhang Z, Lau AK, et al. Exposure to ambient fine particulate matter and semen quality in Taiwan. *Occup Environ Med.* Published Online First: 13 November 2017. doi: 10.1136/oemed-2017-104529.

[106] http://www.ewg.org/research/dirty-dozen-list-endocrine-disruptors

[107] Gore AC, Chappell VA, Fenton SE, et al. EDC-2: The Endocrine Society's Second Scientific Statement on Endocrine-Disrupting Chemicals. Endocrine Reviews. 2015;36(6):E1-E150. doi:10.1210/er.2015-1010.

[108] Are oestrogens involved in falling sperm counts and disorders of the male reproductive tract?" Lancet 341 (8857): 1392–5. doi:10.1016/0140-6736. Sharpe RM, Skakkebaek NE (1993).

[109] http://fabfitover40.com/2014/06/06/soy-protein-friend-foe/

testosterone production[110]. Sperm counts are falling due to exposure to pesticides, endocrine-disrupting chemicals like bisphenol A (BPA)[111], and the many other toxins that are increasingly pervading our water and food supplies. **The most recent study from Hebrew University actually predicts that all men will be infertile by the year 2050[112].**

Phthalates are a problem that exist not just for men, but for women and children as well. There is now enough scientific evidence from animal and human studies to show that exposure to phthalates is associated with reduced testosterone levels and the fertility disorders that come with them[113].

Regardless of the cause, when you are regularly exposed to these endocrine-disrupting chemicals, your testosterone levels will decline and you'll start to feel less energetic over time. This sneaks up on most men in the form of low energy and low vitality, who then accept this as a natural side effect of being "old."

If a man with low levels of testosterone is fortunate enough to be diagnosed by a physician, he can be classified as hypogonadal (i.e. suffering from low levels of testosterone) and be-

[110] How dangerous are phthalate plasticizers? Integrated approach to toxicity based on metabolism, electron transfer, reactive oxygen species and cell signaling Kovacic, Peter. Medical Hypotheses, Volume 74, Issue 4, 626-628.

[111] How safe is bisphenol A? Fundamentals of toxicity: Metabolism, electron transfer and oxidative stress. Kovacic, Peter. Medical Hypotheses, Volume 75, Issue 1, 1-4.

[112] Hagai Levine, Niels Jørgensen, Anderson Martino-Andrade, Jaime Mendiola, Dan Weksler-Derri, Irina Mindlis, Rachel Pinotti, Shanna H. Swan; Temporal trends in sperm count: a systematic review and meta-regression analysis, *Human Reproduction Update*, https://doi.org/10.1093/humupd/dmx022

[113] Urinary phthalate metabolites are associated with decreased serum testosterone in men, women, and children from Nhanes 2011-2012. J Clin Endocrinol Metab. 2014 Nov;99(11):4346-52. doi: 10.1210/jc.2014-2555. Epub 2014 Aug 14.

gin treatment. The most recent data[114] shows that nearly 40% of all men over the age of fifty are classified as hypogonadal (suffering from hypogonadism). But as the science continues to show, this number is significantly underestimated and under-reported.

Defining Hypogonadism

For the purpose of keeping things simple, there are two forms of diagnosed hypogonadism:

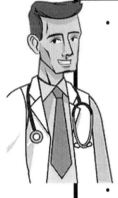

- **Primary Hypogonadism** results from defects of the gonads. This can result from physical defects to the HPTA, and is usually indicated when luteinizing hormone (LH) and/or follicle stimulating hormone (FSH) are elevated. Since these two hormones are produced in the gonads, elevated levels of both hormones likely means the problem of low testosterone is due to issues there.

- **Secondary Hypogonadism** results from hypothalamic or pituitary defects (which may be tied to obesity, insulin resistance, or environmental factors). In this instance, LH and/or FSH are at normal or low levels, suggesting the problem is a disruption within the HTPA/HPGA. This is the diagnosis most normally associated with aging men suffering from a testosterone deficiency.

---

[114] https://www.nebido.com/en/hcp/research/testosterone-research/
testosterone-deficiency-prevalence-and-treatment-rates.php#

Many doctors falsely classify 'normal aging' as the cause of secondary hypogonadism, ignoring the environmental factors that are unique to modern societal living. However, we refuse to accept getting softer, weaker, depressed, and having a low libido as 'normal' and 'healthy' aging.

Why would you, or any man you know for that matter, want to feel this way? Especially knowing that you can optimize your blood levels for life with the power of therapeutic testosterone!

CHAPTER 5 KEY TAKEAWAYS

- Testosterone is a hormone that males and females need in the right amount for optimal mental health and physical performance. It plays many different roles as we age.

- The human body has several regulation systems in place to keep things working properly (ie. maintaining homeostasis), including a system for regulating your testosterone. Through a basic overview of endocrinology, you learned about the importance of the HPTA also known as the HPGA.

- You learn the truth about what is going on in the world, and therefore you know what prevents your body from naturally producing optimal levels of testosterone.

- The modern day environments we live in are catastrophic to our endocrine systems. Being constantly exposed to endocrine-disrupting chemicals and toxins lowers your testosterone levels and you'll start to feel less and less energetic over time. This sneaks up on most men in the form of low energy and low vitality, yet most men accept this as a natural side effect of being "old."

- We defined the two clinical diagnosis terms for Testosterone Deficiency and/or Partial Androgen Deficiency. We also differentiate between Primary and Secondary Hypogonadism. The former is usually due to a medical defect, whereas the latter is normally caused by environmental factors like aging, poor nutrition, obesity, endocrine disrupting chemicals, etc.

CHAPTER 6
Choosing When to Optimize Your Testosterone Levels

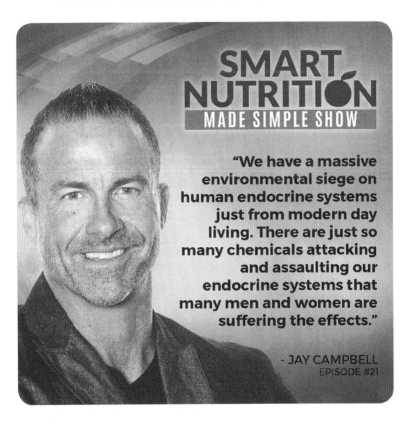

SMART NUTRITION
MADE SIMPLE SHOW

"We have a massive environmental siege on human endocrine systems just from modern day living. There are just so many chemicals attacking and assaulting our endocrine systems that many men and women are suffering the effects."

- JAY CAMPBELL
EPISODE #21

Now that you're aware of the factors decreasing male testosterone levels, and are educated about how crucial the hormone is for your well-being, the next step is to get your own levels checked and investigate if TOT is a good solution for you.

There are some crucial factors you need to take into account before making the decision to proceed with TOT.

Is There an Ethical Dilemma in Choosing to Use Testosterone?

One of the biggest challenges men face today is overcoming the potential moral dilemma of using TOT.

The fact that a naturally occurring hormone, essential to the development of every human being on planet Earth, is being aggressively controlled and demonized is a reflection of the incredible amount of ignorance under which mainstream society lives. There is nothing morally wrong with optimizing your own testosterone levels, any more than taking Lipitor to lower your cholesterol. There are no limits to the factors working AGAINST you and your testosterone levels—stress, diet, pollution, age, popular culture, and so on.

Living with a testosterone deficiency is a silent pandemic because the vast majority of men (and society as a whole) aren't even aware that low testosterone levels are an issue. Most men don't take ownership of their health, and end up walking out of their doctor's offices with a script for a harmful SSRI (which often leads to a worsening of their symptoms and their overall health) and some erectile dysfunction medication (usually Viagra). These medications only treat the symptoms of low testosterone (depressed moods, low sex drive, etc.) but ignore the root cause.

There are dozens of ways in which society accepts the use of drugs for the sake of our health and well-being on a daily basis. Testosterone optimization therapy should be no different.

Think about it:

- If you have a headache, do you think twice about taking Aspirin to stop your head from pounding?

- Do you wake up in the morning with a cup of coffee so you can start the day with a little caffeine?

- If you lose the cartilage in your hips and can only get around in a wheelchair for the rest of your life, would you allow a surgeon to cut you open and replace your joints so you could walk again?

Again, optimizing your levels of testosterone is LITERALLY no different. We have zero doubt that in less than 10 years, TOT will be widely accepted for men who want to live at their highest physical and mental potential.

Testosterone Levels Decline with Age

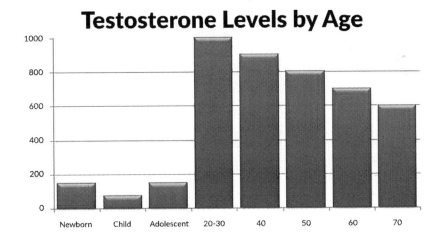

115

---

115   http://www.downtownmedicalservices.com/index.php/low-testosterone-impacts-mens-health/

Ten years ago, we generally would have recommended men to start TOT no sooner than 35 years old, but it's becoming more apparent that low testosterone is a significant problem in men of ALL ages—not just men over 35. We wrote this book as a step-by-step guide for all men, but it's worth emphasizing that younger men need to proceed cautiously and learn as much as possible before seeking out and using TOT. **Daniel Kelly** (who Jay has personally mentored and is one of the smartest people under 35 on the planet in regards to hormonal optimization) is launching his book in the middle of 2018, titled *Optimized Under 35: The Ultimate Hormonal Health Guide for Young Men*[116]. This book will be a MUST HAVE companion book for any younger man looking to fully optimize his life.

If you're under 30 and you have the slightest intention of having children in the future, your doctor should first consider any natural means available for alleviating symptoms of low testosterone - improving your nutrition, reducing body fat and inflammatory markers, and so on. This is preferable to starting TOT, which could interfere with your fertility if you're not working with a doctor who is also prescribing you medications that are designed to retain your reproductive capability. Maintaining your fertility through TOT (which is always possible) is heavily discussed in Chapter 12, where we conduct a "state of the science" interview with **Dr. Merrill Matschke**.

A natural course of action would involve optimizing your lifestyle to get significant sunlight every day, starting a weight training program, and eating a diet rich in healthy fats and low in carbs. In other words, if you're living a sedentary lifestyle, eating tons of cheetos, and spending most of your days playing video games, your FIRST step is to take the necessary steps to

---

[116]   http://danielkelly.eu/

change your lifestyle. TOT is *part* of a healthy lifestyle, not a band-aid solution for an unhealthy one.

Two great sources of information for younger men under the age of 35, as previously mentioned, are Daniel Kelly[117] and also Alexander Juan Antonio Cortes[118]. Both of these men write prolifically on the subject of optimizing health in young males[119].

Today, many young men are suffering from suboptimal testosterone levels, and often times doctors will refuse to acknowledge the problem. Daniel's book will specifically address the issue, challenges and ultimately the solution for hormone optimization therapy for men under 35. If lifestyle changes fail, the next step is doctor-prescribed medications that attempt to raise your testosterone levels (while maintaining your fertility) and are not disruptive (or minimally so) of your body's natural production of testosterone. In Chapters 10 and 12, we will explain how these medications work to raise your natural testosterone levels.

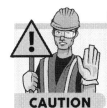

CAUTION

It's important to understand that using TOT productively is a lifelong strategy. And in order to start therapy, you need to be financially stable (We discuss these exact costs in Chapter 8). Being able to pay for your treatment and any additional medications (when necessary) must be factored into your daily life expenses. While we recommend that men in their early 20's pursue natural solutions first, we are also reluctant to recommend TOT

---

[117]   http://www.trtrevolution.com/author/dkelley/

[118]   http://www.trtrevolution.com/author/alexander/

[119]   www.optimizedunder35.com

to this demographic because they may not be financially stable yet. If you happen to be a man in your early 20's, make sure you go to Daniel Kelly's website[120] to find out about his book coming out in 2018.

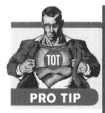

PRO TIP

If you are a much younger man and you believe you are suffering from the symptoms of low testosterone (and would benefit from TOT), we highly recommend that you first go online and pay for an independent blood test[121] to see if your testosterone blood levels are low enough for you to seek out an experienced TOT doctor for guidance. But remember: **low testosterone is a clinical diagnosis, NOT a laboratory one**. It's not simply "low testosterone" on a blood test. What constitutes "low" for you may be different than what is considered low for someone else. It's important to understand that symptoms trump lab results, and we cover what this means later in the book.

Symptoms of Low Testosterone

The most important consideration for choosing to be on TOT is whether or not you're experiencing the symptoms associated with sub-optimal levels of testosterone.

---

120   http://danielkelly.eu/

121   https://www.discountedlabs.com/testosterone-replacement

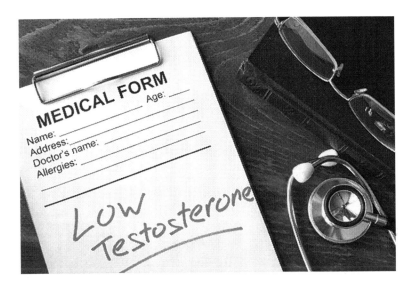

These symptoms can be any of the following:

1. Mental fog or loss of focus
2. Indecisiveness or hesitancy
3. Lack of energy
4. Decreased work performance
5. Decrease in sex drive or ability to reach orgasm
6. Decrease in strength or endurance
7. Decreased "enjoyment of life"
8. Noticeable change in behavior

If you consistently experience any 4 of the previous symptoms, consider further testing and consulting with a doctor about TOT.

There are two commonly used questionnaires which are sometimes used as a diagnostic test in men with symptoms of low testosterone: ADAM and AMS (NOTE: they are always used in conjunction with blood tests to give you the most complete picture of your health).

ADAM (Androgen Deficiency in Aging Males) & AMS (Aging Males Symptoms)

The ADAM survey consists of 10 simple 'yes or no' questions. If you say 'yes' to questions #1, #7, and 3 more, then you may have low testosterone. You can view the survey to see for yourself[122]. The AMS 17-question survey is much more detailed and divided into 3 quadrants: physical, psychological, and sexual symptoms. You can view it here[123].

Both of these questionnaires can be useful for you to gather more data, but they are only an adjunct to a proper clinical diagnosis by an experienced TOT-prescribing physician.

Know Your Testosterone Levels, Understand Your Test Results

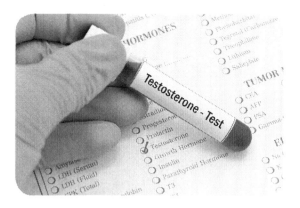

---

122   http://www.prostatehealthnaturally.com/downloads/ADAM_Questionnaire.pdf

123   http://www.aging-males-symptoms-scale.info/documents/question.pdf

The most important objective consideration for TOT is if your measurement of "free" and "total serum" testosterone levels are low, or out of range. Optimally, a man should exhibit testosterone levels at the highest end of the normal range (depending on the total testosterone measuring scale).

The Normal Range Fallacy

There's just one problem: who defines the 'normal' range? There is an infinite amount of hormonal diversity across the male population and there is no real way to compress all men into a rigid 'standard patient' model where the normal range is universally defined. The following chart shows the variance in ranges between the primary blood lab measurement companies:

Laboratory	Normal Range of Total Testosterone
LabCorp	264–1197 ng/dL[124]
Quest Diagnostics	250–1100 ng/dL[125]
Bio Reference Laboratories	300–1000 ng/dL[126]

In July of 2017, LabCorp recently changed its reference range for total testosterone levels. They lowered their normal values of testosterone by roughly 100 ng/dL. The previous reference range was based on a 2011 study of lean healthy males[127]. This

---

[124]   https://www.labcorp.com/assets/11476

[125]   http://www.questdiagnostics.com/testcenter/TestDetail.action?ntc=15983

[126]   http://www.bioreference.com/test-directory/?search=Testosterone

[127]   Bhasin S, Bencina M, Jasuja GK, et al. Reference ranges for testosterone in men generated using liquid chromatography tandem mass spectrometry in a community- based sample of healthy nonobese young men in the Framingham Heart Study and applied to three geographically distinct cohorts. *J Clin Endocrinol Metab.* 2011;96(8):2430-9.

THE TESTOSTERONE OPTIMIZATION THERAPY BIBLE

effectively means that they have arbitrarily lowered their range and re-defined what is "normal."

They cite a new 2017 study[128] as a primary factor for their new reference range:

> "In early 2017, Travison, et al. demonstrated that obesity is directly associated with lower testosterone levels in male patients...The lower numeric range in the new standardized reference interval reflects a difference in average subjects with higher BMIs as well as harmonization with the CDC reference method."

Basically, LabCorp's physician panel had to accommodate a growing population that is now more obese and has lower testosterone levels on average. Remember, there is only a 6 year difference between the studies. In other words, they're lowering their range of 'normal' total testosterone levels to reflect the epidemic of obese men with lower testosterone levels.

Most people have noticed that the lower end of LabCorp's testosterone reference range is now 264 ng/dL, whereas the previous lower end of the 'normal range' was 348 ng/dL.

Previous LabCorp Reference Interval	New LabCorp Reference Interval (effective July 17, 2017)
Adult Male >18 years: 348 – 1197 ng/dL	Adult Male >18 years: 264 – 916 ng/dL
Comment: Adult male reference interval is based on a population of lean males up to 40 years old.	Comment: Adult male reference interval is based on a population of healthy nonobese males (BMI <30) between 19 and 39 years old.

---

128   Travison TG, Vesper HW, Orwoll E, et al. Harmonized reference ranges for circulating testosterone levels in men of four cohort studies in the United States and Europe. J Clin Endocrinol Metab 2017;102(4):1161-73.

So now _if you're 30_ and have the testosterone levels of a geriatric – congratulations, you're normal!

What's even more disconcerting, however, is the fact they've also lowered the top end of the reference range. It was originally 1197 ng/dL and now it is 916 ng/dL. That's almost a 300 ng/dL difference! This is HUGE. Therefore, according to LabCorp, if you're above 916 ng/dL, you have supraphysiological (i.e. above average) testosterone levels.

The biggest issue with these measurement companies is the variance of their assessment between total and free testosterone levels in healthy young men.[129] While variation between laboratories for the same testosterone assay is negligible, the reference ranges for testosterone levels [as well as luteinizing hormone (**LH**) and follicle-stimulating hormone (**FSH**)] differ widely and significantly.[130] In other words, the labs will all give you similarly accurate results, but they will each define whether or not those results are "normal" in a different way.

This means that a physician can't rely entirely on blood levels alone as an indicator of whether or not somebody qualifies for TOT. This presents a conundrum for doctors who might assume that there is a specific testosterone level below which the symptoms appear, and go on to assume that this threshold is the same for everybody.

The reality is that there really is too much variance from person to person. In other words, your body is different from mine

---

[129] Bhasin, S., et al. The impact of assay quality and reference ranges on clinical decision making in the diagnosis of androgen disorders. Steroids, 2008. 73(13): p. 1311-7.

[130] Sikaris, K., et al. Reproductive hormone reference intervals for healthy fertile young men: evaluation of automated platform assays. J Clin Endocrinol Metab, 2005. 90(11): p. 5928-36.

and is also different from someone else's. Therefore, you need to work closely with your doctor to look at the whole picture of your health, rather than rely on a generalized standard.

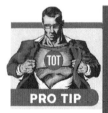

PRO TIP

Physicians should ALWAYS treat the patient's symptoms first before anything else. If you have blood testosterone levels in the normal to high range (usually above 600 ng/dL) then you're likely not a candidate for TOT. There are *always exceptions to the rule*, but under normal circumstances it is not enough for a patient to merely possess low to low-normal blood testosterone levels. They must also demonstrate 4-5 of the accepted low testosterone symptoms before obtaining a prescription for TOT.

Vital Life Markers Necessary for TOT

The purpose of this book is about improving well-being and happiness in every aspect of your life by using TOT as a tool when necessary.

Understanding this, you should meet a minimum of two of these three vital life markers before exploring Testosterone Optimization Therapy:

1) **Age 30 or older:** It is readily apparent that testosterone deficiency is affecting younger men at a higher rate than ever before. If you're in your 20's, proceed with caution. Do your homework and attempt to maximize natural production through improving your lifestyle first. If that fails, make sure

you're financially able to afford TOT. You must also find and work with a progressive TOT-prescribing physician[131] who is willing to work with you, should your presenting symptoms and blood levels warrant a clinical diagnosis of low testosterone.

2) **Testosterone levels lower than 600 ng/dL on a verifiable blood test:**

It depends on your SYMPTOMS if you're at the upper end (500-600 ng/dL) of the normal range. Also, remember that different blood test companies provide a varying range of lab assay values that differ significantly[132]. Physicians should NEVER chase lab numbers, and should clearly evaluate symptoms first and foremost.

3) **Experiencing the symptoms of low testosterone as recognized by your clinician:**

Ultimately, your physician is evaluating your clinical symptoms as their final determinant for diagnosis. Symptoms are the MOST IMPORTANT determinant of whether a man should begin a TOT regimen.

If these all apply to you, it is reasonable to consider yourself a candidate for Testosterone Optimization Therapy.

---

[131]   www.renuehealth.com.

[132]   Bhasin, S., et al. The impact of assay quality and reference ranges on clinical decision making in the diagnosis of androgen disorders. Steroids, 2008. 73(13): p. 1311-7.

How to Get Tested for Low Testosterone

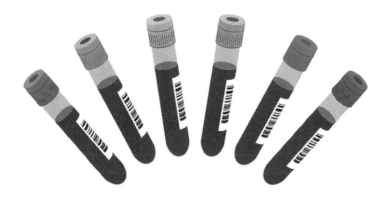

When working with an experienced TOT physician[133], have them order your blood test. Just make sure to inform your doctor about your long term goal of using TOT productively.

Some doctors are more flexible in their criteria for justifying blood tests and will work with you to ensure that everything is evaluated closely. In Chapter 12, we will define and discuss the important lab assays (blood tests) needed in greater detail.

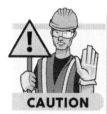

CAUTION

A word to the wise: Any doctor who provides unnecessary resistance to getting a blood test, let alone discussing TOT, is probably going to be resistant to any kind of testosterone therapy. If he or she is unwilling to intelligently discuss your request, or rejects it out of hand, it is your right to seek the counsel of another doctor.

---

[133]   www.bodhd.com

If this happens (and it happens far too often), it usually indicates that your doctor doesn't understand the importance of optimal testosterone levels. As well, you now know that your presenting symptoms can often trump blood values when dealing with low testosterone. It is important that the doctor you work with is able to intelligently discuss your individual condition (respective of both your blood panels and symptoms) and can formulate a sound clinical diagnosis moving forward.

One simple and inexpensive way to measure your serum testosterone levels before having your doctor order comprehensive lab tests is to order a blood test online[134]. *It's easy, fast, convenient* and as simple as ordering a book from Amazon.com. You just go to the website, add the blood test to your cart, and pay for it.

After placing the order, you'll have the option of going to the closest participating blood testing lab in your area (as referred to by the website) and get your blood drawn at your convenience. The lab visit should take less than 10 minutes, and you'll typically receive your results via email within a few days.

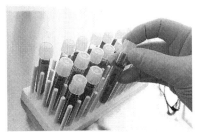

Standard Anti-Aging Tests (Male)

- CBC
- CMP
- Cortisol
- DHEA
- Estradiol
- Homocysteine
- IGF-1
- LH & FSH
- Lipid Panel
- PSA
- SHBG
- Testosterone Free & Total
- Vitamin-D 25
- Thyroid Panel: TSH, Free T3, Free and Total T4
- HBA1-c
- Pregnenolone

---

[134]   https://www.discountedlabs.com/testosterone-replacement

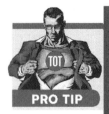

For men in their 20's and 30's undergoing TOT, we recommend you get your blood drawn at least once a year. For those of you in your 40's and up, twice a year is best. Additionally, an Anti-Aging Panel is highly recommended for anybody ages 35 and up. If you are not already doing so, you should begin getting regular blood work done so you can compile and reference all of your blood panel data for life. Having a detailed timeline from your initial blood testosterone panel will provide excellent comparison points as your biomarkers change over time, which they inevitably will as you age.

While your physician will be documenting your lab results, we also recommend you keep your own copies of your blood panels so that you can become intimately aware of the changes you experience. Take responsibility, do your homework, and know your body!

In Chapter 12, we'll discuss the specific types of blood panels that a progressive TOT-prescribing physician should be ordering, along with the importance of monitoring them.

CHAPTER 6 KEY TAKEAWAYS

- There is nothing morally wrong or unethical about optimizing your body's levels of testosterone. It's the same as having Lasix, or an artificial hip replacement surgery.

- Testosterone levels decline with age but this should not stop you from becoming proactive, while seeking to optimize them first via natural means (i.e. through improvement of lifestyle factors like nutrition, exercise, sleep, etc.).

- Understand that using TOT productively is a lifelong strategy. And in order to start therapy, you need to be financially stable. Being able to pay for your treatment and any additional medications (when necessary) must be factored into your daily life expenses.

- We teach you how to recognize the primary symptoms of low testosterone levels (mental fog, indecisiveness, lack of energy, etc.) and show you the questionnaires commonly used as an adjunct to a proper clinical diagnosis.

- We discuss the "Normal Range Fallacy" and how total testosterone levels are being lowered across the board by the lab measurement companies to reflect the increase in obesity, metabolic disorder and insulin resistance in men.

- The 3 vital life criteria necessary to determine whether you should optimize your testosterone levels are as follows: Age 30 or older, testosterone levels lower than 600 ng/dL on a verifiable blood test, and experiencing the symptoms of low testosterone as recognized by your clinician.

- We teach you how to get blood tested (via lab work), with or without a doctor's recommendation.

CHAPTER 7

Testosterone Optimization Therapy - Non-Injectable Options

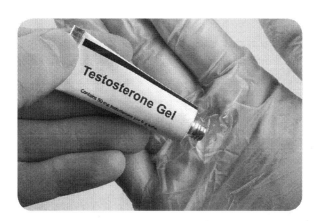

Once you've gotten your blood work collected and your symptoms properly identified, and found a progressive and experienced doctor to prescribe TOT, you get to decide the method of delivery.

There are a number of approved strategies for TOT that differ from one another, almost as much as the physicians administering them. Not all of them are equal. In our experience, we've found the topical delivery methods to be slightly less effective than injectable preparations (which we will cover extensively in the next chapter).

However, we are covering the current and most accepted delivery systems so that you can make an informed decision for yourself. It's crucial that with TOT (and every other aspect of your life), you get the big picture and take full responsibility for your choices.

There are many TOT-prescribing physicians who will disagree with our recommendations regarding injectable testosterone. To be clear, there is nothing wrong with a transdermal strategy. Often times, doctors prescribe transdermals (topicals) over injectables to maintain patient adherence, due to the patient having a fear of needles. This is perfectly acceptable, and ultimately it boils down to the choice of the patient.

After close to 20 years in the trenches, our research strongly indicates that our optimal protocol (discussed in Chapter 8) does the best job of quickly achieving stable blood testosterone levels within the accepted ranges for any age group, while improving health and minimizing side effects. Optimizing blood testosterone levels, while staying within accepted ranges, will provide the ultimate experience that men are looking for when undergoing TOT.

Bio-identical Testosterone

The term 'bioidentical' is often misconstrued, even by physicians who often claim that bioidentical testosterone is "better" or more "natural" than pharmaceutical-grade testosterone. The reality is that all testosterone utilized in TOT possesses an identical molecular structure to your body's naturally-produced testosterone. Pharmaceutical-grade testosterone IS bio-identical to 'natural' testosterone because it is an "esterified" form of testosterone. Esterified testosterone means that the testosterone is attached to a carrier molecule known as an *ester*, which is then enzymatically cleaved (i.e. broken off) in the bloodstream, leaving you with the 'identical' testosterone molecule that your gonads produce (in men).

Creams and Gels

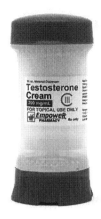

Androgel is the most prescribed TOT protocol in the world[135], and millions of men use it. Many doctors believe in its therapeutic value for raising low testosterone levels. The gels come in either 1%, 2%, 5% or 10% testosterone concentrations. In our opinion, it's sub-optimal for several reasons. The primary drawback is that its concentration is too low and it is also difficult to control the delivery of the dosage. Absorption through the skin is inefficient due to food consumption, sweat glands, and other factors. Often times, this inconsistent absorption rate produces a variance in DHT levels (DHT levels are discussed in much greater detail in Chapter 10) and potentially negative (i.e. estrogenic) side effects like puffy nipples, water retention, and mood swings. It's also too easy to accidentally transfer the cream to women and children when you come in contact with them.

There are doctors who believe that topical delivery systems (when dosed in much stronger compounded concentrations than Androgel) work well. Dr. Crisler, author of *Testosterone Replacement Therapy - Recipe for Success*, believes transdermal delivery systems are superior to injectable formats. This is based on his years of clinical experience with thousands of patients. Dr. Crisler's theory is that transdermal delivery systems produce a serum androgen (base testosterone) profile which will fluctuate during the day, essentially mimicking the normal fluctuations of endogenous testosterone production in a young

---

[135] Yu Z, Gupta SK, Hwang SS, et al. Testosterone pharmacokinetics after application of an investigational transdermal system in hypogonadal men. J Clin Pharmacol. 1997;37:1139–1145. [PubMed][Ref list].

healthy male. In other words, entropy (i.e. randomness) in hormone levels best replicates the feelings of youth. And because they also elevate DHT, the transdermals are better at addressing sexual dysfunction[136]. Dr. Crisler is also interviewed for a landmark discussion about Sex Hormone Binding Globulin later in Chapter 12.

There are now many forms of FDA-approved transdermal testosterone, which you can see in the following chart[137]:

TOPICAL CREAMS/GELS/SOLUTIONS-TESTOSTERONE

BIOIDENTICAL	DOSAGES AVAILABLE	DOSING REGIMEN	COMMENTS/REFERENCES
Testosterone cream, gel or non - alcohol gel (compounding pharmacies) 🈂🈂🈂🈂	Any	25-100 mg once to twice daily	Shippen E. The Testosterone Syndrome, (New York, NY: M. Evans and Company) 1998:197. Brownstein D. The Miracle of Natural Hormones, 3rd Edn. (W. Bloomfield, M I: Medical Alternatives Press) 2003:128.
Androgel® testosterone topical gel (AbbVie Inc.)	10mg/gram packet 16.2mg/gram packet or metered dose pump	25-100 mg daily	Contains 67% ethanol. Each 10 mg/gm packet contains 2.5 grams or 5 grams of gel (25-50mg testosterone) Each 16.2mg/gm packet contains 1.25 grams or 2.5 grams of gel (20.25-40.5gm& testosterone). Each16.2mg/gm pump dispenses 1.25 grams of gel (20.25mg testosterone) Should not be applied to genitals or abdomen. (Androgel [package insert]). AbbVie North Chicago,IL:2014)
Testim® testosterone topical gel (Auxilium. Inc.)	10mg/gram	50-100 mg daily	Contains 74% ethanol. Available in unit dose tubes. Each tube contains 5 grams of gel. Should not be applied to genitals or to the abdomen. (Drug Facts and Comparisons: 2006: 261.)
Axiron® testosterone topical solution (Lily)	30 mg per pump	1-4 pumps to axilla daily	Alcohol based solution. Each pump is 1.5 ml of solution. Use applicator to apply directly to axilla. Apply in 1 pump increments. Alternate axilla for dosing greater than 1 pump. Allow site to dry completely before dressing. Apply deodorant prior to Axiron application. (Drug Facts and Comparisons; 2011:261a-261c.)
Fortesta® testosterone topical gel (Endo Pharmaceuticals Inc)	10 mg per pump	1- 7 pumps daily starting with a dose of 4 pumps.	Alcohol-based gel. Each pump is 0.5 grams of gel. Apply with 1 finger to inner thighs. If dosing more than 1 pump alternate thighs. (Drug Facts and Comparisons; 2011: 261a-261b.)

---

[136] Testosterone Replacement Therapy-A Recipe for Success-Dr. Crisler pg.33 Milestones Publishing (March 13, 2015)

[137] https://www.excelmale.com/showthread.php?1487-Testosterone-Replacement-Treatment-Options

In our experience, it's a nuisance to constantly apply creams or gels throughout the day. On top of that, patients have to avoid swimming, bathing, showering and/or excess sweating for hours after application. As previously mentioned, there is also the very real risk of accidentally transferring the cream to children, women and pets. It is our opinion that most creams and gels don't bring your testosterone levels into the optimal range.

Obviously, there are compounded formulations that work incredibly well. For example, Androgel is 1.62% testosterone by weight. Compounded testosterone cream can be up to 20% testosterone by weight. While both of these branded and compounded products allow testosterone to be dosed transdermally, transdermal creams are recommended over gels for several reasons. For starters, creams offer superior penetration compared to gels. Testosterone creams are compounded in a base that offers a much higher penetration of the testosterone through the skin (40-50%) compared to the 10% penetration of most water-based gels. Since 5 times the amount of drug is being delivered into circulation by using a transdermal cream, versus a gel, a lower amount needs to be applied to achieve optimal testosterone levels. Creams also moisten skin, while alcohol-based gels dry it out. Higher active ingredient loads can be accommodated with creams compared to gels, as most hormones (especially testosterone) are not water soluble and require a lipophillic vehicle to get through the dermis (skin) into systemic circulation. If your insurance doesn't cover branded transdermal testosterone gels, you typically have to pay $300-400 out of pocket every month. Compounded transdermal creams are about ⅛th the cost, so there are significant cost savings.

Many men choose this method of TOT simply because it is the path of least resistance, both from a pain standpoint (i.e. no injections) and because many doctors dispense this form of TOT liberally. Given that TOT has to be administered for life, patient adherence is a primary focus of the treating physician. At the end of the day, some men ultimately prefer to apply cream, rather than inject themselves.

Natesto Nasal Gel

Natesto is a recently FDA-approved intranasal gel (i.e. taken through the nose) for the treatment of suboptimal levels of testosterone. Even though Natesto is a very new medication on the scene, users report a wide variety of side effects with the drug including (but not limited to)[138]:

- Increased Prostate Specific Antigen (PSA) levels. This is a test used to screen for prostate cancer, and a higher PSA potentially indicates an increased risk of cancer.
- Headache
- Runny nose
- Nosebleeds
- Nose pain
- Sore throat, cough
- Upper respiratory infection
- Sinus infection

---

[138] http://www.natesto.com/patient/

Since there is both zero long-term data with the medication and reports of headaches and nasal irritation with usage from many users, we can't recommend this form of therapy.

Oral Forms of Testosterone

There are two new oral forms of testosterone undecanoate currently awaiting FDA review. Both are designed to overcome many of the issues related to TOT products on the U.S. market. These issues are identified on the following chart:

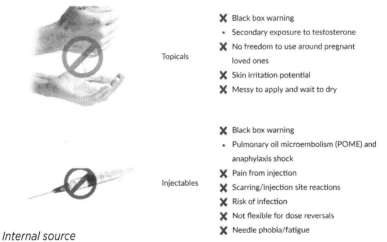

Topicals
✘ Black box warning
• Secondary exposure to testosterone
✘ No freedom to use around pregnant loved ones
✘ Skin irritation potential
✘ Messy to apply and wait to dry

Injectables
✘ Black box warning
• Pulmonary oil microembolism (POME) and anaphylaxis shock
✘ Pain from injection
✘ Scarring/injection site reactions
✘ Risk of infection
✘ Not flexible for dose reversals
✘ Needle phobia/fatigue

Internal source

Each medication is a capsule form of testosterone unde-canoate. The first one was formerly known as **'Rextoro'** but is now known as **'Jatenzo'** of *Clarus Therapeutics* and has recently re-applied for FDA approval[139] after previously getting rejected[140]. In addition, **Tlando**[141] of *Lipocene Inc.* also applied for FDA approval in August of 2017. As of January 11th 2018,

---

[139] https://www.drugs.com/nda/jatenzo_170626.html

[140] http://www.biospace.com/News/fda-panel-denies-clarus-therapeutics-oral/347110

[141] http://bit.ly/2Du2teF

both Jatenzo and Tlando failed to win FDA backing as advisory panels rejected both drugs[142].

In theory, both medications offer great promise when dosed as recommended (twice per day). They are absorbed via the lymphatic system, bypassing the liver (avoiding any potential liver issues). Additionally, many men prefer the convenience of an oral formulation over injections and creams. Other advantages of an oral delivery system exist, as stated by Dr. Theodore M. Danoff, Chief Medical Officer of Clarus Therapeutics (T = testosterone):

> "An oral T-replacement product would not only be convenient, but would avoid many of the safety issues associated with accidental transfer of T to women or children that can occur from transdermal T products. Moreover, published data indicates that men on transdermal T products often do not adhere to their treatment plan and we believe an oral option may improve this."

Most doctors would prefer oral formulations for their patients due to better long-term adherence to their prescribed TOT protocol. In a recent survey of 28 leading endocrinologists and urologists[143], 94% responded that they believed an oral TOT formulation will improve patient compliance.

Previously created oral testosterone formulations of testosterone undecanoate (Andriol, for example) haven't lived up to their promise. Whether these new medications undergoing FDA approval have overcome Andriol's limitations is yet to be determined. The FDA will not be providing an answer until Feb-

---

[142]   http://www.nasdaq.com/article/lipocines-oral-testosterone-drug-fails-to-win-fda-panel-backing-20180111-00006

[143]   https://www.lipocine.com/pipeline/lpcn-1021/

ruary 2018 as to whether they will be granted approval. Because of the lack of clinical data and no insights from experienced long-term users, we'll wait to see the science before saying yay or nay.

Buccal Preparations

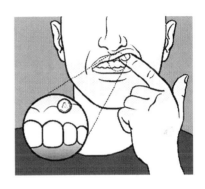

This method involves oral testosterone being absorbed by your gums, which then goes directly into your bloodstream. Known as a "cyclodextrin-complexed testosterone sublingual formulation," or a troche, this form of TOT is rapidly absorbed into circulation while the testosterone is released from the cyclodextrin shell[144].

This is not an efficient method of getting testosterone into your system due to its poor bioavailability and absorption in the body. As well, the potential side effects of dislodged tablets, bleeding gums, mouth sores, toothaches, and headaches make it an ill advised TOT option. There is also the potential risk of transferring the substance to your partner via kissing. This is way too risky. Additionally, when you use this method of TOT, you have to avoid eating and drinking for a while following administration so that you don't negatively affect absorption.

Again, there are more efficient ways to get your TOT.

---

[144] Salehian B, Wang C, Alexander G, et al. Pharmacokinetics, bioefficacy, and safety of sublingual testosterone cyclodextrin in hypogonadal men: comparison to testosterone enanthate – a clinical research center study. J Clin Endocrinol Metab. 1995;80:3567–3575. [PubMed]

Testosterone Pellets

With this form of TOT, small 3 mm x 9 mm pellets containing testosterone are surgically implanted under the skin (usually near the hip) and they slowly release testosterone over the course of 3-6 months[145]. Out of all forms of TOT on the market today, pellets are believed to have the longest duration of action (i.e. the longest-lasting effects). And although the pellets last a long time, this form of therapy is suboptimal.

First of all, there is always a risk of infection and hemorrhage with a surgical procedure, even a simple outpatient one. More importantly, once you've implanted the TOT pellet into your body, it's very difficult to control the concentration of the testosterone dosage being released (according to how your body responds to the treatment). If your blood levels indicate you need more or less of your current dosage, your doctor has to cut you open to add or remove pellets. This is highly invasive, and there are simply safer and more effective ways of receiving TOT.

Patches

Transdermal testosterone is also available as a skin patch. Androderm® is a patch one can apply onto the back, stomach, upper arms, or thighs every night for 24 hours. At the end of the 24-hour period, the used patch is removed and a new one is applied. The manufacturers recommend that users rotate the areas of application, waiting 7 days before reapplying to the same site.

---

[145] Kelleher S, Conway AJ, Handelsman DJ. Influence of implantation site and track geometry on the extrusion rate and pharmacology of testosterone implants. Clin Endocrinol.2001;55:531–536. [PubMed]

The manufacturer claims it is OK to swim or shower with the patch, but you have to wait 3 hours after applying it. Users are allowed to maintain normal activities, including sexual activity while wearing the patch, but strenuous exercise or excessive perspiration (sweating) may loosen the patch or cause it to fall off.

This form of TOT can also cause skin irritation at the place of adhesion (normally identified as a pink or red area that is inflamed). The manufacturer recommends using hydrocortisone skin cream to soothe the area. It's also a challenge to get the patch to stick unless one regularly shaves the area of application. For men with lots of body hair, this is extra work that must be done regularly to maximize patch adherence.

All of these topical TOT options can work, but our experience shows them to be far from optimal. Their benefits do not outweigh their potential side effects nor their many inefficiencies in preparation for application, especially when compared with injectable testosterone therapies.

CHAPTER 7 KEY TAKEAWAYS

- We explain how the term "bio-identical" testosterone is structurally identical to pharmaceutical-grade testosterone and 'naturally' produced testosterone.

- Transdermal creams and gels may emulate normal fluctuations of the body's production of testosterone. However, it is an impractical delivery system. Patients have to avoid common everyday activities for hours following application, the absorption rate of testosterone is inefficient, and there's the risk of accidentally transferring the cream to women, children and pets.

- Nasal gels have a high frequency of negative side effects, in addition to the lack of long-term data demonstrating the effectiveness of this TOT option.

- The newest oral formulations show promise as they can improve long-term patient adherence and compliance due to a common fear of needles. There is insufficient clinical data on these TOT options, and they are still awaiting FDA approval.

- Buccal preparations (absorption via gums) come with a high occurrence of negative side effects, in addition to the poor absorption of testosterone into the body. You also have to avoid eating, drinking and kissing for a while after administering the preparation.

- Testosterone pellets inserted surgically come with the risk of infection, plus the dosage of testosterone is extremely difficult to control and adjust.

- Skin patches like Androderm cause skin irritation at the place of adhesion, produce high levels of dihydrotestosterone, and are inconvenient due to the frequency of body preparation (shaving, etc.) for proper application.

- All of these topical TOT options can work, but our experience shows them to be far from optimal. Their benefits do not outweigh their potential side effects, and they are inefficient when compared with superior forms of testosterone therapy.

CHAPTER 8

The Optimal TOT Protocol: Injectable Testosterone

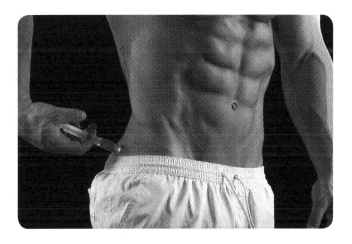

Based on our experience with every TOT method of delivery, the single most effective form of TOT to optimize testosterone levels is via injection[146]. This chapter outlines the four main types of injectable testosterone formulations found on the market today. As with the rest of the book, we include the science so that you're empowered to do your own research and make the right call for your body.

---

[146] Injection of Testosterone May be Safer and More Effective than Transdermal Administration for Combating Loss of Muscle and Bone in Older men. Stephen E. Borst and Joshua F. Yarrow. Am J Physiol Endocrinol Metab (April 21).

Testosterone Undecanoate

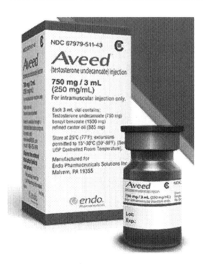

This injectable testosterone preparation is better known as Nebido, and is used in Europe and Scandinavian countries. Recently, Aveed of Endo Pharmaceuticals has become available in the U.S.[147]. In theory, it is a perfect formulation because it has a very long half-life (the length of time the ester is bioactive in the body) and needs to be injected only once every 10 to 14 weeks[148]. But in practice, many men who have used it report 'the effects of valleys' (i.e. lows in mood, sex drive and assertiveness associated with lower levels of testosterone). These can be expected from a longer-acting testosterone ester that often loses its effectiveness around weeks 7–10 of a standard 14-week injection protocol.

Each user is biochemically unique in the way his body will metabolize the testosterone ester into his bloodstream. Some break it down much faster than others, which causes these noticeable valleys (drops) at 7-10 weeks into the injection protocol. Anecdotally, Nebido has rarely been found to raise testosterone levels above the mid-range of 'normal' when measured between 4-8 weeks into therapy.

---

[147]   NOTE: This preparation is known as Aveed in the US, and Nebido in every other part of the world.

[148]   Von Eckardstein, Nieschlag E. Treatment of male hypogonadism with testosterone undecanoate injected at extended intervals of 12 weeks: a phase II study. J Androl. 2002;23(3):419–425. [PubMed]

Most concerning, however, is the potential of having higher estrogen levels, with very little testosterone left from the original undecanoate injection. In other words, a patient will have to experience side effects from the lack of balance that exists due to low testosterone levels and higher estrogen levels, all while waiting for the next injection to come! Thankfully, as of 2017, clinicians are now allowed to adjust the therapeutic dosage by decreasing the time between injections.

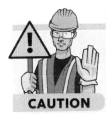

CAUTION

Also note that Aveed's website offers a very stern warning of the risk of "serious pulmonary microembolism (POME) reactions and anaphylaxis" upon injection. In other words, there is a risk of a user experiencing a severe negative reaction from the injection. This is due to the chemical particulates in the injectable formulation (which are used to extend its half-life) being potentially harmful upon injection to some users. This should scare most potential users away.

In practice, most users of Aveed/Nebido complain about the issues mentioned above.

This form of TOT looks great from a theoretical standpoint[149], but real-world experience tells a different story. Based on the existing documented results, we can't recommend this form of injectable therapy, especially in comparison to the next 3 injectable options we are going to discuss.

---

[149] Edelstein D, Basaria S. Testosterone undecanoate in the treatment of male hypogonadism. Expert Opin Pharmacother. 2010;11(12):2095-2106.

Testosterone Propionate

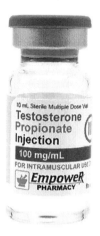

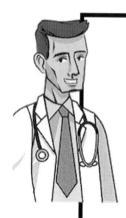

Testosterone propionate is a fast-acting, short half-life (1.75-2.25 days) testosterone ester. The length of the testosterone ester determines how long it takes your body to dispose of the hormone in question, and propionate is one of the shortest esters available with a testosterone base. There are enzymes in the body called 'esterases' which are responsible for removing the ester from testosterone. Once the ester is removed, all that is left is the testosterone molecule itself. The longer the ester clings to the testosterone, the longer testosterone is active in the body. If testosterone is active in the body for a longer period of time, a smaller amount of the overall testosterone dosage is absorbed.

Because of testosterone propionate's short half-life, peak blood levels of testosterone can be effectively controlled via injection frequency. When dosed daily or every-other-day (EOD), propionate can mimic the testosterone your body naturally produces. Its half-life is shorter than the longer-acting esters of cypionate, enanthate and undecanoate. After a single 50 mg injection of testosterone propionate, the maximum concentration of blood testosterone is reached after approximately 14 hours following the injection[150].

The chart below shows how much testosterone is absorbed and used for each 100 mg injected of various testosterone compounds. Depending on the weight of the ester, the injectable formulations deliver different net bioavailable amounts (in milligrams). For example, if you inject 100 mg of testosterone undecanoate, only 63 mg of it will be available for use by the body.

100 mg of injectable as:	Approximate Free Equivalent (how much actually gets used by the body from a 100 mg dosage):
Testosterone Propionate	83 mg
Testosterone Enanthate	72 mg
Testosterone Cypionate	70 mg
Testosterone Undecanoate	63 mg

[151]

[150] Behre HM, et al. Pharmacology of testosterone preparations. In: Nieschlag E, Behre HM, editors.Testosterone, action, deficiency, substitution.Cambridge University Press; 2004. pp. 405–44.

[151] Simons SS. What goes on behind closed doors: physiological vs. pharmacological steroid hormone actions. BioEssays: news and reviews in molecular, cellular and developmental biology. 2008;30(8):744-756. doi:10.1002/bies.20792.

Testosterone propionate is the strongest injectable testosterone formulation (from a peak effectiveness standpoint, as seen in the table) found on the market today.

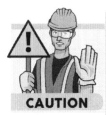

CAUTION

With testosterone propionate, there is a small percentage of men who will experience an unfavorable reaction due to pain at the injection site. If the propionate ester causes skin irritation upon injection, it will lead to pain and an uncomfortable feeling. For these men, propionate is not an option anymore.

Testosterone Cypionate and Testosterone Enanthate

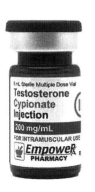 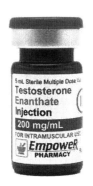

Many progressive, experienced TOT-prescribing physicians in North America prescribe the following: An *80–200 mg dose of injectable testosterone cypionate and/or testosterone enanthate to be administered every 7 days.* These weekly dosage amounts vary depending on the doctor, their individual methodologies and the patient's response (determined from measuring blood testosterone levels).

This is the tried and true protocol of many of the best TOT-prescribing clinicians for the following reasons:

• Cypionate and enanthate have longer half-lives, allowing the user to minimize their injection frequency. For the men who have an aversion to injections (i.e. 'needle phobia'), reducing the amount of shots taken per month provides better long-term patient adherence.

• Enanthate and cypionate are also produced by compounding pharmacies[152], and their cost is more economical than any other testosterone product. Compounding pharmacies are able to make them in bases such as grapeseed oil, whereas commercial testosterone injections are only available in cottonseed oil. Grapeseed oil is normally better tolerated (when injected) when used to stabilize injectable testosterone formulations.

• 200 mg of injectable ester is normally the maximum dosage that keeps serum (total) testosterone levels within clinically acceptable ranges when measured over a 7-day moving average.

What primarily differentiates testosterone cypionate and testosterone enanthate are the vehicles they are compounded in. Testosterone cypionate requires 20% benzyl benzoate in order to solubilize it. Testosterone enanthate melts slightly above room temperature, so benzyl benzoate is not required in this formulation. Since they both have the same half life, the advantage of using one over the other is typically patient-specific. If you are sensitive to benzyl benzoate, then testosterone enanthate is your best option.

Testosterone cypionate and enanthate are virtually identical in their pharmacokinetics and pharmacodynamics, and there is little difference between the two, from a chemical standpoint. The ester found in both forms has an active half-life between

---

[152]   https://www.empowerpharmacy.com/

5 (enanthate) and 6 (cypionate) days, but blood levels of both compounds fall sharply 4 days after administration[153].

Unfortunately, there are still too many primary care physicians who are inexperienced with TOT and prescribe doses of inject-able *testosterone cypionate* and *testosterone enanthate* once every 14–21 days. Again, their dosage amounts vary depending on the doctor and their individual methodologies. In fact, this is still listed as the standard practice in many endocrinology textbooks[154].

Spacing injections too far apart shows a fundamental misun-derstanding of the testosterone ester's half-life when it breaks down in the bloodstream. This creates wide swings in blood testosterone levels, which means you have too many highs and lows between the levels of both testosterone and estrogen[155]. This leads to emotional ups and downs because those hor-mones are fluctuating too much, throwing your body out of balance. Remember: The primary goal of TOT is feeling great, which results in an optimal balance between your levels of T (testosterone) and E (estrogen).

A much more effective TOT injection protocol, when using testosterone cypionate or testosterone enanthate, is injections done twice per week while providing the correct dosage (80-200 mg TOTAL throughout the week, depending on patient

---

153   Dobs AS, Meikle AW, Arver S, Sanders SW, Caramelli KE, Mazer NA. Pharmacokinetics, efficacy, and safety of a permeation enhanced testosterone transdermal system in comparison with bi-weekly injections of testosterone enanthate for the treatment of hypogonadal men. J Clin Endocrinol Metab. 1999;84:3469–3478. [PubMed].

154   Jones, Hugh T. Testosterone Deficiency in Men. 2nd Edition. Oxford Endocrinology Library Press 2013.

155   Behre HM, et al. Pharmacology of testosterone preparations. In: Nieschlag E, Behre HM, editors. Testosterone, action, deficiency, substitution. Cambridge University Press; 2004. pp. 405–44.

response) to maintain the peak (2-3.5 days post-injection) and avoid the bottom (4 days post-injection) associated with the half-lives of testosterone cypionate and enanthate.

Patients are often prescribed an *aromatization inhibitor* (AI) medication like Arimidex (Anastrozole) to fix the problem of increased estrogen inadvertently created from a suboptimal dosing schedule. On a proper dosing schedule, it's very rare (except in highly specific cases of older men, men with high levels of body fat, or those with a pre-established clinical need before starting TOT) that any patient should start out on an AI. **The need for estrogen control must be proven first via blood tests.** Follow-up labs are crucial to understand what is really going on in that individual's endocrine (i.e. hormone) system as a response to using supplemental testosterone.

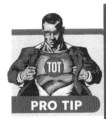

PRO TIP

It is also IMPERATIVE, when first beginning a TOT protocol, that no other medications which manipulate hormone levels (**Aromatase Inhibitors [AIs]** or **Selective Estrogen Receptor Modulators [SERMs]**) be dosed (except for the use of **hCG** for men looking to retain their fertility) to find out how the testosterone dose *alone* affects that person's endocrine system. It is critical to establish baseline patient blood levels to one exogenous medication (i.e. testosterone) to understand how their body responds to the prescribed dosage. Adding in other medications that also potentially raise testosterone and/or raise (or lower) estrogen will prevent the physician from having a clear picture of what medication is having what effect(s) when measuring the blood work in follow-up labs.

Once follow-up blood labs are received, it may be practical to start a patient on an AI if aromatase inhibition is warranted. For instance, there might be noticeable estrogenic side effects the patient complains of, such as sensitive nipples, tissue growth around the nipple, water retention/feeling bloated, or an overall irritability and/or a sense of malaise. There are exceptions to this rule that we will discuss in Chapter 10.

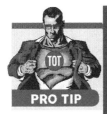

PRO TIP

There are experienced TOT physicians who are coming forward and discussing the risks associated with bone mineral density when using Arimidex as an AI medication for long periods of time. **Dr. Rob Kominiarek D.O., FACOFP** is a board-certified fellow of the American College of Osteopathic Family Physicians with an advanced certification in Age Management Medicine and Bioldentical Hormone Replacement Therapy. He is the medical director of ReNue Health® in Springboro Ohio[156]. Dr. Kominiarek specifically states that men on Arimidex for periods of 12 months or longer while on TOT normally reveal bone mineral degradation when undergoing DEXA scans. There are multiple studies confirming his assertion[157,158].

---

[156]   http://www.renuehealth.com/about-renue-health/

[157]   Bone Mineral Density and Response to Treatment in Men Younger Than 50 Years with Testosterone Deficiency and Sexual Dysfunction or Infertility. Kacker, Ravi et al. The Journal of Urology, Volume 191, Issue 4, 1072 - 1076.

[158]   Finkelstein JS, Lee H, Leder BZ, et al. Gonadal steroid–dependent effects on bone turnover and bone mineral density in men. The Journal of Clinical Investigation. 2016;126(3):1114-1125. doi:10.1172/JCI84137.

It is for this very reason that we are militant about not placing a patient on an AI medication unless absolutely necessary. And even when there is a medical need, the patient and physician should make every effort to fix things (including lifestyle changes such as losing body fat, lowering the dose of testosterone and modulating the frequency of the delivery system) before starting the use of an AI. Once the AI has been initiated, the minimum effective dose (MED) principle should be followed (normally 0.25 mg, 1-2x per week) with a specific goal of weaning the patient off of the AI as soon as possible.

Our Recommended TOT Protocols

After close to 20 years of using injectable testosterone in the context of health and longevity, we present our recommended protocols in order of preference for lifelong TOT administration. Each option works extremely well and it is our opinion that as long as one of them is consistently adhered to (depending on the needs/wants of the patient), the differences between them are miniscule in relation to establishing stable blood testosterone levels, overall patient happiness and long-term success with TOT.

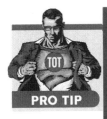

PRO TIP

Option 1A: 10-30 mg of testosterone injected daily.

This provides the most stable testosterone levels (i.e. mimicking endogenous production of testosterone as closely as possible), and it will also help to minimize aromatization and erythrocytosis. Normally, this type of therapy works well in Type A personality types. Dr. Rob Kominiarek discusses this in his interview in Chapter 17.

Option 1B: 50- 70 mg of testosterone injected every other day (EOD)

This is a nice compromise between daily and twice-a-week administration if you cannot bring yourself to administer daily injections.

Option 2: 50-100 mg of testosterone injected twice weekly (preferably every 3rd day)

This option is the most popular choice (preferred by most patients due to the lack of injection frequency) and still more advantageous than once per week therapy.

The "right dosage" is an individual thing, and it will require collaborating with your doctor to regularly test your levels of testosterone and estrogen in order to establish and maintain optimal hormonal balance. **A general baseline upper range dosage limit is 200-250 mg every 7 days.** Balance will correspond to the right hormonal levels, but it will ultimately come down to feeling great with little to no side effects. We are big proponents of the minimum effective dosage principle (**MED**). Always start low and go slow.

For patients who are extremely fearful of needles, one intramuscular (i.e. into the muscle) injection of 100-250 mg every 7th day (once per week) is acceptable. However, acceptable is not optimal. We highly recommend the once per-week dosing as your last resort. If you have a prescribing physician that insists on making this your only option (meaning you have to come to the office once per week to get your dose administered), you should consider other options and find another doctor.

NOTE: Our recommendations are based on the use of multidose vials, commonly prescribed in the United States. However, if you are based outside of the United States, it's likely that you will be prescribed glass ampoules that will hamper your ability to customize your dosage. This is because once the glass ampoules have been opened and exposed to air, the contents must be used or discarded immediately for sterility reasons. The work around is to fill up one syringe with the contents of the ampule and then dispense into insulin syringes, or just fill up multiple insulin syringes from the ampule. This would prevent the contents of the ampule from being lost and also preserve them for later usage.

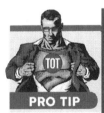

PRO TIP

Sustanon is an oil-based injectable preparation found mostly in the UK and Europe. Sustanon is a trade name owned by Organon Pharmaceuticals for oil-based injectable blends of esterized testosterone compounds. Esterization of the testosterone molecules theoretically provides for a sustained (i.e. longer-lasting) release of testosterone into the bloodstream. **Sustanon 250** is a blend of four esterized testosterone compounds: 30 mg testosterone propionate, 60 mg testosterone phenylpropionate, 60 mg testosterone isocaproate and 100 mg testosterone decanoate. The issue with this preparation is the lack of multi-dose vials. Users must score an ampule (in other words, break off a piece of glass) to insert the injection needle into the bottle. This can cause an unhygienic condition from microscopic shards of broken glass getting into the injectable preparation.

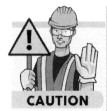

CAUTION

As we have stated previously: if you live in a country or state where it is illegal to administer testosterone without a doctor's prescription, then choosing the route of self-administration without a legitimate prescription is breaking the law. We urge all of our readers to educate themselves on the laws of their respective country and/or state.

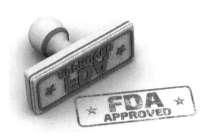

The FDA and Testosterone Therapy

The United States FDA (Food and Drug Administration) is an agency whose actions and motives are sometimes difficult to predict. In 2014, it appeared they were trying to "narrow down" the official approval guidelines for TOT when their expert panels[159] urged them to limit the diagnosis for prescribing TOT "to men whose low testosterone stems from an acute medical problem such as damaged testicles or thyroid disease."

In 2015, they released a ruling stating that testosterone products must have a black box warning label[160] placed on them "to

---

[159] http://www.mdmag.com/medical-news/will-the-fda-tighten-the-use-of-testosterone-replacement-therapy

[160] http://www.latimes.com/science/sciencenow/la-sci-sn-testosterone-heart-stroke-risk-20150303-story.html

clarify that the prescription hormone is meant for use by men whose low testosterone levels are caused by certain medical conditions," such as "genetic disorders and conditions affecting the testicles, pituitary gland, and brain."

It turns out the data upon which the FDA based its ruling is only relevant to a narrow group of individuals: men over 65 years of age with pre-existing heart conditions[161]. Obviously, this shouldn't be applied to the general population of men who are supplementing with testosterone.

The bottom line is this: It is not only appropriate, but also safe to place warnings on medications to alert those who may be at risk for side effects. Do ALL MALES fall into this high-risk category? Are the millions of Americans currently on testosterone therapy destined to develop heart disease? Of course not! In fact, there are hundreds of studies[162] demonstrating testosterone's profound cardioprotective (heart-protecting) effects. Links to some of the most recent data are provided and thoroughly discussed in Chapter 12.

TOT will probably remain under FDA scrutiny as a gray area of male hormone replacement therapy (HRT) for the foreseeable future. This only reinforces the need for the care and guidance of a highly qualified physician who can help you optimize your health.

Vetting your TOT doctor is critical to make sure they are a concerned and helpful advocate on your lifetime journey of TOT.

---

[161] Vigen R, O'Donnell CI, Barón AE, Grunwald GK, Maddox TM, Bradley SM, Barqawi A, Woning G, Wierman ME, Plomondon ME, Rumsfeld JS, Ho PM. Association of Testosterone Therapy With Mortality, Myocardial Infarction, and Stroke in Men With Low Testosterone Levels. *JAMA*. 2013;310(17):1829–1836. doi:10.1001/jama.2013.280386

[162] http://www.ncbi.nlm.nih.gov/pmc/?term=Testosterone+is+Cardio+Protective

Choosing the Right TOT-Prescribing Physician

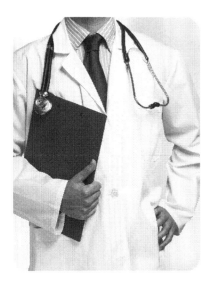

Much of the time, the primary objective of our medical industry is to treat disease by medicating the symptoms instead of the the root cause. If you're reading this book, you're learning the importance of optimizing your overall health from the ground up, with TOT being just one key factor. An essential part of optimizing your health is finding an experienced TOT doctor who can optimize your hormones to run as efficiently as possible (alongside your entire body) and for as long as possible.

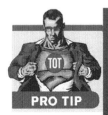

PRO TIP

When taking advice from a doctor for your health, take a look at their own results. If someone is giving you advice about how to optimize your health, a reliable indicator of credibility is their own physical condition. Would you take financial advice on how (or where) to invest your money from a college graduate who has a bachelor degree, OR from an investor with a multi-million dollar investment portfolio? Skin in the game is everything, and this is a key principle to follow for areas outside of your health as well.

Vetting Your TOT Doctor

Because it's critically important for you (as the patient) to work with the right physician, we offer you 10 key questions to ask your doctor to find out if they are qualified to treat you and ultimately optimize your testosterone levels.

Ideally, you need to respect that the physician will have certain practice-based preferences based on their own professional experience. However, they should be open to being a partner in managing your health instead of being a "White Lab-Coat God Complexed Dictator."

These questions will give you an idea of those practice-based preferences and their willingness to be a partner with you in your TOT.

1) How long have you been managing patients on TOT, and how much of your total practice do those patients represent?

2) Do you have a preferred form of therapy (injections, gels, etc.)?

3) How do you determine your dosing schedule for a new patient (Testosterone, AIs, etc.)?

4) What is your opinion on the usage of AIs?

5) What blood labs are you going to draw before initiating TOT? When do you draw labs again, once TOT starts?

6) How many times will you want to draw labs per year?

7) What is your preferred therapy for maintaining fertility (hCG, hMG, Clomid, etc.)?

8) Will you use these medications with or without concomitant TOT (i.e. at the same time as TOT)? Explain the dosage strategy to me.

9) How long does it typically take until I start seeing results, or feeling different?

10) Will you allow me to administer my own TOT injections, upon scripting injectable testosterone?

The Costs of TOT

On the more expensive side, an anti-aging clinic can charge as much as $250-1,250 for an initial consultation, along with a monthly membership fee ($99-350) to allow their patients to obtain a prescription for testosterone, various anti-aging medications, and concierge (VIP) access to the physician.

Other clinics will simply charge a fee to speak with a doctor or nurse, and medications will be prescribed so that you can be reimbursed through your health insurance (when covered). In some instances, medical treatments are offered conveniently through a telemedicine platform[163], allowing the patient to consult with expert TOT physicians virtually via webcam,

---

[163]   www.bodhd.com

phone, and email. That way, you don't have to travel far to get affordable treatment.

As the telemedicine industry evolves, Jay and Jim will be highly involved in creating global treatment solutions for men and women seeking effective and affordable hormonal optimization. If you are interested in working with a doctor we recommend, visit TOTDoctors.com[164].

NOTE If you are a physician who would like to list your practice on TOTDoctors.com, please fill out the intake form found here[165].

---

[164] www.totdoctors.com

[165] http://www.totdoctors.com/providers/

CHAPTER 8 KEY TAKEAWAYS

- We discuss the various injectable testosterone delivery systems (Undecanoate, Propionate, Cypionate and Enanthate) in depth and how they differ with respect to their behavior in the bloodstream.

- We give you our recommended TOT protocol and provide you with various options, based on your personal lifestyle and other factors.

- We provide insights into the relationship between the FDA and the prescribing physician community. We also give you the details on why there are Black Box warning labels on testosterone products.

- We discuss the importance of choosing the right TOT physician and why vetting them is critical to find out whether they are qualified to help you.

- We tell you explicitly how much TOT will cost, based on your individual wants and needs, and direct you to our recommended physicians.

How to Properly and Safely Inject Yourself for Life

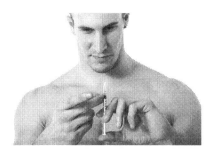

Here's something you already know: Needle phobias are very common, and the thought of regularly injecting oneself with anything can freak some people out.

Most men on TOT self-administer their TOT, as well as their **hCG** injections (hCG will be discussed in greater depth in Chapters 10 and 12). Regular injections (daily, every-other-day or bi-weekly) simply become a part of your day-to-day existence, just like brushing your teeth or walking your dog.

There is no need to worry about injecting yourself. After all, millions of diabetics inject themselves with insulin on a daily basis. Once you perform a couple of injections, your fear will quickly dissipate. When you perform your first successful injection, you will realize how simple and painless it actually is.

Syringe, Needle Gauge, and Withdrawing

Syringes come in lots of sizes, so to keep the math of your testosterone dosage simple, we recommend your physician to provide you with 1 mL syringes. This will help you easily prepare the correct testosterone dosage every time. The barrel portion of the syringe will have units of measure from ½ - 3 mL in the form of tick marks along the side (see the picture on next page).

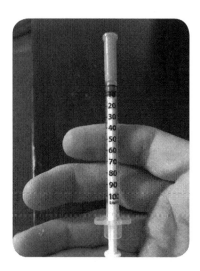

In terms of the actual size (i.e. diameter) of the needle, a 26-28 gauge (the higher the gauge, the thinner the needle), inch-long needle syringe is optimal for intramuscular injections.

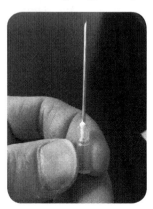

When withdrawing the testosterone solution from the vial, it's much easier to use an 18 gauge, 1½" needle because the injectable solution is relatively viscous (i.e. thick) and will flow easier through a larger gauge (thicker) needle. You then replace the 18 gauge needle attached to the syringe with a thinner (smaller) 26-28 gauge injection needle (while the solution is still in the barrel) prior to injecting yourself.

For an incredibly informative website on safe and proper injection techniques, along with the correct use of syringes and needles, visit Vitality Medical[166].

---

[166]   https://www.vitalitymedical.com/blog/selecting-syringes-and-needles.html

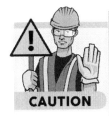

CAUTION

For men who have higher body fat percentages (over 20%), you are likely going to have to inject yourself with a **longer needle that's 1.0-1.5 inches long**. You'll have to penetrate the needle beyond your visceral fat to ensure you inject the testosterone solution into your muscle. This is another reason to focus on losing excess body fat: Being lean makes your injections far easier!

Where To Inject The Needle, and How to Inject Yourself Safely

It is safest to inject testosterone into the following muscle areas: deltoids, gluteus, or upper/outside quadriceps. We recommend rotating your injection sites (i.e. do deltoids one time, gluteus the next, and so on) to minimize scar tissue formation in one area. With three different areas on each side of the body, you'll have up to 6 different places where you can routinely inject your testosterone.

TRT University[167], launching mid 2018, will have excellent videos demonstrating propert injection procedures and techniques. In fact, we're still gathering insights into what type of information you'd like to see from us. Please take this online questionnaire to provide us with your feedback[168].

---

[167]   www.trtuniversity.org

[168]   http://www.surveygizmo.com/s3/4161097/TRT-University-Questionnaire

Intramuscular (IM) Injection Sites

Deltoid Site

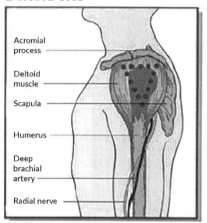

Acromial process

Deltoid muscle

Scapula

Humerus

Deep brachial artery

Radial nerve

Ventrogluteal Site

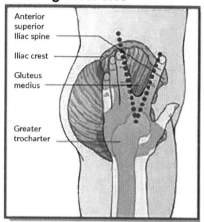

Anterior superior Iliac spine

Iliac crest

Gluteus medius

Greater trocharter

Vastus Lateralis Site

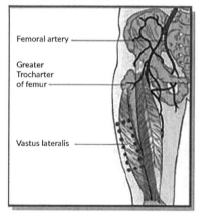

Femoral artery

Greater Trocharter of femur

Vastus lateralis

Dorsogluteal Site

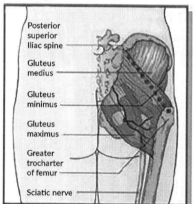

Posterior superior Iliac spine

Gluteus medius

Gluteus minimus

Gluteus maximus

Greater trocharter of femur

Sciatic nerve

Source: http://medictests.com/

TOT Via Subcutaneous Administration

Subcutaneous vs. Intramuscular Injections

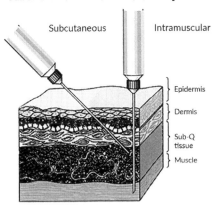

Subcutaneous injections involve injecting the needle into the fat tissue of the lower stomach, or the buttocks area with an insulin syringe (similar to how things are done with hCG[169]).

There is solid research indicating that subcutaneous TOT injections produce therapeutic serum concentrations at lower doses than intramuscular injections (i.e. lower amounts needed for optimal health effects)[170].

According to one study, less testosterone needs to be injected subcutaneously to achieve optimal testosterone blood levels than what needs to be injected if you use intramuscular TOT. Both Dr. Eugene Shippen and Dr. Crisler are successfully using subcutaneous injection protocols with hundreds of patients. In some patients, Dr. Crisler has found that 40 mg of testosterone cypionate injected subcutaneously twice a week is just as effective as 100 mg injected intramuscularly (IM)[171].

---

[169] Evaluation of the efficacy of subcutaneous administration of testosterone in female to male transexuals and hypogonadal males — Olshan et al. 34 (3): MON-594 — Endocrine Reviews.

[170] Ibid.

[171] Testosterone Replacement Therapy-A Recipe for Success-Dr. Crisler pg.99 Milestones Publishing (3-13-05).

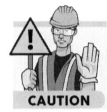

CAUTION

Due to the potential aromatization of the testosterone (i.e. conversion into estrogen) in adipocytes (fat tissue), we believe subcutaneous injections should initially be done as an experiment. This means that one would have to try this form of therapy out for himself to see how his body responds. Remember: aromatase loves to hang out in fat tissue[172]. Injecting testosterone subcutaneously into men with higher body fat levels *might* lead to greater estradiol (E2) conversion, and the resulting side effects that come with greater levels of estrogen.

Things have changed since *The Definitive TRT MANual* was written nearly 4 years ago. Although we were reluctant to support this delivery system back then, subcutaneous injections are now a well-recognized delivery system backed by solid research data[173]. If you're taking control of your health and want to see if this method works for you, we recommend you experiment with that delivery method under the supervision of a qualified physician, evaluate how you feel and monitor your blood work for significant before-and-after changes.

NOTE Jay and Jim have tried subcutaneous administration but find that it leads to irritation at the point of injection. For this reason, we both prefer IM injections. We both acknowledge

---

[172]   Intra-adipose sex steroid metabolism and body fat distribution in idiopathic human obesity. Clin Endocrinol (Oxf). 2007 Mar;66(3):440-6.

[173]   Kovac JR, Rajanahally S, Smith RP, Coward RM, Lamb DJ, Lipshultz LI. Patient satisfaction with testosterone replacement therapies: the reasons behind the choices. *The journal of sexual medicine.* 2014;11(2):553-562. doi:10.1111/jsm.12369.

subcutaneous injections as a viable alternative for a lot of men. We also know that for some men, frequent IM shots with a smaller gauge needle are ineffective due to the significant amount of body fat they possess. In higher body fat men, a larger needle is needed to perform an IM shot correctly. For these men, subcutaneous injection is a viable alternative.

Needle Disposal

Once you're done injecting, properly dispose of your used syringes after a single use. Reusing syringes is simply unhealthy and could lead to an infection. The most hygienic way to dispose of your used syringes is by purchasing a Sharps Container Biohazard Needle Disposal container (or check[174] container), or check with your local waste management company as they sometimes have suggestions. Keep your syringes out of the reach of children for obvious reasons.

Minimizing Scar Tissue Formation with Foam Rolling and Myofascial Release

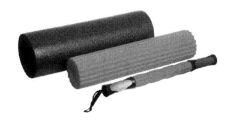

A foam roller[175] and/or a Beastie Ball[176] are essential home tools to break up scar tissue that forms at injection sites. Just a couple times a week[177] for 2-5 minutes each

174   http://www.amazon.com/exec/obidos/ASIN/B003V5LZBY/trtrevbook-20

175   http://www.amazon.com/exec/obidos/ASIN/B0040EGNIU/trtrevbook-20

176   http://www.amazon.com/exec/obidos/ASIN/B00ECASXA8/trtrevbook-20

177   https://youtu.be/FWf9wZStDAk

session is enough. But as you work out and build larger muscle fibers, you'll definitely want to use them more frequently to relieve muscle tightness and assist post-workout recovery so that your muscles stay flexible, healthy, and supple[178].

Whenever possible, supplement your at-home treatment with a deep tissue massage - **Active Release Technique (ART)** - by a professional massage therapist a couple times a month. ART massage is an incredible way to improve full-body muscle elasticity while speeding up tissue recovery and healing. It is also a great way to enhance strength and flexibility[179].

Don't let the words "scar tissue" scare you. We're just talking about fascial adhesions here[180], which are just tiny micro-traumas that can build up from years of local injections into the muscle. They are rarely noticeable (or felt), but it's still an excellent course of action to have an ART-trained massage therapist break them up so they don't harden and solidify over time. Again, using foam rollers and the Beastie Ball will also help as a personal form of therapy.

---

[178] http://fabfitover40.com/2014/06/25/key-to-remaining-fit-over-40/

[179] DiGiovanna, Eileen; Schiowitz, Stanley; Dowling, Dennis J. (2005) [1991]. "Ch. 12: Myofascial (Soft Tissue) Techniques." *An Osteopathic Approach to Diagnosis and Treatment* (3rd ed.). Philadelphia: Lippincott Williams & Wilkins. pp. 80–2.

[180] http://destroychronicpain.wordpress.com/fascial-adhesions-2/

CHAPTER 9 KEY TAKEAWAYS

- We teach you everything you'd ever want to know about injecting yourself safely, including how to select the right-sized syringes and needle gauges.

- We also provide instructions and videos on where and how to inject testosterone into your body, along with safely disposing of needles.

- We go into great detail about the differences between subcutaneous and IM (intramuscular) injections.

- We discuss how you can minimize the formation of scar tissue with ART (Active Release Technique) and foam rolling.

CHAPTER 10
Potential Side Effects, Their Likelihood, and How to Alleviate Them

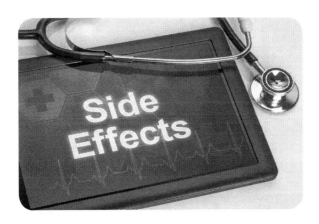

It's time to talk about the potential side effects of TOT, all of which are minimal and typically easy to spot and treat.

Again, your primary goal is to achieve balance (defined as feeling good without side effects) between your levels of testosterone (both free and total) and estrogen (E2). This is also why working closely with an experienced TOT physician as your body evolves over time is critically important.

Many men have received (and continue to receive) ineffective care from their TOT-prescribing physicians. Often times, an inability to alleviate side effects forces men to prematurely end their treatment altogether. Frankly, there is *NEVER A REASON* for this to happen, especially when you utilize the services of a progressive and experienced TOT-prescribing physician[181].

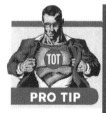

PRO TIP

As we stress throughout this book (and will continue to do so), it is crucial that you keep detailed records of your blood panels in order to best understand your test results as they change over time. Know your own body, compile your blood panel data, and do your homework to ensure your TOT is successful over the long term. Take full responsibility for your therapy. Study your reactions. Take notes. Be vigilant in knowing your body and what allows it to work optimally.

Remember, doctors are said to have *practices* for a reason. They are human beings just like you and me, and sometimes they make mistakes. You are the only one who truly knows your body, so do the work, pay attention, and you'll stay optimized.

Before discussing what we believe are the optimal supporting medications to manage potential side effects, we'll cover the primary issues and potential side effects men may face when undergoing TOT.

---

181   www.bodhd.com

Estradiol (E2)

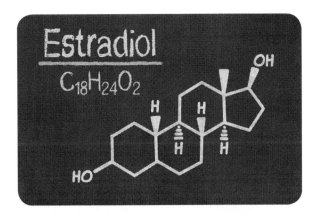

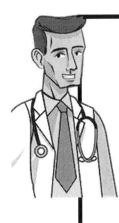

Monitoring and managing estrogen is an important topic in TOT, and recent studies have shown that estrogen is just as important to male brain and sexual function as testosterone itself[182]. Most of you probably think of estrogen as the "female hormone" and the substance that makes women "emotional." As with anything in the human body, there are many systems of interactions at play. Estrogen is actually composed of three different forms[183], including one that plays a huge role in how men feel: estradiol (E2).

---

[182]   Jankowska, E.A., Rozentryt, P., and Ponikowska, B. (2009). Circulating estradiol and mortality in men with systolic chronic heart failure. Journal of the American Medical Association. 2009 May 13;301(18):1892-901.

[183]   Sinchak K, Wagner EJ. Estradiol Signaling in the Regulation of Reproduction and Energy Balance. Frontiers in neuroendocrinology. 2012;33(4):342-363. doi:10.1016/j.yfrne.2012.08.004.

So why is estradiol so important? It has profound implications for general health and has the potential to cause some very unpleasant symptoms if its levels are unbalanced. As testosterone levels decrease and estradiol levels increase, the ratio of free testosterone to estradiol reaches a critical point where high estrogenic side effects are more noticeable[184]: Sexual dysfunction (poor erectile strength), lack of libido/arousal, poor sleep and reduced insulin sensitivity are just some of them.

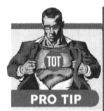

PRO TIP

In our experience, both personally and in consulting with many men who are on TOT, the biggest reason why TOT doesn't "work" is because of poor estrogen (E2) management. Often times, it's out of balance due to a lack of physician observation and/or management. Unfortunately, a man can have side effects when suffering from both low and high levels of estrogen. Believe it or not, the single biggest determinant of whether estradiol (E2) is out of balance or not is erectile strength. When a man is unable to maintain a strong erection, this is normally the sign of excess E2 (estrogen) production. On the other hand, when E2 levels are too low (normally due to overdosing of an aromatase inhibitor (AI) medication), it causes sexual dysfunction (lack of interest) and an inability to get an erection. There is nothing more psychologically damaging to a man than being unable to perform sexually when the opportunity arises.

---

[184] The role of estradiol in the maintenance of secondary hypogonadism in males in erectile dysfunction. Cohen, P.G. Medical Hypotheses, Volume 50, Issue 4, 331 - 333.

Another obvious and noticeable side effect of high E2 levels is water retention. Some men genetically overproduce aromatase (the enzyme necessary for the conversion of testosterone to estrogen), leading to increased estrogen production and its potentially negative side effects. In a later section of this chapter, we will discuss aromatase in great detail.

It is extremely important to work with an experienced physician to dial in your estradiol levels as you begin TOT. Normally, a good doctor will take an initial blood estradiol (E2) panel to establish a baseline, and then take future readings after starting TOT to figure out what level of estradiol is best for you. There is a narrow therapeutic estrogen (E2) range in which a patient feels good when balancing estrogen and testosterone, while initiating and adhering to lifelong optimization at the same time. Therefore, it is CRITICALLY important for you (the patient) and your doctor to understand the optimal range of estradiol for your body.

In recent research[185] from urologist Dr. Ranjith Ramasamy, he recommends that estradiol should be kept below 80 pg/mL, and that the optimal Testosterone-to-Estradiol ratio to maintain is 10 to 1 ("total testosterone level @ ng/dL" to "estradiol level @ pg/mL"). However, we do not agree with this 10 to 1 ratio. In our opinion, there is no cookie-cutter range of values within which men should attempt to keep their E2 levels. How a patient feels, along with qualitative symptoms, is a far more important factor to examine when attempting to dial in a patient's optimal therapeutic level of estrogen.

It is important that a TOT physician orders a 'sensitive' or 'enhanced' estradiol assay[186] (lab work) before and after a

---

[185]   https://youtu.be/PY2NBkHTZvY

[186]   https://www.labcorp.com/test-menu/24871/estradiol-sensitive-lc-ms

patient initiates TOT. This is important because the standard estradiol test is designed for women, and tends to greatly overestimate a patient's actual estrogen levels. It is critical for both the patient and the doctor to establish accurate baseline levels of estrogen (E2) before starting TOT AND during TOT. This is also why it's important for your physician to initiate therapy with testosterone in isolation (i.e. with no other medications alongside it) to understand how your body responds to it by itself. Doing so will help establish a legitimate baseline between testosterone and estrogen.

NOTE A sensitive estradiol assay is a luxury few TOT prescribing physicians outside the United States have. In Europe it's virtually non-existent. Therefore, they should be aware that the normal E2 test overestimates estradiol in men.

DHT

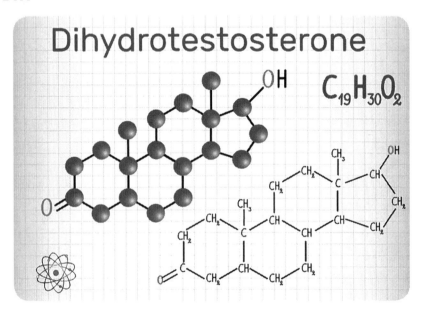

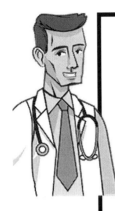

Even though the main androgen (hormone) secreted by the testes is testosterone, the main testosterone signal comes from **di-hydrotestosterone (DHT)**. DHT is responsible for sending this signal to your brain, central nervous system, skin and the genitals - practically everything in your body but your muscles. Testosterone is converted to the active androgen DHT by the action of the enzyme 5-alpha-reductase (5-AR). Because DHT binds about 3-5 times more strongly to the androgen receptor than testosterone does, it is much more anabolic in nature[187]. In other words, DHT is a modified, more active form of testosterone.

You're probably still wondering: What the hell is DHT? To simplify things, DHT is what helps develop your genitals at birth. It's the sex steroid responsible for lowering your voice and putting hair on your chest during puberty.

DHT is also largely responsible for male pattern baldness, and can cause benign (harmless) growth of the prostate, increased oiliness of the skin, and acne[188].

When we think about DHT only in terms of these negative side effects, it is easy to believe that your goal should involve eliminating or reducing it. But DHT is essential for proper brain chemistry and proper sexual function, including libido.

---

[187] Androgen receptor signaling induced by supraphysiological doses of dihydrotestosterone in human peripheral blood lymphocytes. Proteomics. 2010 Sep;10(17):3165-75.

[188] Dihydrotestosterone and the concept of 5alpha-reductase inhibition in human benign prostatic hyperplasia. Eur Urol. 2000 Apr;37(4):367-80.

Because of this odd duality, DHT is NOT something you want to reduce or eliminate in the body. We explain the reason for this in the next section. Furthermore, if you recall, earlier in the book we mentioned that one of the main reasons Dr. Crisler preferred topical testosterone delivery systems was due to the improvement in sexual function it gave men from the rise in DHT levels.

However, due to varying biochemistry amongst individuals, some men will need to keep DHT levels under control in order to avoid the previously mentioned side effects. Your physician should carefully monitor your DHT levels relative to both your initial baseline blood panel and your ongoing blood panels over time.

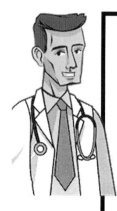

If you utilize TOT transdermally (cream or gel), it is very important to monitor your DHT levels as transdermals often convert testosterone to DHT and will elevate PSA (Prostate Specific Antigen) values in the short term (usually until an effective dose of testosterone is established). A very recent landmark research study[189] on DHT found that "the preponderance of available clinical data indicates that modest elevations in circulating levels of DHT in response to testosterone therapy should not be of concern in clinical practice." Elevated DHT has not been associated with increased risk of prostate disease (e.g., cancer or benign hyperplasia, evidenced by growth of the

[189] DIHYDROTESTOSTERONE: BIOCHEMISTRY, PHYSIOLOGY AND CLINICAL IMPLICATIONS OF ELEVATED BLOOD LEVELS. Endocr Rev. 2017 May 2. doi: 10.1210/er.2016-1067. Swerdloff RS1, Dudley RE2, Page ST3, Wang C1,4, Salameh WA1.

prostate) nor does it appear to have any systemic effects on cardiovascular disease (CVD) or safety parameters (including increased risk of erythrocytosis) beyond those commonly observed with available testosterone preparations.

In other words, using a testosterone gel or cream MAY cause a temporary but ultimately harmless rise in both your DHT and PSA levels until your doctor establishes an effective dose of testosterone necessary to achieve an optimal balance between testosterone and estrogen (the primary goal of TOT). To reiterate, if you use transdermal delivery systems for your TOT, make sure to measure DHT and PSA levels upon initiating therapy, and 4-6 weeks after starting to account for any transient (i.e. short-term) elevations.

Baldness and Acne

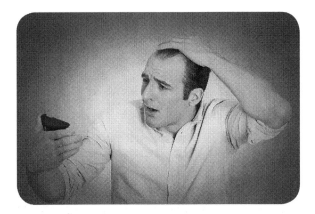

Baldness, otherwise known as 'male pattern baldness' (**MPB**), is genetic. Using TOT can definitely exacerbate or speed up hair loss via testosterone converting into *dihydrotestosterone* (**DHT**).

The idea of losing hair is very difficult to deal with for many men, but we believe that accepting symptoms of low testosterone in order to retain a receding or thinning hairline doesn't make sense. Shave your head and enjoy the rest of the benefits that TOT brings to your life.

There are numerous medications men take to prevent thinning hair from receding entirely. The most popular is **Propecia**, also known as **Proscar**. The active ingredient in Propecia is **Finasteride**, which is a *5-alpha-reductase* (**5AR**) *inhibitor*. It works by blocking the enzymes that naturally convert testosterone into DHT. With that being said, there are several problems with **5AR** inhibitors. Not only do they inhibit the testosterone molecule itself (effectively blocking many of the positive effects of TOT), but they also reduce libido (sex drive), weaken the strength of your erections[190] and reduce your fertility by reducing your motile sperm count[191].

What kind of man wants to lose erectile strength in the middle of sex? If your hair is that important to you, we recommend you try a topical application to directly affect the hair at its root. You can read much more about the causes of hair loss and available topical treatments on the Excel Male forums[192]. There are exciting new developments in regard to hair transplants, such as 'Hair Cloning' (which is likely to be available soon).

---

[190]   Finasteride and male infertility: a case for prospective collaborative research databases? Fertility and Sterility, Volume 100, Issue 6, December 2013, Pages 1528-1529.

[191]   The dark side of 5α-reductase inhibitors' therapy: sexual dysfunction, high Gleason grade prostate cancer and depression. Traish AM1, Mulgaonkar A2, Giordano N2. Korean J Urol. 2014 Jun;55(6):367-79. Epub 2014 Jun 16.

[192]   https://www.excelmale.com/showthread.php?6407-Testosterone-and-Hair-Loss-What-You-Need-to-Know&highlight=Hair+Loss+Remedies

One of the best places online to read about the upcoming advancements in hair cloning is Bernstein Medical[193].

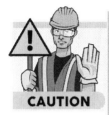

CAUTION

There are men who report very nasty side effects from the usage of Finasteride. *Post-Finasteride Syndrome* (**PFS**) describes persistent sexual, neurological, and physical adverse reactions in patients who have taken finasteride. Unfortunately, PFS is a condition with no known cure and few, if any, effective treatments. As more and more men continue to report these side effects to health and regulatory agencies worldwide, medical and scientific communities are only beginning to realize the scope of the problem. For much more information on PFS, we recommend you visit the PFS Foundation's website[194].

DHT is also known to have negative effects on the skin and hair follicles. **DHT** increases the production of oil in the skin's sebaceous glands, which often leads to bouts of acne. For those men who were prone to incidences of acne in their teen years, testosterone can cause flare-ups on their backs and shoulders later on.

It's also important to understand that diet is often the source of acne. Eating a diet high in essential fatty acids (EFA's), along with reducing refined and processed food consumption, can make a big difference in clearing up the oily skin that leads to acne. Fasting via the lifestyle protocols found in our book *The Metabolic Blowtorch Diet: How to Optimize Intermittent Fasting*

---

[193] https://www.bernsteinmedical.com/medical-treatment/hair-cloning/

[194] http://www.pfsfoundation.org/

to Burn Fat, Preserve Muscle, Enhance Focus and Transform Your Health[195] has also been shown to clear up acne[196]. We discuss what constitutes a 'clean' diet in Chapter 13. There is also a genetic component to acne and some men may do well by consulting a dermatologist for severe issues. A great source of information regarding acne and the usage of TOT is the Excel Male Forums[197].

Prolactin

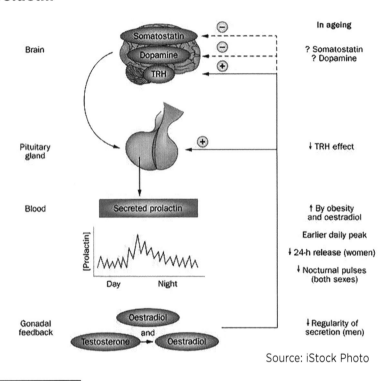

Source: iStock Photo

---

[195]   www.metabolicblowtorchdiet.com

[196]   Please refer to this article for more information: http://bradpilon.com/weight-loss/intermittent-fasting-and-acne/

[197]   https://www.excelmale.com/showthread.php?6487-Testosterone-and-Acne-What-You-Need-to-Know&highlight=Hair+Loss+Remedies

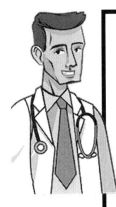

Prolactin is a hormone found in your bloodstream that can interfere with testicular function, ultimately lowering your testosterone levels and interfering with your sex life. Excessively high prolactin levels are also associated with gynecomastia (i.e. "man boobs")[198]. Studies have found that high prolactin levels in men (>30 ng/dL), a condition known as hyperprolactinemia, are linked to low sexual desire, erectile dysfunction and galactorrhea (i.e. milk production)[199]. Men with severe hyperprolactinemia frequently show mild hypogonadism (low testosterone), and complain of a loss of libido and sexual dysfunction[200].

If you are using TOT long-term and start suffering an unusual decline in libido, we encourage you to get your serum prolactin levels measured. In rare circumstances, an extremely elevated reading (> 300 ng/dL) may require an MRI of your pituitary gland to determine if the issue is a *pituitary adenoma*. This is a benign (i.e. non-cancerous) pituitary tumor that may cause vision problems and headaches if left untreated. It is either monitored regularly over time while prolactin levels are controlled via medication, or surgically

[198] Bromocriptine monotherapy of a prolactinoma causing erectile dysfunction. Arch Esp Urol. 1997 Jun;50(5):526-8.

[199] Hyperprolactinemia and Erectile Dysfunction. Rev Urol, 2000 Winter, 2(1):39–42,

[200] Prolactin and testosterone: their role in male sexual function. Carani C1, Granata AR, Fustini MF, Marrama P. Int Androl. 1996 Feb;19(1):48-54

removed through an amazingly routine procedure known as transsphenoidal surgery[201]. For men who have total testosterone levels below 150 ng/dL before starting TOT, it is important that an experienced physician runs tests to ensure that a pituitary adenoma is the root cause.

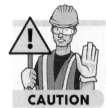

CAUTION

The medication used to control elevated prolactin levels is Cabergoline. Cabergoline is a potent dopamine receptor agonist that directly has a suppressive effect on prolactin cells[202]. Many age-management practices are using Cabergoline regularly in their practices with men to boost libido and/or improve sexual function[203]. Anecdotal studies show **that a 0.5 mg Cabergoline tablet taken twice a week** improves the quality and intensity of your sex drive, arousal, and orgasms[204]. This is clearly an "off label" usage of this medication due to the lack of peer-reviewed research data pertaining to these specific benefits. Multiple

---

201 Nishioka H. Recent Evolution of Endoscopic Endonasal Surgery for Treatment of Pituitary Adenomas. *Neurologia medico-chirurgica.* 2017;57(4):151-158. doi:10.2176/nmc.ra.2016-0276.

202 Wakil, A.; Rigby, A. S; Clark, A. L; Kallvikbacka-Bennett, A.; Atkin, S. L (2008). "Low dose cabergoline for hyperprolactinaemia is not associated with clinically significant valvular heart disease." *European Journal of Endocrinology.* 159 (4): R11–4. PMID 18625690. doi:10.1530/EJE-08-0365.

203 Six months of treatment with cabergoline restores sexual potency in hyperprolactinemic males: an open longitudinal study monitoring nocturnal penile tumescence. J Clin Endocrinol Metab. 2004 Feb;89(2):621-5.

204 Krüger TH, Haake P, Haverkamp J, Krämer M, Exton MS, Saller B, Leygraf N, Hartmann U, Schedlowski M. Effects of acute prolactin manipulation on sexual drive and function in males. *J Endocrinol.* 2003;179(3):357-65.

studies[205] have shown, however, that the long-term use of Cabergoline on prolactinomas (i.e. pituitary adenoma)[206] is safe[207].

To learn more about Prolactin, read this article from SelfHacked called "Everything to Know about Prolactin and How to Increase or Decrease it"[208].

SERM's (Selective Estrogen Receptor Modulators) and AIs (Aromatase Inhibitors) to Treat Side Effects

The authors of this book have used almost every **SERM** and **AI** available.

We have chosen the optimal ancillary medications for physicians to treat and correct the potential side effects of TOT. These ancillaries are quite potent, so there must be a specific diagnosed medical need to use them. Some men, due to the uniqueness of their biochemistry, will need stronger TOT side-effect medications than others.

---

[205] Auriemma RS1, Pivonello R, Perone Y, Grasso LF. Safety of long-term treatment with cabergoline on cardiac valve disease in patients with prolactinomas. Eur J Endocrinol. 2013 Aug 28;169(3):359-66. doi: 10.1530/EJE-13-0231.

[206] Gu H1, Luck S, Carroll PV. Cardiac valve disease and low-dose dopamine agonist therapy: an artefact of reporting bias? Clin Endocrinol (Oxf). 2011 May;74(5):608-10.

[207] Vallette S1, Serri K, Rivera J, Santagata P. Long-term cabergoline therapy is not associated with valvular heart disease in patients with prolactinomas. Pituitary. 2009;12(3):153-7. doi: 10.1007/s11102-008-0134-2.

[208] https://selfhacked.com/blog/prolactin/

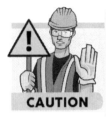

CAUTION

Because these **SERM's** and **AIs** have not been FDA-approved for use in men, TOT physicians prescribe them for 'off-label' use. Due to the fact that some of them are now manufactured as generic medications in most markets, it is unlikely that a drug company would pursue FDA approval for using these drugs in men because of the limited profit incentive.

FDA approval is expensive to obtain, so without the motivation for profitability, a drug company is unlikely to seek approval despite the obvious therapeutic benefits that exist for a given drug. With that being said, just because something isn't FDA-approved doesn't mean you and your doctor can't discuss a medication's potentially therapeutic benefits. In the USA, doctors have some dispensation to prescribe non-FDA approved drugs at their discretion if they feel it will benefit the patient.

SERM's and **AIs** were initially designed to treat breast cancer in women, and so when these medications are used in male endocrine systems, the patient needs to be closely monitored. However, they are usually well tolerated. Work with a TOT physician who is familiar with how these drugs interact with the human body.

NOTE Recent studies on Arimidex[209] (an AI), along with patient data from progressive physicians, indicate that this medication may pose a long-term risk to bone mineral density in select patients. Understanding this, you should insist that your doctor

---

[209]   De Ronde W, de Jong FH. Aromatase inhibitors in men: effects and therapeutic options. *Reproductive Biology and Endocrinology : RB&E.* 2011;9:93. doi:10.1186/1477-7827-9-93.

performs regular DEXA scans[210] to assess any bone mineral loss or spinal degradation if you are using Arimidex while also on TOT. We are not fond of AI medications and recommend the minimum effective dose (MED) principle is followed. You should ALWAYS act with the primary goal of weaning off the AI completely, as soon as there is a therapeutic range of E2 established (absent of side effects).

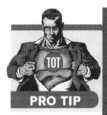

PRO TIP

Your doctor will analyze your lab work and symptoms, and prescribe you any necessary ancillary medications recommended in the chart below (when your symptoms and/or blood values warrant it). They will also discuss the potential side effects of these medications and their ramifications before you start taking them.

---

[210] https://www.bodyspec.com/what-is-dxa

Drug Classification	Name of Drug	Normal Dosage and Side Effects Addressed
SERM (Selective Estrogen Receptor Modulator)	*Nolvadex*[211] (Tamoxifen) 10–20 mg Tablet	Nolvadex actually has quite a few applications for TOT users. First and foremost, its most common use is for the prevention of gynecomastia (i.e. male breast tissue growth). Nolvadex binds to the receptor site in breast tissue, safely preventing estrogen formation. The advantage of Nolvadex is that it doesn't completely reduce estrogen in your body, ensuring that some estrogen is still floating around.

Estrogen is important for a properly functioning immune system, while maintaining healthy joints. It has also been shown to improve lipid profiles while using testosterone[212]. |

---

[211]   https://pubchem.ncbi.nlm.nih.gov/compound/2733526

[212]   Furr BJ, Jordan VC (1984). "The pharmacology and clinical uses of tamoxifen." Pharmacol. Ther. 25 (2): 127–205. doi:10.1016/0163-7258(84)90043-3.

Drug Classification	Name of Drug	Normal Dosage and Side Effects Addressed
SERM (Selective Estrogen Receptor Modulator) *continued...*	*Nolvadex* (Tamoxifen) 10–20 mg Tablet *continued...*	Normal dosage of Nolvadex is **10-40 mg per day or EOD (every other day) until symptoms disappear.** The half life of Nolvadex is between 5 and 7 days. Most progressive TRT physicians will taper the medication (i.e. gradually reduce the dose over time).
SERM (Selective Estrogen Receptor Modulator)	*Clomid*[213] (Clomiphene Citrate or Omifin) 25-50 mg Tablet	Clomid works by blocking estrogen's actions in the pituitary gland[214]. The pituitary thereby 'sees' less estrogen and secretes more luteinizing hormone (LH). In turn, increased LH levels stimulate the Leydig cells in the testis to synthesize more testosterone. Clomid binds to estrogen receptors and

---

[213] https://pubchem.ncbi.nlm.nih.gov/compound/60974

[214] Kim, E.D., et al., The treatment of hypogonadism in men of reproductive age. Fertil Steril, 2013. 99(3): p. 718-24.

Drug Classification	Name of Drug	Normal Dosage and Side Effects Addressed
SERM (Selective Estrogen Receptor Modulator) *continued...*	*Clomid* (Clomiphene Citrate or Omifin) 25-50 mg Tablet *continued...*	also restores the body's natural production of testosterone[215]. Low-dose Clomid therapy is now preferred by a number of TOT physicians like **Jeffrey Dach MD, Rob Kominiarek DO, John Crisler DO,** and **Dr. Eugene Shippen** to be the preferential SERM used as 'monotherapy' for hypogonadal men looking to remain fertile (i.e. retain normal levels of motile sperm). These doctors have had great results using ***Clomid at 12.5 to 25 mg EOD (every other day)*** to restore normal testosterone production. The half life of clomid is between 4-6 weeks. In some men, however, clomid increases Sex Hormone Binding Globulin (SHBG) and this ultimately decreases

215 Tan, RS; Vasudevan, D. (Jan 2003). "Use of clomiphene citrate to reverse premature andropause secondary to steroid abuse." *Fertil Steril* 79 (1): 203–5.

Drug Classification	Name of Drug	Normal Dosage and Side Effects Addressed
SERM (Selective Estrogen Receptor Modulator) *continued...*	*Clomid* (Clomiphene Citrate or Omifin) 25-50 mg Tablet *continued...*	free testosterone. Some men do not respond well to Clomid (i.e. they experience a minimal testosterone increase) and others experience significant side effects with it. For an excellent summary on understanding the pharmacodynamics of Clomid, see Lee Myer's article "The Half Life of Clomid[216]." As always, careful evaluation of your blood work is paramount.
SERM (Selective Estrogen Receptor Modulator)	*Toremifene Citrate*[217] (Fareston) 60 mg Tablet	Toremifene, while chemically similar to Nolvadex, has several other well-known effects that include acting as an estrogen antagonist in the Hypothalamus-Pituitary-Testes-Axis (HPTA). Because its testosterone to estrogen

Drug Classification	Name of Drug	Normal Dosage and Side Effects Addressed
SERM (Selective Estrogen Receptor Modulator) *continued..*	*Toremifene Citrate* (Fareston) 60 mg Tablet *continued..*	ratio is 5x that of Nolvadex, Toremifene is probably capable of increasing total testosterone[218]. We find Toremifene to be a good supporting medication to use after long periods of TOT usage, whereby an increase in libido is needed. It has been known to deliver a 'jolt' to your HPTA, improving sexual desire and feelings of intimacy. A daily dose of **30 mg for two to three days in a row** (until libido and feelings of sexual desire are restored) has been effective for some patients. This is another SERM rarely prescribed by TOT doctors.

---

[218] Price N, Sartor O, Hutson T, Mariani S. Role of 5a-reductase inhibitors and selective estrogen receptor modulators as potential chemopreventive agents for prostate cancer. Clin Prostate Cancer 2005;3:211-4. PMID 15882476.

Drug Classification	Name of Drug	Normal Dosage and Side Effects Addressed
SERM (Selective Estrogen Receptor Modulator)	*Raloxifene*[219] (Evista) 60 mg Tablet	Raloxifene is the newest SERM at the disposal of TOT physicians and their patients. Raloxifene is in the same family of compounds as Novaldex. Raloxifene has about 10x the binding affinity for the estrogen receptor in breast tissue compared to Nolvadex[220]. In other words, it binds much more strongly to the receptor site and virtually eliminates the possibility of any estrogen reaching a receptor and exerting an undesired effect[221]. If you're reading between

---

[219] https://pubchem.ncbi.nlm.nih.gov/compound/raloxifene

[220] J Pediatr. 2004 Jul;145(1):71-6. Beneficial effects of raloxifene and tamoxifen in the treatment of pubertal gynecomastia. Lawrence SE, Faught KA, Vethamuthu J, Lawson ML. Source Department of Pediatrics, University of Ottawa, Ontario, Canada.

[221] Vogel, Victor; Joseph Constantino, Lawrence Wickerman et al. (2006-06-21). "Effects of Tamoxifen vs. Raloxifene on the Risk of Developing Invasive Breast Cancer and Other Disease Outcomes." The Journal of the American Medical Association 295 (23).

Drug Classification	Name of Drug	Normal Dosage and Side Effects Addressed
SERM (Selective Estrogen Receptor Modulator) *continued...*	*Raloxifene* (Evista) 60 mg Tablet *continued...*	the lines, you can see how effective Raloxifene might be in the treatment and prevention of gynecomastia (if caught early enough). An optimal dosing protocol is **60 mg daily until the gynecomastia is gone, which ends up working for most patients.** The half life of Raloxifene is 27 hours[222].
AIs (Aromatase Inhibitors)	Arimidex[223] (Anastrozole) Tablet 1 mg Tablet	Arimidex is known as a "competitive inhibitor," which means it competes with estrogen for binding to the aromatase enzyme. Arimidex works by actively blocking the aromatase enzyme from binding to an androgen (testosterone), thereby blocking the body's ability to produce estrogen. It is the most frequently prescribed AI due to its

---

[222] http://www.aafp.org/afp/1999/0915/p1131.html

[223] https://pubchem.ncbi.nlm.nih.gov/compound/2187

Drug Classification	Name of Drug	Normal Dosage and Side Effects Addressed
AIs (Aromatase Inhibitors) *continued...*	Arimidex (Anastrozole) Tablet 1 mg Tablet *continued...*	wide availability and its effectiveness. An optimal dosing protocol of Arimidex while on TOT is **0.25 mg once per day, between 1-3 days a week depending on one's estrogen levels and need to reduce estrogen levels into a therapeutic range. Some men will need to go as high as 0.5 mg EOD** in order to prevent side effects such as moodiness, water retention and lowered libido. The half life of Arimidex is about 46 hours[224]. Some men with higher body fat percentages *potentially* need **0.5 mg of Arimidex twice a week** when starting TOT as a good failsafe to prevent potential side effects caused by the aromatase enzyme

---

[224] https://dailymed.nlm.nih.gov/dailymed/archives/fdaDrugInfo.cfm?archiveid=5257

Drug Classification	Name of Drug	Normal Dosage and Side Effects Addressed
AIs (Aromatase Inhibitors) *continued...*	Arimidex (Anastrozole) Tablet 1 mg Tablet *continued...*	(found in their fat tissue) converting testosterone into estrogen.

Unfortunately, Arimidex can and does reduce HDL (i.e. 'good') cholesterol levels, and therefore its use needs to be monitored closely[225]. Reducing HDL levels can lead to an increased risk of heart disease, and lead to bone mineral density issues. In fact, very recently published studies[226-227] prove that Arimidex, as an AI medication, is detrimental |

---

[225] Rubinow KB, Tang C, Hoofnagle AN, et al. Acute Sex Steroid Withdrawal Increases Cholesterol Efflux Capacity and HDL-Associated Clusterin in Men. Steroids 2012;77(5):454-460. doi:10.1016/j.steroids.2012.01.002.

[226] Bone Mineral Density and Response to Treatment in Men Younger Than 50 Years with Testosterone Deficiency and Sexual Dysfunction or Infertility. Kacker, Ravi et al. The Journal of Urology, Volume 191, Issue 4, 1072 - 1076.

[227] Effect of Anastrozole on Bone Mineral Density: 5-Year Results From the Anastrozole, Tamoxifen, Alone or in Combination Trial 18233230. Richard Eastell, Judith E. Adams, Robert E. Coleman, Anthony Howell, Rosemary A. Hannon, Jack Cuzick, John R. Mackey, Matthias W. Beckmann, and Glen Clack. Journal of Clinical Oncology 2008 26:7, 1051-1057.

Drug Classification	Name of Drug	Normal Dosage and Side Effects Addressed
AIs (Aromatase Inhibitors) *continued...*	Arimidex (Anastrozole) Tablet 1 mg Tablet *continued...*	to long-term bone health. Understanding this, the most progressive TOT doctors believe minimizing the usage of Arimidex is the optimal strategy.
AIs (Aromatase Inhibitors)	Aromasin[228] (Exemestane) 25 mg Tablet	Aromasin is considered a "suicide inhibitor" AI, which means it attaches to the aromatase enzyme and permanently disables it. Aromasin at 12.5–25 mg a day will raise testosterone levels by about 60%. It also increases the free testosterone (i.e. bioavailable testosterone) to bound testosterone ratio by lowering levels of SHBG in the body by 20%[229]. The benefits of lowering SHBG are discussed in much greater detail in Chapter 12.

---

[228] https://pubchem.ncbi.nlm.nih.gov/compound/60198

[229] De Ronde W, de Jong FH. Aromatase inhibitors in men: effects and therapeutic options. *Reproductive Biology and Endocrinology: RB&E* 2011;9:93. doi:10.1186/1477-7827-9-93.

Drug Classification	Name of Drug	Normal Dosage and Side Effects Addressed
AIs (Aromatase Inhibitors) *continued...*	Aromasin (Exemestane) 25 mg Tablet *continued...*	Aromasin is also compatible with Nolvadex, and in some instances has beneficial effects on bone mineral content and lipid profiles. It suppresses estrogen more strongly than Arimidex, but as a Type 1 AI, it deactivates the aromatase enzyme and renders the enzyme inactive, thus allowing other ancillary medications to work[230]. This medication is rarely prescribed by TOT physicians. It needs to be studied more closely due to its unique ability to raise testosterone levels via its reduction of SHBG levels. It should also be more rigorously examined because Arimidex, as the primary alternative, is being shown in recent

[230] Simpson ER (2003). "Sources of estrogen and their importance." The Journal of Steroid Biochemistry and Molecular Biology 86 (3–5): 225–30. doi:10.1016/S0960-0760(03)00360-1. PMID 14623515.

Drug Classification	Name of Drug	Normal Dosage and Side Effects Addressed
		studies[231] to be detrimental to bone mineral density (BMD) over time. There have been some rare cases of hepatoxicity[232] (i.e. liver toxicity) found with its use. As previously stated with Arimidex, we believe it is prudent to minimize the usage of all AIs when undergoing TOT.

The Usage of AIs and SERM's as TOT

More and more physicians are using a **SERM** (such as *Clomid*, *Nolvadex* or *Toremifene*) or even an **AI** (such as *Arimidex*) as the entirety of a "TOT" protocol. These medications will elevate luteinizing hormone (LH) and overall total testosterone levels[233], so it's easy to see why such an approach would be

---

[231]   Finkelstein JS, Lee H, Leder BZ, et al. Gonadal steroid–dependent effects on bone turnover and bone mineral density in men. The Journal of Clinical Investigation. 2016;126(3):1114-1125.

[232]   Bao T, Fetting J, Mumford L, et al. Severe prolonged cholestatic hepatitis caused by exemestane. *Breast cancer research and treatment.* 2010;121(3):789-791. doi:10.1007/s10549-009-0576-x.

[233]   Short-term aromatase-enzyme blockade unmasks impaired feedback adaptations in luteinizing hormone and testosterone secretion in older men. Veldhuis JD1, Iranmanesh A. J Clin Endocrinol Metab. 2005 Jan;90(1):211-8. Epub 2004 Oct 13.

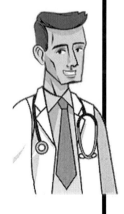

taken. From our experience and the most prominent research done to this date on **AIs** in men[234], patients rarely report long-term benefits from these strategies (increased lean body mass, libido, less fatigue, etc.) for the following reasons:

1. A major risk of using an AI alone is the possibility of driving estrogen levels too low. This could have terrible consequences for your good cholesterol profile, bone mineral density, libido, and overall feelings of well-being. Talk to any man who has dealt with having his estrogen levels pushed too low. It feels terrible! There is no sex drive or function, and you often experience lethargy and overall lifelessness.

2. A serious limitation of the use of aromatase inhibitors in isolation in aging men is that the stimulating effect on testosterone levels may be too weak, especially in men with the lowest baseline testosterone levels who would potentially benefit the most from stimulation[235].

234 De Ronde W, de Jong FH. Aromatase inhibitors in men: effects and therapeutic options. *Reproductive Biology and Endocrinology: RB&E.* 2011;9:93. doi:10.1186/1477-7827-9-93.

235 De Ronde W, de Jong FH. Aromatase inhibitors in men: effects and therapeutic options. Reproductive Biology and Endocrinology : RB&E. 2011;9:93. doi:10.1186/1477-7827-9-93.

3. There is normally a narrow therapeutic window in reg-ulating estrogen (estradiol/E2) levels before you even-tually start negatively impacting your health and your libido. Less, in terms of estrogen levels, is rarely better and these values need to be monitored on a regular basis with an experienced TOT physician. Remember, it is all about balance for the individual patient.

If your doctor has you on a SERM or AI as a 'sole form of TOT', we encourage you to show them this book so they can better understand why using testosterone is a much more effective strategy.

However, combining TOT with a SERM or an AI (when there is an observed clinical need, due to symptoms being reflective of higher E2 levels) is often a necessary short-term option for achieving the optimal balance between testosterone and estrogen. **The notable exception is for TOT patients (normally between 30-50 years old) who want to stay fertile**. These patients should consider using low doses of clomid, or hCG monotherapy, to help restore and improve low rates of natural testosterone production. Please see the eye-opening interview with **Dr. Merrill Matschke** in Chapter 12 on maintaining fertility through hormonal optimization.

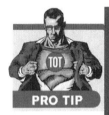

PRO TIP

Due to scientific studies[236] showing the negative consequences to bone mineral density[237] from long-term use of AI medications[238], we adamantly recommend that AIs are ONLY used for short periods of time. This is to get estrogen levels within an acceptable therapeutic range where hormonal balance is achieved and side effects are alleviated. A much safer and effective strategy is to either reduce the testosterone dosage, or alter the dosing schedule to deal with the symptoms of excess estrogen. **Dr. Robert Kominiarek** sees patients in his practice with osteoporosis (breakdown of the bones) in the spine and hips after being on Arimidex for 6-12+ consecutive months (or longer). This is a terrible situation for a TOT patient, and one that physicians attempt to avoid at all costs.

The dosing of these AI medications is highly variable as all men are biochemically different from one another. As aromatase inhibition is dose-dependent, it has been suggested that aromatase is less suppressed in the testes than in adipose and muscle tissue, which explains the incomplete effectiveness of aromatase inhibition in men. Again, that is why it is crucial to have a competent TOT

---

[236] Changes in bone mineral density at 3 years in postmenopausal women receiving anastrozole and risedronate in the IBIS-II bone substudy: an international, double-blind, randomised, placebo-controlled trial. Sestak, Ivana et al. The Lancet Oncology, Volume 15, Issue 13, 1460 - 1468.

[237] Alleviating anastrozole induced bone toxicity by selenium nanoparticles in SD rats. Kiritkumar K. Vekariya Jasmine Kaur Kulbhushan Tikoo.

[238] Finkelstein JS, Lee H, Leder BZ, et al. Gonadal steroid–dependent effects on bone turnover and bone mineral density in men. The Journal of Clinical Investigation. 2016;126(3):1114-1125.

prescribing doctor[239] who can evaluate lab values and attend to symptoms, if and when they arise. Additionally, ongoing blood draws done regularly and honest patient feedback are crucial for both the patient and the doctor to achieve (and maintain) an optimal hormonal balance. With some men, hormonal balance can take time to achieve.

Metabolic Syndrome, Obesity, Insulin Resistance, Aromatase and Estrogen

Testosterone levels are lower in men with obesity, metabolic syndrome, and type 2 diabetes[240]. You can see this just by looking around, as obesity is increasing dramatically across most of the world. We all know the reasons behind this: poor diet, and a lack of exercise are literally killing us.

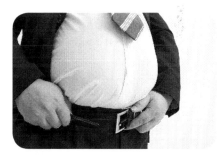

Recent studies indicate that TOT in men with type 2 diabetes has beneficial effects on decreasing insulin resistance and lowering visceral body fat[241], both of which play a key role in cardiovascular

---

[239] www.bodhd.com

[240] Wang C, Jackson G, Jones TH, et al. Low Testosterone Associated With Obesity and the Metabolic Syndrome Contributes to Sexual Dysfunction and Cardiovascular Disease Risk in Men With Type 2 Diabetes. *Diabetes Care*2011;34(7):1669-1675. doi:10.2337/dc10-2339.

[241] Jones TH, Arver S, Behre HM, et al., TIMES2 Investigators. Testosterone Replacement in Hypogonadal Men With Type 2 Diabetes and/or Metabolic Syndrome (the TIMES2 Study). *Diabetes Care* 2011;34(4):828-837. doi:10.2337/dc10-1233.

disease. If you want to do a quick calculation as to your risk of cardiovascular disease, check out CVRiskCalculator[242].

TOT has been proven to increase lean body mass (LBM), reduce fat mass, reduce waist circumference and BMI[243], and produce sustained and significant weight loss. Wouldn't TOT in obese men with low levels of testosterone be a unique and effective therapeutic approach to the management of obesity? Of course it would. And if you're already an obese man, a very recent study[244] says that being testosterone deficient will dramatically increase your risk of death.

It would also make sense for men with Type 2 diabetes and metabolic syndrome to consider having their testosterone levels measured. If testosterone levels were found to be low or low-normal, a well-designed TOT protocol (along with a proper diet and exercise program fully structured to reduce body fat) might be a reasonable strategy for optimizing their health. There are many physicians now advocating TOT as a possible front-line treatment for men suffering from Type 2 diabetes, due to testosterone's profound ability to improve most health markers.

Aromatase, the enzyme responsible for converting testosterone to estrogen, is more abundant in fat tissue[245]. The higher

---

[242] www.cvriskcalculator.com

[243] Traish AM. Testosterone and weight loss: the evidence. *Current Opinion in Endocrinology, Diabetes, and Obesity* 2014;21(5):313-322. doi:10.1097/MED.0000000000000086.

[244] Double Trouble: co-occurrence of testosterone deficiency and body fatness associated with all-cause mortality in US men.Clin Endocrinol (Oxf). 2017 Oct 25. doi: 10.1111/cen.13501. [Epub ahead of print].

[245] The hypogonadal–obesity cycle: role of aromatase in modulating the testosterone–estradiol shunt – a major factor in the genesis of morbid obesity. Cohen, P.G. Medical Hypotheses, Volume 52, Issue 1, 49 - 51.

your body fat percentage, the more aromatase enzymes you have floating around and the more likely you are to convert supplemental testosterone into estrogen (estradiol, E2). This conversion happens more often in stubborn body fat[246] deposit areas (which contain specific stubborn fat receptor cells with poor blood flow), such as the fat tissue found in the love handles, chest, and upper and lower back.

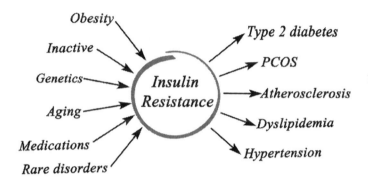

In other words, the higher your body fat percentage, the more likely you are to be susceptible to negative estrogen-induced side effects like poor erectile strength, moodiness, water retention, increased fat deposition, and so on (from high estrogen levels). For men with high body fat percentages who are starting TOT, it **may be** prudent to use a minimum effective dose of an AI medication after initiating testosterone therapy to minimize potential estrogen-induced side effects. This is a temporary solution, due to the potential damage to HDL and bone mineral density that the AI medications can cause. Always discuss this with your physician and make sure to regularly monitor sensitive E2 (estrogen) levels throughout therapy until balance (i.e. feeling good with no side effects) is achieved.

---

[246]   http://fabfitover40.com/2014/03/09/struggle-removing-stubborn-body-fat/

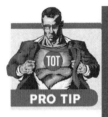

PRO TIP

*If your **body fat is above 20%** and you want to ensure that you are minimizing potential aromatization and estrogenic side effects, you should prioritize losing body fat while undergoing TOT.* We discuss strategies for losing body fat[247] and optimizing your fitness[248] while on TOT in Chapter 16.

Dr. Rob Kominiarek[249] loves using transdermal testosterone delivery systems in a lipiderm base for obese men suffering from metabolic disorder and insulin resistance. He uses it to drive up DHT levels, thereby improving sexual function. This melts the highly inflammatory subcutaneous fat off the midsection, ultimately increasing HDL and reducing insulin levels. When this is combined with the use of peptide hormones like Tesamorelin[250], the fat-burning effect is greatly enhanced. We discuss **Tesamorelin** more in *Chapter 15: Agents of Change.*

---

[247] www.metabolicblowtorchdiet.com

[248] www.advancedforgedtraining.com

[249] http://www.renuehealth.com/

[250] Stanley TL, Grinspoon SK. Effects of Growth Hormone Releasing Hormone on Visceral Fat, Metabolic and Cardiovascular Indices in Human Studies. Growth hormone & IGF research : official journal of the Growth Hormone Research Society and the International IGF Research Society. 2015;25(2):59-65. doi:10.1016/j.ghir.2014.12.005.

CHAPTER 10 KEY TAKEAWAYS

- The potential side effects of TOT (when managed by the right TOT physician) are minimal in scope, easy to spot and easy to safely correct.

- It's crucial to maintain ongoing and consistent blood work to best understand your test results as they change over time. Know your own body, compile your blood panel data, and do your homework to ensure your TOT is successful over a long period of time.

- We go into depth about the side effects of out-of-range E2 (estradiol) levels, whether too high or too low. The biggest reason why TOT doesn't "work" is because of poor estrogen (E2) management. Often times, it's out of balance due to a lack of physician observation, or even an over reliance on using AI medications that push E2 levels too low. Therefore, it is critical for both the patient and the doctor to establish accurate baseline levels of E2 (estrogen) before starting AND while undergoing TOT.

- We discuss DHT and what it's responsible for, while reminding you that DHT levels should be managed (NOT reduced or eliminated). We also discuss baldness and acne in relation to DHT.

- We also let you know why monitoring your prolactin levels is important, especially when you experience potential side effects from excessively high values (and suffer from low testosterone levels).

- We go deep down the rabbit hole of explaining the differences between all the existing AI and SERM medications commonly used alongside TOT. We tell you the normal dosages used by physicians, and the side effects associated with each of them.

- We talked about metabolic syndrome and insulin resistance, and tell you how obesity and high aromatase levels go hand in hand with low testosterone levels.

CHAPTER 11
Eliminating Gynecomastia Permanently

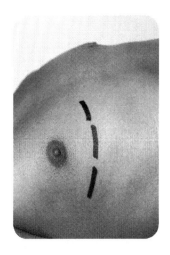

Gynecomastia, commonly known as 'gyno' or more crudely as "bitch tits," is the over-development of the male breast. It is a growing epidemic in Western society.

There are estimates saying that 60% of all men[251] are affected by gyneco-mastia. Read that sentence again: More than 60% of men suffer from gynecomastia! Why do we not hear more about this?

With the average male becoming more overweight over time, men are experiencing breast tissue growth that is made worse by poor nutrition, stress, additional body fat and a combination of high estrogen and low testosterone. This is an issue that extends way beyond aesthetics and looking good without your clothes on.

Unfortunately, most men will suffer from gynecomastia in silence because of how growing breasts negatively affects a man's self-confidence. With confidence completely stripped away, many men are too afraid to remove their shirt in public.

---

[251]   http://www.gynecomastia.org/

Most gyno sufferers deal with emotional and psychological trauma that dramatically impacts their lives.

Men need to physically recover from this condition, while treating the psychological component at the same time. There is no reason that modern-day men dealing with the shame and taboo surrounding gyno shouldn't be able to work with elite physicians who can treat and eliminate this condition for good.

To provide you with insights from the world's foremost subject matter expert on gynecomastia, we interviewed Dr. Joseph Cruise. Dr. Cruise is a Board Certified Plastic Surgeon in Newport Beach, California and a recognized world authority[252] in the treatment of gynecomastia. Dr. Cruise has worked with more than 3000 gyno patients and successfully performed more than 2000 gyno removal surgeries.

During our interview with Dr. Cruise, we were floored by how bad the problem actually was. His stories about the emotional devastation suffered by many of his patients was heartbreaking.

Types of Gynecomastia

There are 6 different types of gynecomastia[253]. For men using TOT, Dr. Cruise focuses on Types 1-3 because they are the most common forms found in individuals who are on TOT (see images below). For more information on types 4-6, please visit his website[254].

---

[252] http://www.trtrevolution.com/interview-worlds-leading-plastic-surgeon-gynecomastia-dr-joseph-cruise/

[253] http://www.LAgynecomastia.org

[254] https://lagynecomastia.org/gynecomastia-overview/

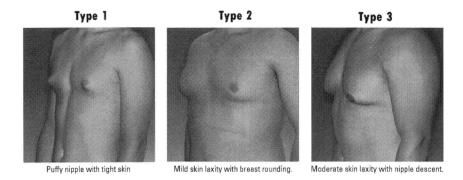

Type 1	Type 2	Type 3
Puffy nipple with tight skin	Mild skin laxity with breast rounding.	Moderate skin laxity with nipple descent.

Gynecomastia is technically defined as excess breast tissue that has been present for 2 years or more. Over time, the surrounding skin loses its elasticity. If there is no excess breast tissue left to hold, this loss of elasticity is relatively unnoticed. However, if that skin is holding the weight of gynecomastia, it will eventually fail. In this case, a patient has gone from a Type 1 or 2 (which requires incisions that are not noticeable) to Type 3 or Type 4 (which requires progressively higher levels of skin tightening and hence, longer incisions are necessary).

Dr. Cruise was kind enough to offer some important take away points regarding gyno treatment.

Before discussing the two most effective options to treat gynecomastia, we need to unfortunately mention the most common option – *Conceal and/or Avoid*, also known as the "Gynecomastia Routine." Dr Cruised coined this term to describe a way of life that gyno patients often fall into without even realizing it. Often times, this leads them to be bullied, teased, and sometimes become suicidal.

Option 1 - Conceal/Avoid

This is always the most common option. Not uncommonly, gyno sufferers find out about TOT and/or surgery through their research, yet become frustrated over the chaos Google has to offer. There are stories of bad outcomes, useless medications, contradictory opinions, and it's hard to make sense of it all. Unfortunately, just like there are numerous physicians dispensing TOT incorrectly, there are just as many surgeons who are not skilled in the removal of gynecomastia.

Not surprisingly, gynecomastia and testosterone deficiency have a lot in common.

- Despite both conditions being defined as medical problems, they are tragically dismissed and often viewed with a "that's just how it is" perspective.

- They are both non life-threatening, yet they are capable of taking the life out of you.

- Both erode quality of life, and slowly emasculate you over time.

- Fortunately, both have effective and predictable treatments available!

Gynecomastia Routine

Dr. Cruise originally coined this term to highlight what he would often see in his gyno patients. They dress to hide, not to impress. They often wear 2 shirts at the same time, and have the outer shirt oversized to make sure their chest contour is not revealed. No tight shirts or white shirts. Their shoulders are slightly hunched to cover the chest, and they often pull at the shirt to make sure it does not cling to their chest.

Unknowingly, this "Gynecomastia Routine" emasculates even the most masculine of men. Even more tragic are the joys of life one misses to avoid putting themselves in a potentially revealing position. Imagine living with the shame of not being able to remove your shirt when you're at the gym, a pool party, or even taking your kid to the beach!

Option 2 - Lose Fat, Build Muscle, & Balance Hormones through TOT

> *"Unquestionably, the single best way to 'treat' gyno is to avoid it altogether, or minimize it before it becomes a problem," says Dr. Cruise.*

Unfortunately, due to the lack of evidence-based information found online, most men struggle to find answers. Not to mention that their eyes catch stories of men who have had horrific experiences with failed surgeries.

Dr Cruise, like us, is a big believer in the therapeutic usage of testosterone:

> *"I have zero doubts about the positive effects of optimizing your testosterone under the supervision of an experienced physician, and it's certainly possible to lose fat in (and around) the chest area by building muscle. But it's only in rare instances where I've seen this achieved in men with previous existing conditions of gynecomastia."*

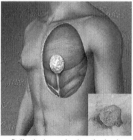
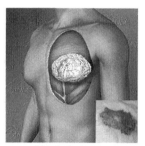
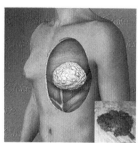

| Puffy nipple, predominantly gland. | High gland to fat ratio. | High fat to gland ratio. |

Dr. Cruise indicated there is one small caveat men should be aware of when undergoing TOT: Some men will be over-sensitive to the conversion of testosterone to DHT, leading to mild gland growth around the nipple. This will happen for a small subset of men. This is what likely happened to Jay, as you'll see later on in this chapter.

Option 3 - Surgical Removal

Despite doing all the 'right things', some men are simply over sensitive to evenly balanced estrogen and testosterone ratios, such as those found in people following optimized TOT protocols. These men still end up with enlarged, sensitive and puffy nipples.

More commonly, many men have had enlarged breast glands for a long period of time, going all the way back to the onset of puberty. Over time, several processes occur that make it impossible to get rid of gyno without surgery. Some of these processes are self-inflicted, such as in bodybuilders who use supraphysiologic (i.e. extremely high) doses of testosterone and/or anabolic steroids (AAS). Unfortunately, many men often discover there is no defined cause of these processes.

On the bright side, surgical removal of Type 1 and Type 2 gynecomastia (i.e. gynecomastia without skin laxity) is a life-changing procedure when performed by a competent gynecomastia surgeon. In fact, once the gland is removed, it is gone forever.

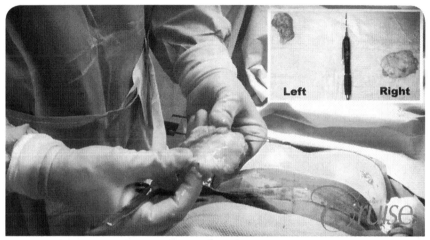

Gynecomastia gone forever.

Despite being a conservative surgeon by nature and living by the motto "If it isn't broke, don't fix it," Dr. Cruise believes there IS solid reasoning behind the surgical removal of excess breast tissue when non-surgical methods are not working.

However, there are many plastic surgeons who are unwilling to treat the issue of gynecomastia in males. While this greatly limits your choices, Dr. Cruise believes it is an advantage for gyno sufferers. At the end of the day, gynecomastia removal is a highly specialized and nuanced surgery. It requires a surgeon with technical skills, practice-based experience and a deep understanding of what the patient wants.

In his own words:

> "Gynecomastia is more than a mere aesthetic concern. The emotional and psychological effects of this condition run deep and strip away self-confidence like cancer. It's scary how unknown and mysterious this condition is. There is a psychological component to the suffering that should not be overlooked. The world is more concerned about hiding it than learning about how to fix it. I feel a sense of obligation to shine a spotlight on gynecomastia, so that all men affected can seek treatment."

The story of gynecomastia hits close to home for Jay. He had a form of glandular gyno in his right breast that came out of nowhere after 15 years of successful TOT in 2015. The causes were investigated, but ultimately determined to be unknown. Hormonal fluctuations, stress, cortisol/IGF-1, and varying insulin levels may have all played a role.

It was very painful and caused him great suffering when hugging his wife or children in day-to-day living. It also started to become noticeable in a tank top or tight-fitting clothing. After treating it with various ancillary medications (AIs and SERM's) prescribed by his doctor and not having any success, he decided to have it surgically removed in May of 2016.

After a couple of hours of searching online, it was clear that Dr. Joseph Cruise was the best choice for getting the procedure done correctly. It was a surprisingly easy and quick surgery – less than 70 minutes, and the whole thing was done under local anesthesia as an outpatient procedure in his clinic in Orange County, California. Jay was back to work in 4 days, and back to the gym in less than a month. The surgery could not have gone any better! See the before and after pictures below.

There is no reason to suffer in silence any longer. If you or someone you know is suffering from this condition, have them watch this video[255] and send them to the websites LAGynecomastia[256] and Gynecomastia[257].

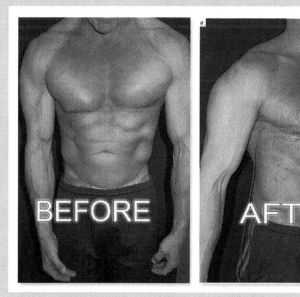

---

255   https://youtu.be/WCEeTsfNWBA

256   www.lagynecomastia.org

257   http://www.Gynecomastia.org

CHAPTER 11 KEY TAKEAWAYS

- We talked about what gynecomastia is and how more than half of men around the world are silently suffering from it. It requires physical and psychological treatment.

- We briefly discussed the 6 different types of gyne-comastia, and the process through which an individual can go from Types 1-2 to Types 3-4.

- Through insights gained from Dr. Joseph Cruise, the world's foremost subject matter expert on gynecomastia, we outlined three possible options for treating gynecomastia and went into detail about the effectiveness of each one. We also talked about the role of TOT in relation to gynecomastia.

- Finally, Jay shares his personal story about suffering from glandular gynecomastia and how he was able to treat it through quick, easy and painless surgery from a trusted and qualified surgeon.

CHAPTER 12
Monitoring TOT for Optimum Health

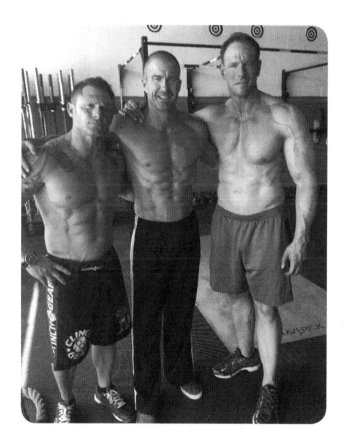

If you look at most people, you may notice they spend more time and energy on their cars than they do on their own bodies. Beginning TOT means you're going to be different, and you're going to invest the time it takes to learn what works for your body to stay optimized[258] until your very last breath.

---

[258]   www.90days2optimized.com

That begins when you make it an unfailing priority to familiarize yourself with the biomarkers we cover in this chapter to understand how lifelong TOT administration will affect them. You should become acutely aware and educated on each marker so both you and your doctor can minimize and/or avoid issues before they arise.

TOT is simply supplementing a natural hormone in your body, but you are also adding something external to your endocrine system. This will change things in your body, and therefore it's now your responsibility to get regular blood work done and stay on top of how your body responds to this new input.

Your physician must work with you to alleviate any concerns you have and resolve any potential side effects. And for those of you living in a country/state/city where it is legal to be your own doctor[259], you'll need to take full responsibility to do the necessary research and become intimately aware of your body's individual response to TOT. Remember, you are a biochemically unique human being and your body will respond in ways specific to you. Track your body's health markers over time to set your own benchmarks.

Understanding Your Blood Panels

After gathering your medical history, an informed TOT-prescribing physician will measure your blood work by running the following assays.

- **Testosterone, Free and Total**
- **CBC, specifically Hemoglobin/Hematocrit**

---

[259]   www.trtuniversity.org

- **Sex Hormone Binding Globulin (SHBG)**
- **Homocysteine**
- **Estradiol (Sensitive or Enhanced)**
- **Vitamin D, 25-Hydroxy**
- **Prolactin**
- **C-Reactive Protein Quant (hs-CRP preferred)**
- **Thyroid Panel**
- **Basic Metabolic Panel**
- **Lipid Panel**
- **DHEA-S**
- **Prostate Specific Ag Serum**
- **HbA1c**
- **Pregnenolone**

While all of them are important to monitor for out-of-range values (i.e. extreme highs and lows), we're going to focus on what we believe are the assays (lab tests) that TOT users MUST keep a watchful eye on for the entire duration of their therapy. Since TOT is a lifetime therapy, this means you'll be tracking these assays for the rest of your life.

BioMarker cheat sheet

Here is a Cheat Sheet for the most important biomarkers (and their respective ranges, where applicable) and tests for men to monitor regularly while undergoing lifelong TOT.

Test & Ranges	How Often/Where to Get It
Total Testosterone > 600 ng/dL (Remember that symptoms are <u>always</u> more important than lab values)	***2-3 times per year, depending on age and whether one is on TOT or not.*** *Levels over 1500 ng/dL accompanied by high Hematocrit, low HDL and/or other side effects may require dosage reduction.*
Free Testosterone > 2% of Total Testosterone	*If low, test for SHBG. Higher TOT dose may increase free testosterone by decreasing SHBG. Low SHBG levels may be from diabetes.*
Blood Pressure (especially if you have too much body fat) **< 135/85 mmHg**	***Weekly or semi-monthly*** *via purchase of an over-the-counter cuff[260], visiting a pharmacy or an office visit with your physician. If your blood pressure is high, focus on fat loss and exercise (i.e. resistance and cardiovascular training).*
Complete Blood Count (CBC)	***Twice during your first year on TOT (6 months apart), and then annually.***
Hemoglobin & Hematocrit	***2-3 times per year depending on age and whether one is no TOT or not.*** You need to make sure your numbers don't exceed 20 g/dL (Hemoglobin) / 52-54% blood volume (Hematocrit). Anything

---

[260] http://www.amazon.com/exec/obidos/ASIN/B004D9P1A8/trtrevbook-20

Test & Ranges	How Often/Where to Get It
Hemoglobin & Hematocrit *continued...*	beyond those numbers (a likely explanation is **erythrocytosis, i.e. blood thickening**) is an indication to have your platelets measured while also considering the option of donating your blood (via a phlebotomy). You could also withhold TOT until RBC (red blood cell) count is increased. Some patients may need to be phlebotomized multiple times a year while undergoing TOT.
Comprehensive Metabolic Panel This panel measures the blood levels of albumin, blood urea nitrogen, calcium, carbon dioxide, chloride, creatinine, glucose, potassium, sodium, total bilirubin and protein, and liver enzymes (alanine aminotransferase, alkaline phosphatase, and aspartate aminotransferase).	**Once a year.** Many strength trainers and weight lifters consume extra protein, along with supplements like creatine monohydrate. This can create false positive elevations in Blood Urea Nitrogen (BUN) and Creatinine (i.e. your reading shows up as something higher than what it actually is). Intense weight lifting can also cause a false positive increase in BUN and Creatinine as well. An informed TOT physician will account for this in their patients to avoid kidney or liver problems.

Test & Ranges	How Often/Where to Get It
Lipid Panels HDL > 40 mg/dL	*At least once a year, via a fasted blood test.* Higher TOT dosages may decrease HDL levels.
Estimated Glomerular Filtration Rate (eGFR), Kidney Function > 60 mL/min/1.73 m²	*Once a year. If low, then good hydration, use of blood pressure medications and/or stopping oral supplements may improve eGFR.* *Resistance exercise, high protein intake and higher muscle mass can also decrease eGFR.*
Prostate Specific Antigen (PSA) Value < 4 ng/mL	*Baseline (before starting TOT), and then yearly* (consult with your physician for further details). When utilizing transdermal testosterone delivery systems, it is especially important to monitor this marker as DHT can increase PSA rapidly upon starting therapy. As stated previously, this is only a temporary rise. An experienced TOT physician needs to be aware of the most recent research showing that DHT elevation DOES NOT lead to cancer[261]. Please refer back to Chapter 10 for more information.

---

[261] Dihydrotestosterone: Biochemistry, Physiology and Clinical Implications of Elevated Blood Levels. Endocr Rev. 2017 May 2. doi: 10.1210/er.2016-1067. Swerdloff RS1, Dudley RE2, Page ST3, Wang C1,4, Salameh WA1.

Test & Ranges	How Often/Where to Get It
(PSA) *continued...*	If PSA is higher than 4 ng/mL, talk to your doctor about the possibility of a prostatic infection, or ask for a referral to a urologist. NOTE: TOT is contraindicated if PSA is higher than 4 ng/dL.
Thyroid Stimulating Hormone (TSH) **< 2.5 units/mL**	**1-2 times per year.** If high, perform additional thyroid hormone tests such as free T3 (triiodothyronine), free T4 (thyroxine) and other antibodies to detect possible subclinical hyperthyroidism.
Free T3 > 3.7 pg/mL	1-2 times per year. *If low, hyperthyroidism may be present. See previous comment on TSH. If high (>5 pg/mL), explore hyperthyroidism.*
Digital Rectal Exam (DRE)	*Once a year after age 45* (especially if you have a family history of prostate cancer).
Estradiol (E2) **Sensitive Test** **20-50 pg/mL**	*After a baseline is obtained (before starting TOT), and during TOT (1-2x per year)* to ensure proper hormonal balance (dependent on side effects or

Test & Ranges	How Often/Where to Get It
Estradiol (E2) **Sensitive Test** **20-50 pg/mL** *continued...*	symptoms). It's best to order 'enhanced', 'sensitive', or 'ultra sensitive' to better evaluate male symptomatology regarding estrogen levels. If E2 levels are high, a short-term minimum effective dose of an AI can bring E2 into therapeutic levels, where no side effects are present (or the patient feels good). If E2 levels are low, increase testosterone dosage or stop AI altogether.
Prolactin <30 ng/dL	***After baseline is obtained (before TOT) and during TOT (1x per year)*** based on perceived symptoms and side effects (such as a loss of libido, feelings of moodiness or depression, etc.). Elevated prolactin over 300 ng/dL should result in an MRI to check for a pituitary adenoma.
Ferritin 55-270 ng/mL **Iron 55-160 g/dL**	**Once a year after 40.** *If low (both Ferritin & Iron), reduce frequency of blood donations or phlebotomies, and supplement with iron until levels are normal again. If high, get therapeutic phlebotomy ASAP.*

Test & Ranges	How Often/Where to Get It
C-Reactive Protein (CRP)< 3.0 mg/dL	***Once a year after age 40.*** As written in Chapter 2, CRP is a test to measure for systemic inflammation levels. Be careful when measuring CRP, as the lab values can be changed by variable lifestyle factors (intense training, a flu/virus, cold, etc.).
Homocysteine between 4.4 and 10.8 micromoles per liter of blood.	***Twice a year*** (Much more on Homocysteine later in this chapter).
DHEA (dehydroepiandros-terone)	***Once a year for men over 40.*** Make sure to test DHEA-S, as there is much more 'S' in the body (which provides more to measure). DHEA is a tricky hormone, but it has a lot of potential life-enhancing qualities. Read this amazing article about DHEA[262] and consider whether you should start supplementing with it. The most important takeaway is whether or not the blood work indicates a

---

[262] http://suppversity.blogspot.de/2013/09/suppversity-science-round-up-seconds.html

Test & Ranges	How Often/Where to Get It
DHEA (dehydroepiandros-terone) **Age (20-29)** **280-640 mcg/dL** **Age (30-39)** **120-520 mcg/dL** **Age (40-49)** **95-530 mcg/dL** **Age (50-59)** **70-310 mcg/dL** **Age (60-69)** **42-290 mcg/dL** **Over 69** **28-179 mcg/dL**	clinical need for supplementation. This is not a supplement to start randomly using because you feel like it.

Our recommendations about frequency of blood work in Chapter 4 are worth repeating here:

*For men in their 20's and 30's fortunate enough to be undergoing TOT, we recommend you get your blood drawn **at least once a year.***

*For those of you in your 40's and up, **twice a year is best.** An Anti-Aging Panel[263] is also highly recommended for anybody 35 and up.*

---

[263] www.bodhd.com

Each time you get blood work, review it and keep it in a file so you can compile and reference all of your data for life. Having a detailed timeline from your very first blood testosterone panel will provide you with a reliable baseline as your values and biomarkers change over time. Your physician will be documenting this, but you should keep copies of your blood panels yourself. If you do your homework and know your body, you'll be able to speak intelligently with your doctor.

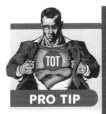

PRO TIP

We can't stress how important it is for every man reading this book to take control of his health while undergoing TOT via regular and methodical collection of blood panels. Order the Hormone and Wellness Panel for Men first[264], and if you're already a lifelong TOT patient, make sure to proactively get follow-up blood panels done.

Beyond drawing blood and pulling a serum testosterone panel, there is no other biochemical test which can precisely measure testosterone levels in your body (including salivary testing).

---

[264] https://www.discountedlabs.com/pre-trt-male-hormone-wellness-panel/

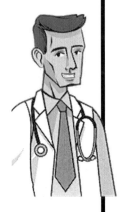

It's important to examine why saliva tests used to measure blood testosterone levels are wholly inaccurate. We're seeing a small number of doctors use a patient's saliva for bio-marker testing, along with a greater number of at-home testing kits[265] that use salivary testing. These at-home kits are often marketed online as a cheap way to determine whether one has testosterone deficiency.

The only hormone that most doctors and researchers agree can accurately be measured by saliva testing is cortisol. Progressive and experienced practitioners DO NOT order saliva testing for testosterone for the following reasons[266]:

- It's limited to immunoassay techniques
- Much less sensitivity
- Less specificity due to cross-reaction sensitivities
- Certain foods, and smoking, alters results
- Adequate volumes are difficult to collect, especially past 40 years of age
- Any artificial stimulation of saliva flow alters concentrations of saliva solutes, including hormones

---

[265] https://livewelltesting.com/all-products/zrt-8-hormone-imbalance-saliva-home-test-kit/

[266] Dr. Crisler Laboratory Lecture 2017 AMMG Fall Conference Tucson AZ

- Certain drugs, such as cholinergic and dopaminergic agonists and antagonists, affect secretion rate of saliva
- Buccal microbleeds will noticeably distort salivary results

In fact, there are a limited number of reasonable studies[267] supporting its use at all. Due to the reasons listed above and the extremely limited research to support salivary testing as a reliable form of blood testosterone measurement, you should avoid any doctor who recommends it.

Also, most health insurance companies do not cover salivary testing for testosterone. If your healthcare provider recommends a salivary test for testosterone or tells you that you have abnormal levels of testosterone based solely on a salivary test, request a SERUM blood test to confirm the findings. Serum testosterone levels are the gold standard when measuring both bioavailable (free) and total testosterone levels.

Evaluating Blood Testosterone

So now that you know what to expect when you get your labs done, take a look at an anonymized blood test from a healthy and fit 33-year-old male with low body fat. Shockingly, he still suffers from low testosterone levels. This is a very common occurrence that's happening right now in doctors' offices all across the world.

---

[267] The use of saliva as a biological fluid in relative bioavailability studies: comparison and correlation with plasma results. Biopharm Drug Dispos. 2010 Nov;31(8-9):476-85. doi: 10.1002/bdd.728. Epub 2010 Sep 27.

Take a look at the Serum and Free Testosterone levels on the chart below.

Ordered Items
CBC With Differential/Platelet; Testosterone,Free and Total; Prostate-Specific Ag, Serum; Venipuncture

TESTS	RESULT	FLAG	UNITS	REFERENCE INTERVAL	LAB
CBC With Differential/Platelet					
WBC	4.5		x10E3/uL	3.4 - 10.8	01
RBC	4.61		x10E6/uL	4.14 - 5.80	01
Hemoglobin	14.6		g/dL	12.6 - 17.7	01
Hematocrit	44.6		%	37.5 - 51.0	01
MCV	97		fL	79 - 97	01
MCH	31.7		pg	26.6 - 33.0	01
MCHC	32.7		g/dL	31.5 - 35.7	01
RDW	13.6		%	12.3 - 15.4	01
Platelets	211		x10E3/uL	150 - 379	01
Neutrophils	50		%		01
Lymphs	39		%		01
Monocytes	7		%		01
Eos	3		%		01
Basos	1		%		01
Neutrophils (Absolute)	2.3		x10E3/uL	1.4 - 7.0	01
Lymphs (Absolute)	1.7		x10E3/uL	0.7 - 3.1	01
Monocytes(Absolute)	0.3		x10E3/uL	0.1 - 0.9	01
Eos (Absolute)	0.1		x10E3/uL	0.0 - 0.4	01
Baso (Absolute)	0.0		x10E3/uL	0.0 - 0.2	01
Immature Granulocytes	0		%		01
Immature Grans (Abs)	0.0		x10E3/uL	0.0 - 0.1	01
Testosterone,Free and Total					
Testosterone, Serum	**332**	**Low**	ng/dL	348 - 1197	01
Comment:					
Adult male reference interval is based on a population of lean males up to 40 years old.					
Free Testosterone(Direct)	**7.4**	**Low**	pg/mL	8.7 - 25.1	02
Prostate-Specific Ag, Serum					
Prostate Specific Ag, Serum	0.9		ng/mL	0.0 - 4.0	01
Roche ECLIA methodology.					
According to the American Urological Association, Serum PSA should					

Date Issued: 10/05/14 1703 ET   **FINAL REPORT**   Page 1 of

Serum testosterone is the total concentration of testosterone in your blood stream and **free testosterone** is the small amount of testosterone floating around that your body can actually use. Usually, only about 2% of the testosterone found in the body at any point in time is 'free/active'[268] and **bioavailable** (i.e. available for your body to use).

Although the normal range varies depending on the lab running the tests, accepted total testosterone levels are generally in a range of around **264–916** nanograms of testosterone per deciliter of blood (ng/dL), according to LabCorp[269]. The scale varies depending on the blood laboratory performing the tests, and the range between labs can be wide[270]. It's worth noting that the "normal" range used to be **348-1197 ng/dL** but was changed in July of 2017 to **264-916 ng/dL** in order to reflect the epidemic of obese men with lower testosterone levels as previously discussed in Chapter 6.

These new numbers are what the labs will say is the normal range for all men of any age. If you're in your 30s or 40s, you won't get an age-specific range because those values remain unclear. This means you could be 35 with testosterone levels that are actually "within range" of a 70-year-old, but low for your age and your body. This is a reminder of why it is imperative for progressive TOT physicians[271] to treat the actual symptoms of their patients instead of solely relying on the findings of a single lab report.

---

[268] 54. Vermeulen A, Verdonck L, Kaufman JM. A critical evaluation of simple methods for the estimation of free testosterone in serum. J Clin Endocrinol Metab. 1999;84:3666–3672.

[269] (It's important to consider these ranges were just lowered on the low and high end by LabCorp in July of 2017, as already discussed in Chapter 6).

[270] Endocrinology: Wide Variability in Laboratory Reference Values for Serum Testosterone. Lazarou, Stephen et al. The Journal of Sexual Medicine. Volume 3, Issue 6, 1085 - 1089.

[271] www.checkmybloodwork.com

The Importance of Sex Hormone Binding Globulin (SHBG)

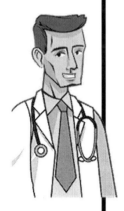

In a healthy young male, 60% of testosterone is attached to Sex Hormone-Binding Globulin (SHBG)[272]. SHBG is primarily produced by the liver and then released into the bloodstream.

Hormones bound to SHBG can't be used by the body, and therefore they lose their anabolic effect. As men age, SHBG levels rise and bind strongly to the testosterone molecule. This lowers the body's absorption of free testosterone[273]. We want to have as much FREE (usable) testosterone available as possible to enjoy the benefits it provides.

SHBG is also an important marker of insulin resistance, and studies have shown that it is an independent predictor of metabolic syndrome and Type 2 diabetes[274]. In aging men, the rise in SHBG and associated maintenance of total testosterone values may mask low levels of free testosterone. For the reasons stated, SHBG is a critical component of proper TOT evaluation. It is imperative for your doctor to be vigilant in tracking your SHBG levels and free testosterone levels while you are on TOT.

---

[272] Hammond GL (2011). "Diverse Roles for Sex Hormone-Binding Globulin in Reproduction." *Biology of Reproduction* 85 (3): 431–441. doi:10.1095/biolreprod.111.092593.ISSN 0006-3363. PMID 21613632.

[273] 56 Diabetes Care. May 2004 v27 i5 p1036(6), "Testosterone and sex hormone-binding globulin predict the metabolic syndrome and diabetes in middle-aged men."

[274] Stanworth RD, Jones TH. Testosterone for the aging male; current evidence and recommended practice . Clinical Interventions in Aging 2008;3(1):25-44.

In short, Sex Hormone Binding Globulin (**SHBG**) is the foundation of proper hormonal evaluation. To further discuss the critical importance of SHBG in hormonal optimization, Jay interviewed Dr. Crisler.

Jay: Let's discuss the role of SHBG in TOT, and even more importantly, the critical need of its proper evaluation during therapy.

Dr. John: Sex Hormone Binding Globulin [SHBG] is the first thing I look at when evaluating labs, and probably spend the most time thinking about. SHBG is unquestionably the centerpiece of every proper sex hormone evaluation. It's what hands out the cards. If your SHBG is high, then it's going to take more testosterone to get over top of it in order to have enough free and bioavailable testosterone left over. Remember, nearly half of all testosterone is very tightly bound to the SHBG that is floating around in our bloodstream, and is therefore unavailable to be used by your body.

Higher SHBG levels would probably rule out our new LD [low dose] clomiphene therapy, because you just can't produce enough testosterone with clomiphene to compensate for all that SHBG. And clomiphene can actually elevate SHBG on its own, by virtue of the fact that half of clomiphene is an estrogen mimicker. However, I have several patients who do very well on clomiphene therapy, even in the face of higher SHBG. So it's important to remember that everybody is biochemically unique. As such, experimentation and close monitoring by a progressive physician is critical.

About 15 years ago, I decided to stop being surprised by anything I see in this field of medicine. If a guy tells me he's happy, he's happy. That's how we roll. It doesn't matter what the numbers are on the laboratory printout. So there's a quantum quality to Interventional Endocrinology in that the numbers on labs, and how the guy feels, often don't match up at all. There is just too much going on here globally with a person's hormonal milieu and its optimization. I like to say that I'm treating a living, breathing human being, not ink on a piece of paper.

But then again, if the SHBG levels are high, you do get some buffering action (i.e. blocking of the effects of high E2) with respect to high estrogen levels, because that estrogen is being eaten up too. But this happens to a lesser degree, because the affinity for SHBG is less with estrogen than testosterone, and therefore SHBG will preferentially grab on to androgens (i.e. testosterone) over estrogens. So as SHBG goes up, it grabs more and more of the testosterone, so your ratio between your testosterone and estrogen will go down. Conversely, if testosterone levels are lower, you can get away with a lower SHBG level because more testosterone will be free and bioavailable for your body to be used.

Jay: Dr. John, what do you think of total testosterone and free (bioavailable) testosterone levels? Does the ratio between the two matter?

Dr John: I don't think much of ratios. Their use is to help describe clinical symptoms. They are not a treatment goal. Without getting any more technical, it helps to remember that this is a bell-shaped world. Again, if a guy comes in at 415 ng/dL and he's happy, he's happy. You also have to keep in mind the variability of hormone levels throughout the day, pre-TOT or after, and especially when clomiphene therapy is added into the mix, which more closely mimics natural testosterone production patterns.

We have known for some time that SHBG has its own actions. There are receptors for it on the outside of the cell. Usually, these hormones have to enter the cell before they do anything. But if SHBG is not already bound to a sex hormone, it can bind to these SHBG receptors [SHBG-R], and then a sex hormone (either androgen or estrogen - the opposite of androgen is estrogen, as estrogen is actually a group of about 40 hormones) binds to the anchored SHBG. This initiates a mechanism inside the cell.

So, obviously, if we have a higher SHBG level, more of this is going on. But, as I just said, both testosterone and estrogen also do this—and that is a can of worms to think about. By the way, no one I have heard of has quantified exactly how much effect this really has.

This might be a good time to point out that the results of the SHBG blood test are a combination of that which is freely floating around, plus that which is bound to hormones in the blood sample. The SHBG bound to its own receptor on the outside of the cell is not measured routinely, yet. I probably should add that the SHBG blood test seems to be a rather tricky test to run properly, and results may vary.

Additionally, it's been shown that many tissues make their own SHBG. There is even a special kind made in the testicles. Maybe these SHBG molecules are produced by the cell to act on itself, or even on its neighbors. But the majority of the SHBG in the body - and what we test for on labs - is made in the liver, then released into the bloodstream. It's basically a protein, as the liver makes many of our proteins.

So now let's consider the other end of the scale, when SHBG is low, or even just lower. The real problem with low SHBG is that sometimes the patient can tolerate almost no levels of estrogen because so much of it will be free. And also, the patient tends to be what we call a "hyper-excreter," which means that he excretes a lot of testosterone into his urine. We normally excrete a certain amount of hormones into the urine. That is why the 24-hour urine test is so useful, as it indicates how much testosterone was made over the entire day.

For guys with lower levels of SHBG, when comparing their blood testosterone to their urine testosterone, the urine will be way higher (within their respective ranges). The kidneys can excrete extra testosterone in the urine, perhaps trying to drive it down, especially after a big spike in serum testosterone. Unfortunately for us, they don't excrete more estrogen in the same way. So guys with lower SHBG (and therefore a higher percentage of free testosterone, or after a concentrated dosage of testosterone) are basically leaving the testosterone in the urine.

Jay: So following this, how does this affect injection therapy for men with lower levels of SHBG?

Dr John: This is EXACTLY why splitting your weekly dose of testosterone cypionate into two shots will leave you feeling better: it's still left in the body, but a lower amount is flushed down the toilet. I've seen this make as much as a 20% difference in well being! It's also why guys with low[er] SHBG levels tend to do less well on transdermal testosterone. The direct infusion from the subdermal capillary bed (i.e. blood vessels in your skin) to the bloodstream, along with more constant changes in testosterone levels (ironic, as being younger and healthier leads to testosterone being more variable) means that more testosterone is lost. This also results in a greater probability of an anxiety issue for those who are predisposed to it. Again, as always, everybody is different.

But this SHBG-R (i.e. SHBG bound to its receptor) may have something to do with why adult male patients who have anxiety issues are more likely to have low (or lower) SHBG levels. I've never seen a study proving that, but have seen it hundreds of times over the years in clinical practice.

We've all read posts from guys on the 'boards' who report that their first dose of testosterone gave them nervousness, anxiety, heart palpitations, and so on. Maybe this SHBG-R action has something to do with that. The answer then is to lower the dose down, somewhere around 50 mg per week for testosterone cypionate as a starting point.

The guys who have lower SHBG levels need multiple smaller doses of testosterone because they're basically peeing it out as soon as it's released from the cypionate ester from shots, or as it's absorbed from a transdermal gel or cream. Therefore, those guys are definitely going to need twice-a-week shots. Whereas guys with higher SHBG levels might be able to get away with once-per-week shots (i.e. a bigger single dose), then they'd be fine for the rest of the week. This can really determine what kind of protocol they're going to do. And of course this is also in combination with their associated lifestyle choices, and how much time they are going to commit to optimizing their health.

And with lower SHBG levels, there will naturally be less of this extracellular (i.e. "outside the cell") mechanism with the SHBG receptors on the cell wall. Again, we don't yet know all that much about that, but we do know it is important.

Jay: Wow, that's some awesome information! Let's stay there. You and I are seeing such a degradation in our environment - there's obviously endocrine disruption everywhere. It's inescapable. The bigger the city, the more endocrine disruption there is. It's just what plays a role in a guy having naturally higher SHBG levels, vereus having lower SHBG levels.

Dr. John: Honestly, if I knew for sure, I'd be manipulating my own levels. My own SHBG levels are now over 90 nmol/mL, and I have no idea why. It could be something I'm taking, or maybe it's something I'm taking after my heart attack, some antioxidant. Either way, I have no idea.

There are probably hundreds of different influences simultaneously pushing SHBG levels up and down. It finds its own level based on all those inputs. We do know that SHBG levels decrease in the presence of androgens like testosterone, insulin (such as seen in Type II diabetics), growth hormone, IGF-1, and prolactin. Estrogen tends to increase SHBG levels, and so can ANY form of Thyroid Replacement Therapy. For those who enjoy the antioxidant properties of green tea, I'd limit it to a couple of cups a day as it's been shown to elevate SHBG levels too.

SHBG levels tend to go up as we age. One problem with this is that testosterone production simultaneously tends to fall. In that case, you have less total testosterone in the body and (due to the increased SHBG levels) even less free testosterone.

The pre-lab instructions I email my patients always directs them to not work out the day before (and the morning before) getting their blood drawn. Not only can a workout increase liver function test results (especially alanine transaminase), it also increases SHBG levels. This could completely change the regimen I put them on.

I should note that caloric restriction can also increase SHBG levels. Strangely, so does liver failure. You can drive SHBG down by taking 50 mg of Danazol per day. But why take - and pay for - an extra medication when we can simply adjust our TOT protocol to compensate? And I have never seen lowering SHBG levels lead to an increase in testosterone levels for any length of time. I've tried it numerous times with labs. That's because, with normal feedback mechanisms in place, the body just lowers Luteinizing Hormone (LH) to compensate and therefore testosterone production is also lowered. You end up right back where you started, except your wallet is lighter. This is known in medicine as "wallet diuresis."

Jay: Yes, many men have dealt with wallet diuresis. So ultimately, what is a progressive physician to do when trying to evaluate SHBG levels for their patient?

Dr John: We must treat SHBG like a cork floating on the top of the water. Wherever it bobs, that's where we play it. We just monitor it regularly. It can change drastically in a month or so, which is about how long it takes to re-establish its new baseline after a change.

And also, no matter what people say, there is a variability in the "stickiness" of SHBG. Sometimes it grabs onto testosterone "harder', other times less. I know this because you see such differences in free testosterone levels (compared to total testosterone) in a lot of these tests. Why would we not have variability in the force of the binding of sex hormones to SHBG? We see such variability in everything else in our body that it only makes logical sense.

The SHBG molecule has two "pockets" where the sex hormones bind. Some claim that one pocket holds an estrogen while the other holds an androgen. If that is true, maybe this variability also has something to do with which kind of hormone binds first, serum concentrations, the strength of the hormone's binding to SHBG (known as "affinity"), or some other factor. I don't know.

But I have also read that SHBG, even with two binding sites for sex hormones, is more likely to bind to a single hormone molecule. This kind of thing is why I remind myself, every day, that we have only begun to scratch the surface of this exciting field of medicine.

This would also be where the relative ratios of testosterone to estrogen, for instance, may come into play. That conversation is beyond the scope of this interview, but it's one of the reasons why I started this talk. I probably spend more time thinking about SHBG than any other topic. By the way, as I already mentioned, androgens have greater affinity for SHBG than estrogens.

And strangely, DHEA binds to SHBG but DHEA-S does not. More things to think about as we administer DHEA sublingually (i.e. under the tongue) through what we call a troche (which is the best way to do it) or by applying it to the skin. As my old pal Dr. Eugene Shippen pointed out, doing so by these routes increases the ratio of DHEA to DHEA-S; something that seems to make a difference.

Hematocrit and Hemoglobin

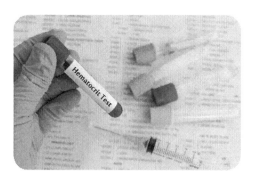

There is a noticeable correlation between high testosterone levels and high hemoglobin (the protein inside red blood cells) levels because testosterone stimulates erythropoietin production, which increases RBC (red blood cell) count and oxygen saturation[275]. This increased production of RBC's is called **erythrocytosis**. Erythrocytosis is the most common adverse reaction to testosterone therapy, occurring in up to 40% of users[276]. Patients using an injectable testosterone delivery system experience higher rates of erythrocytosis than those using transdermal delivery systems or pellets[277].

---

[275] Wang C, Nieschlag E, Swerdloff R, et al. Investigation, treatment and monitoring of late-onset hypogonadism in males: ISA, ISSAM, EAU, EAA and ASA recommendations. Eur J Endocrinol. 2008;159:507–514.

[276] Testosterone induces erythrocytosis via increased erythropoietin and suppressed hepcidin: evidence for a new erythropoietin/hemoglobin set point. Bhasin S4. J Gerontol A Biol Sci Med Sci. 2014 Jun;69(6):725-35. doi: 1093/gerona/glt154. Epub 2013 Oct 24.

[277] Layton JB, Meier CR, Sharpless JL, Stürmer T, Jick SS, Brookhart MA. Comparative safety of testosterone dosage forms. *JAMA internal medicine.* 2015;175(7):1187-1196. doi:10.1001/jamainternmed.2015.1573.

The good news is that this condition is easily treatable through therapeutic phlebotomy.

Work with your physician to monitor your hemoglobin/hematocrit levels[278] to make sure they stay under **20 g/dL (Hemoglobin) / 52-54% blood volume (Hematocrit)**. If they are elevated above these reference ranges, periodically giving blood (via therapeutic phlebotomy) will lower hemoglobin/hematocrit levels and keep them within the reference ranges[279]. Currently, the Endocrine Society Guidelines state that Hematocrit levels over 54% warrant discontinuation of TOT[280]. At the optimal dosage levels of TOT referenced in Chapter 8, however, it is rare to have chronically elevated hematocrit values. With that being said, it is still a crucially important biomarker for you and your physician to stay on top of (and treat where appropriate).

Dr. Neil Rouzier[281] is a well known clinician and respected thought leader in the TOT space. He is very outspoken regarding his belief that many doctors are confused regarding whether testosterone causes polycythemia (a blood thickening disorder that increases the risk of blood clots). He is adamant in his opinion that TOT DOES NOT cause polycythemia, nor does it

[278] Billett HH. Hemoglobin and Hematocrit. In: Walker HK, Hall WD, Hurst JW, editors. Clinical Methods: The History, Physical, and Laboratory Examinations. 3rd edition. Boston: Butterworths; 1990. Chapter 151. Available from: https://www.ncbi.nlm.nih.gov/books/NBK259/

[279] Nieschlag E. Testosterone treatment comes of age: new options for hypogonadal men. Clin Endocrinol (Oxf)2006;65:275–281. [PubMed].

[280] Shalender Bhasin, Glenn R. Cunningham, Frances J. Hayes, Alvin M. Matsumoto, Peter J. Snyder, Ronald S. Swerdloff, Victor M. Montori; Testosterone Therapy in Men with Androgen Deficiency Syndromes: An Endocrine Society Clinical Practice Guideline, *The Journal of Clinical Endocrinology & Metabolism*, Volume 95, Issue 6, 1 June 2010, Pages 2536–2559, https://doi.org/10.1210/jc.2009-2354.

[281] https://www.rejuvinage.com/dr-neal-rouzier

cause an increase in arterial or venous thrombosis. As such, he believes that many physicians are over-phlebotomizing their patients and lowering ferritin levels too far. Ferritin levels are a measure of your iron storage, which should remain above 100 ng/mL. Iron is used for much more than making blood, as it is also important for proper thyroid function. When iron gets too low, so will your RBC count.

Rouzier states that the erythrocytosis which testosterone causes is commonly extrapolated to be just as harmful as polycythemia. This is both an incorrect and inappropriate extrapolation due to a misunderstanding of both erythrocytosis and polycythemia. In spite of the widespread use of phlebotomy to treat erythrocytosis, erythrocytosis is NOT the same thing as polycythemia. Rouzier offers currently conducted studies which demonstrate no harm of physiologic erythrocytosis caused by either testosterone or living at high altitudes, and this elevation of red blood cells does not require treatment (via phlebotomy) in spite of the rest of the world thinking that it does. In fact, he unequivocally states that there is no increased risk for blood clotting when using TOT. Dr. Rouzier has pointed out there is not one single example of TOT causing a blood clot in people who do not have a genetic disease which puts them at risk for blood clots.

Dr. Rob Kominiarek provides a much more concise breakdown of the difference between erythrocytosis and polycythemia in men who are prescribed injectable TOT.

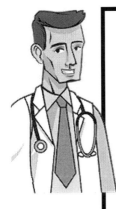

Elevated RBC counts are quite common, and almost universal, in those who take injectable testosterone. It is more prevalent in those individuals taking injectable testosterone (about 67% of users) and less so in those using the creams or gels (about 13%). Most physicians become concerned about this elevation of hemoglobin and hematocrit because they associate and confuse this elevation with a blood condition called polycythemia vera, which causes hyperviscosity and potential for heart attacks and strokes. However, this is definitely not the case with those that use testosterone and have elevated red blood cell counts. The two conditions are commonly confused with each other, and mistakenly many physicians use the medical terms interchangeably and incorrectly, yet they are entirely different in their cause, treatment, and outcomes.

POLYCYTHEMIA: ALL BLOOD CELLS ARE ELEVATED, INCLUDING PLATELETS

Also known as: polycythemia vera, polycythemia rubra vera, erythremia, vaquez disease, osler-vaquez disease. It is a stem cell disorder characterized as a panhyperplastic, malignant, and neoplastic marrow disorder. Its most prominent feature is an elevated absolute red blood cell mass because of uncontrolled red blood cell production.

ERYTHROCYTOSIS: ONLY HEMOGLOBIN AND HEMATOCRIT ARE ELEVATED

The condition that men injecting testosterone often develop is termed erythrocytosis, and is simply an increase in the red blood cells due to the stimulation of hematopoietic growth factors from testosterone therapy. In addition, serum testosterone levels are related to erythrocytosis, rather than erythropoietin (EPO) levels in hypogonadal men. Testosterone was shown to dose-dependently increase the hemoglobin and hematocrit rate (i.e. depending on the dose), but does not show an increase in EPO. Testosterone stimulates erythropoiesis through the production of hematopoietic growth factors and is suggested to act directly on bone marrow, specifically on the polychromatophylic erythroblast. This is a similar phenomenon that occurs when athletes use Epogen or Procrit to raise their blood count to enhance their endurance.

This is also the same process that causes people who live at high altitude to have an increase in red blood cell counts. This is because it is a physiologic yet harmless increase in RBCs alone, not in any other cells or clotting factors.

Treatment is not necessary for anyone with erythrocytosis that lives at high altitude, as it does not cause any problem whatsoever and is quite beneficial. Over 400 million people worldwide live at high altitudes and have higher blood counts, and yet no treatment is necessary, nor is there ever any harm. In fact, athletes train at high altitudes to raise their blood cell counts and increase their exercise endurance at sea level. Why do you think the Olympic Training Center is in Colorado?! It gives them an advantage. Colorado has the

8th lowest mortality rate, the 3rd lowest cardiovascular rate in the US and the longest life expectancy at 87 in the high ski country, all despite having the highest average altitude and hematocrit rates. People with chronic lung problems such as COPD also have high blood counts and we never treat them as the response is physiologic. In other words, the response is normal, expected, and not harmful in order for their blood to carry more oxygen.

Many physicians confuse erythrocytosis with a blood disorder called polycythemia rubra vera. This is a harmful blood condition that causes an increase in clotting, which can lead to strokes and heart attacks. The difference is that erythrocytosis only causes increased red blood cells and no harm. Polycythemia causes an increase in platelets, which causes increased clotting. More importantly, polycythemia is associated with a defect in the blood vessel wall, which stimulates the clotting cascade of thrombosis, in addition to increasing platelet count. These two factors cause an increased risk of blood clots and strokes, thereby requiring treatment by phlebotomy or blood donation to lower blood counts and prevent the complications of polycythemia. Hydroxyurea is also a possible form of therapy. Additionally, a JAK-2 V617F Gene mutation test can simply be performed to make the polycythemia diagnosis.

Polycythemia is classically defined as an increase in red blood cells, white blood cells, platelets, splenomegaly, and clotting disorders. In addition, the literature clearly demonstrates that TOT causes erythrocytosis only, and not polycythemia vera. Testosterone administration has never been associated with any risk of clotting or stroke in any of the studies over the last 40 years. Therefore, the erythrocytosis itself requires no treatment. Nearly all men using injectable testosterone have the same erythrocytosis that people have who live at high altitudes, and they should receive the same treatment as they do, which is nothing! For any physician uncomfortable with this data, refer your patient to a hematologist who will hopefully understand this very well.

Due to working with a number of men over the last 10 years who have experienced elevated values of both hemoglobin and hematocrit, both Jim and Jay also recommend improving body composition[282] (i.e. reducing body fat) and cardiovascular efficiency via regular cardiovascular exercise. In our experience, this often takes care of out-of-range values. The optimal types and forms of cardiovascular exercise are discussed in-depth in Chapter 16.

Liver Health

Unfortunately, many people still believe that elevated testosterone levels may lead to liver toxicity. This assumption is patently false, and it is not based on any real world data.

There have been no documented cases of benign or malignant hepatic (liver) tumors with the use of injectable or transdermal TOT[283]. After nearly 15 years of active physician-guided TOT, we have never once had elevated (i.e. out of range) liver panels. We believe that detrimental lifestyle habits such as over consuming alcohol, eating diets high in saturated fats, and failing to exercise will stress your liver far more than TOT ever could. There is a

---

[282] https://www.amazon.com/exec/obidos/ASIN/B075YB3GQT/trtrev-71-20

[283] Gurakar A, Caraceni P, Fagiuoli S, Van Thiel DH. Androgenic/anabolic steroid-induced intrahepatic cholestasis: a review with four additional case reports. J Okla State Med Assoc.1994;87:399–404. [PubMed].

deeper analysis about the usage of alcohol and its negative effects in relation to TOT in Chapter 13.

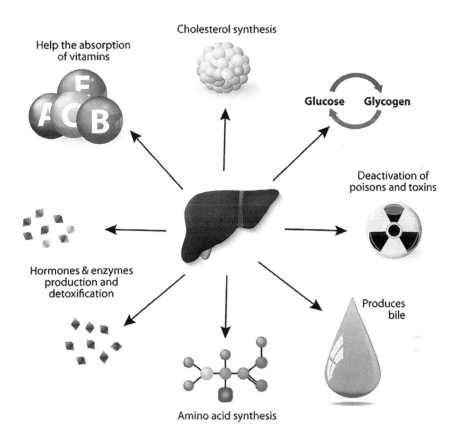

At the same time, those very same detrimental lifestyle habits dramatically increase the prevalence of **Fatty Liver Disease**, more specifically known as **Non-Alcoholic Fatty Liver Disease** (NAFLD). To learn more about NAFLD, read Dr. Aaron Grossman's article *"Why 30% of You Have the Liver of an Alcoholic"*[284]. You

---

[284] http://aarongrossmanmd.com/fattyliverdisease/

do NOT want to be diagnosed with NAFLD. You can avoid this by living an insulin-controlled lifestyle, minimizing alcohol consumption and focusing on your physical fitness. All of these things are discussed in great detail in Chapters 15 and 16.

So whether you're currently living a 'clean' lifestyle or not, you can see the importance of having your liver enzymes measured once a year. If you experience any elevation in your liver enzymes, supplementing with **N-Acetyl-Cysteine (NAC)** and **Tauroursodeoxycholic acid (TUCA)** is an optimal approach to lowering elevated panel readings (We discuss **NAC** more in *Chapter 13: The Critical Role of Nutrition in TOT*).

PSA (Prostate-Specific Antigen) & Prostate Health

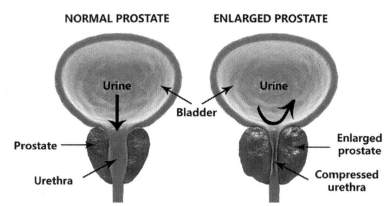

Source: Istock Photo

It's also important to have a yearly PSA screening while on TOT. Even with all the sensationalist claims in the media about how testosterone causes prostate cancer and benign prostatic hyperplasia (BPH), there is no conclusive evidence that TOT increases the risk of either prostate cancer or BPH[285].

The most influential research data on TOT and prostate cancer[286] destroys the long held belief that greater total testosterone concentrations lead to cancer growth. The recent findings[287] of Dr. RM Coward and Professor CC Carson appear to disprove the theory entirely.

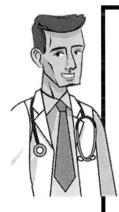

The most plausible explanation for what is observed clinically in the current era of TOT (i.e. low testosterone levels are supposedly the cause of prostate cancer) is supported by the recently re-evaluated saturation model which states that secondary to limited androgen receptor binding sites, prostate cancer growth is sensitive to variations in total testosterone levels that are only below castrate range (supremely low levels). In other words, optimized levels of testosterone are NOT the culprit - low testosterone levels are[288]!

[285]   Marks LS, Mazer NA, Mostaghel E, et al. Effect of testosterone replacement therapy on prostate tissue in men with late-onset hypogonadism: a randomized controlled trial. JAMA. 2006;296:2351-2361.

[286]   Coward RM, Simhan J, Carson CC. Prostate-specific antigen changes and prostate cancer in hypogonadal men treated with testosterone replacement therapy. BJU Int 2009;103:1179–83.

[287]   Ibid.

[288]   Morgentaler A, Traish AM. Shifting the paradigm of testosterone and prostate cancer: the saturation model and the limits of androgen-dependent growth. Eur Urol 2009;55:310–20.

Dr. Coward and Professor Carson go on to say the following:

"Based on all available data, as well as our personal experience, it is our opinion that testosterone deficiency syndrome can be safely treated with TOT after successful prostate cancer treatment."

Although this positive data is more than 6 years old (at the time of writing this), it HAS NOT gotten the exposure it deserves amongst the community of TOT-prescribing physicians. There are still far too many doctors who are unaware of the role of therapeutic testosterone in men with prostate cancer. The Life Extension Foundation (LEF), citing Dr. Abraham Morgentaler in his landmark research article "Destroying the Myth About Testosterone Replacement and Prostate Cancer"[289], offers this positional stance on the risks of testosterone[290] and prostate cancer[291].

Low blood levels of testosterone do not protect against prostate cancer and, indeed, may increase the risk.

High blood levels of testosterone do not increase the risk of prostate cancer.

Treatment with testosterone does not increase the risk of prostate cancer, even among men who are already at high risk for it.

This data represents a revolutionary change with regard to the use of TOT in men with prostate cancer (known as **PCa** in the

---

[289] http://www.lef.org/magazine/2008/12/destroying-the-myth-about-testosterone-replacement-prostate-cancer/page-01.

[290] Morgentaler A. Testosterone and the prostate: is there really a problem? Contemporary Urol. 2006;18:26-33.

[291] Testosterone and prostate safety. Front Horm Res. 2009;37:197-203. doi: 10.1159/000176054.

medical literature) over the last 10–15 years. The long-held belief that raising total testosterone levels necessarily causes rapid and universal growth of existing PCa has not been supported by the existing data[292].

Clearly, the paradigm continues to shift as the medical community's knowledge of the role testosterone plays in men who are survivors of prostate cancer (and currently diagnosed with the disease) improves. This impact of this cannot be understated, and is good cause for celebration for men who suffer from (or have survived) prostate cancer and can now reclaim their vitality with TOT.

Because it has been confirmed that serum androgens (i.e. hormones) like testosterone and DHT are unrelated to prostate cancer risk[293], the most recent research[294] is now focused on the usage of TOT as an actual treatment for prostate cancer[295]. Even though there are presently not enough clinical studies done to draw definitive conclusions, the data sets currently available[296] are highly encouraging. Here are summaries of the most notable ones:

---

[292] Morgentaler A, Conners III WP. Testosterone therapy in men with prostate cancer: literature review, clinical experience, and recommendations. *Asian Journal of Andrology.* 2015;17(2):206-211. doi:10.4103/1008-682X.148067.

[293] Ibid.

[294] Kaplan AL, Hu JC. Use of testosterone replacement therapy in the United States and its effect on subsequent prostate cancer outcomes. Urology. 2013;82:321-326.

[295] Denmeade SR, Isaacs JT. Bipolar androgen therapy: the rationale for rapid cycling of supraphysiologic androgen/ablation in men with castration resistant prostate cancer. Prostate. 2010;70:1600-7.

[296] Atan A, Tuncel A, Yesil S, Balbay D. Serum Testosterone Level, Testosterone Replacement Treatment, and Prostate Cancer. Advances in Urology. 2013;2013:275945. doi:10.1155/2013/275945.

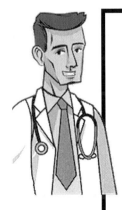

Presenting at the Sexual Medicine Society of North America's 18th Annual Fall Scientific Meeting in October 2017, Ahmad Haider, MD (in private urology practice in Bremerhaven, Germany) and his colleagues studied[297] 400 hypogonadal men (i.e. testosterone level of 350 ng/dL or less) who received 1000 mg of testosterone undecanoate every 3 months for up to 10 years (the TOT group), and 376 hypogonadal men who opted against TOT (the control group). During a median follow-up of 8 years, 9 men in the TOT group (2.3%) were diagnosed with PCa compared with 26 (6.9%) in the control group. The incidence was 31 per 10,000 years in the TOT group, compared with 95 per 10,000 years in the control group.

In March of 2017, Stacy Loeb, MD (of New York University) and her colleagues published the results of a case-control study[298] showing that men who received TOT had a decreased risk of aggressive PCa. In fact, patients who received TOT had significantly increased odds (35%) of more favorable-risk PCa in general and decreased odds (50%) of aggressive PCa when compared with patients not exposed to TOT.

[297] Haider A, Haider K, Saad F. Prostate cancer incidence and severity in testosterone-treated vs. untreated hypogonadal men: Real-life experience from more than 5500 patients years. Poster presented at the Sexual Medicine Society of North America 18th Fall Annual Meeting in San Antonio, October 26-29, 2017. Poster 1.

[298] Loeb S, Folkvaljon Y, Damber JE, et al. Testosterone replacement therapy and risk of favorable and aggressive prostate cancer. *J Clin Oncol* 2017;35:1430-1436.

In a population-based matched cohort study of men aged 66 years or older in Ontario, Canada, Christopher J.D. Wallis, MD, PhD, and his colleagues from the University of Toronto found that TOT recipients in the highest tertile of testosterone exposure had a significantly decreased risk (40%) of a PCa diagnosis when compared with controls (i.e. people not exposed to testosterone)[299].

Finally, in a study[300] published in the *Aging Male* journal (2017;20:125-133), Aksam Yassin, MD (from the Institute of Urology and Andrology, Segeberger Kliniken, Norderstedt, Germany) and his colleagues found that hypogonadal men (i.e. men with low levels of testosterone) who received TOT had a lower rate of PCa upon performing a prostate biopsy when compared with hypogonadal men not exposed to TOT and eugonadal (i.e. normal gonadal functioning) men - 16.7% vs 51.8% vs 37.8%, respectively. They were also less likely to have less severe PCa, as determined by grading and staging.

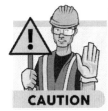

CAUTION

There is a possibility that TOT could cause prostatitis (irritation of the prostate), prostate infection or inflammation over long-term use. While this is not dangerous, it can be troublesome as it causes restricted urine flow and frequent nighttime urination symptoms. For this, there are a number of potential treatments to consider.

[299]   Wallis CJ, Lo K, Lee Y, et al. Survival and cardiovascular events in men treated with testosterone replacement therapy: an intention-to-treat observational cohort study. Lancet Diabetes Endocrinol. 2016;4:498-506.

[300]   Yassin A, Salman M, Talib RA, Yassin DJ. Is there a protective role of testosterone against high-grade prostate cancer? Incidence and severity of prostate cancer in 553 patients who underwent prostate biopsy: a prospective data register. *Aging Male*. 2017;20:125-133.

5-alpha reductase inhibitors such as **Flomax** or **Uroxatral** relax the smooth muscle of the prostate wall and bladder neck, often improving urine flow[301]. A more radical but efficient approach is the use of a laser[302] to eliminate any prostate tissue obstruction[303].

NOTE: PSA levels have been shown to temporarily rise in men at the start of using transdermal testosterone delivery systems, due to their elevation of DHT levels[304]. Normally, once testosterone levels have stabilized, PSA will drop back down into a baseline range.

Recently, the usage of the erectile dysfunction drug **Cialis (Tadalafil)** at 2.5 - 5.0 mg every day has also been approved for the treatment of BPH[305]. Cialis is truly an amazing medication in relation to its improvement of **endothelial dysfunction** (i.e. systemic inflamed state of the inner lining of the endothelium, also known as your blood vessels). To many progressive physicians, endothelial function is the primary indicator of cardiovascular health. We discuss Cialis and its many amazing medical applications in much greater detail in *Chapter 15: Agents of Change.*

---

[301] The efficacy and safety of alpha-1 blockers for benign prostatic hyperplasia: an overview of 15 systematic review-J, Liu, Y, Yang Z, Qin X, Yang K, Mao C. Curr Med Res Opin. 2013 Mar;29(3):279-87.

[302] http://www.amsgreenlight.com/HPS_intro.html

[303] Photoselective laser vaporization of the prostate (PVP) for the treatment of benign prostatic hyperplasia (BPH): 12-month Results from the First United States Multi-center Prospective Trial. J Urol 2004; 172:1404-1408.

[304] Glenn Cunningham, Laurence Belkoff, Gerald Brock, Mitchell Efros, Marc Gittelman, Dario Carrara, Anders Neijber, Masakazu Ando, and Jules Mitchel (2017) EFFICACY AND SAFETY OF A NEW TOPICAL TESTOSTERONE REPLACEMENT GEL THERAPY FOR THE TREATMENT OF MALE HYPOGONADISM. Endocrine Practice: May 2017, Vol. 23, No. 5, pp. 557-565.

[305] Latest pharmacotherapy options for benign prostatic hyperplasia. Expert Opin Pharmacother. 2014 Epub 2014 Aug 28th.

Blood Pressure

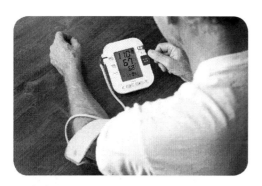

It is always important to monitor blood pressure (BP) as it remains the world's #1 "silent killer" due to its ability to cause strokes and heart attacks. As previously stated throughout the book, men with higher body fat percentages tend to convert testosterone into estrogen (estradiol) more readily. Some men also have genetically higher levels of aromatase enzymes[306], which will also negatively impact testosterone levels through their over-conversion of testosterone to estrogen.

High levels of estrogen can cause water retention, which can lead to high blood pressure. Most studies indicate that clinical TOT dosing protocols rarely affect blood pressure in a negative way. As an important failsafe, you should get your BP measured in the first month of TOT to see whether it has risen higher than your normal baseline BP.

You can purchase a blood pressure cuff[307] over-the-counter and measure your BP at home, or you can choose to visit your local pharmacy to measure your BP regularly. This is in addition to having it monitored with regular office visits to your physician. Be aware of your normal blood pressure values, both systolic (below 120) and diastolic (below 80) or **120/80 mm/Hg** and understand when your readings are elevated beyond normal.

---

[306]   Czajka-Oraniec I, Simpson ER (2010). "Aromatase research and its clinical significance." Endokrynol Pol 61 (1): 126–34. PMID 20205115.

[307]   http://www.amazon.com/exec/obidos/ASIN/B004D9P1A8/trtrevbook-20

Sleep Apnea and TOT

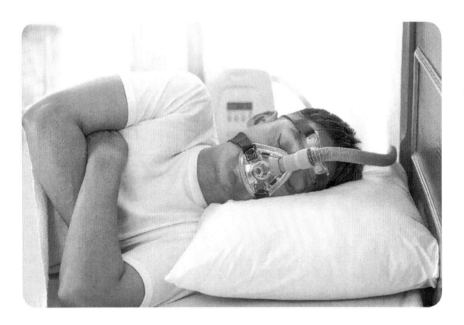

Men of all ages with testosterone deficiency generally don't sleep well. They often sleep less efficiently, enjoy less rapid-eye movement (REM) sleep and wake up more frequently. Recent research into Obstructive Sleep Apnea[308] (OSA) has found a relationship between hormonal health and OSA: Men who sleep poorly also tend to have suboptimal levels of testosterone. Even worse, treating low testosterone levels with various TOT delivery systems may actually aggravate underlying sleep breathing problems or lead to the development of OSA[309].

---

[308] https://www.somnosure.com/obstructive-sleep-apnea-information

[309] The effects of testosterone on ventilatory responses in men with obstructive sleep apnea: a randomised, placebo-controlled trial. Killick R, Wang D, Hoyos CM, Yee BJ, Grunstein RR, Liu PY. J Sleep Res. 2013 Jun; 22(3):331-6.

Unfortunately, the lack of research makes this a difficult topic for us to weigh in on. It is our opinion that the majority of men using TOT with sleep apnea can do so without significant risk. This statement assumes that these men are also reducing body fat, exercising (both resistance and cardiovascular training) and wearing their prescribed treatment apparatus (Cpap mask) as instructed.

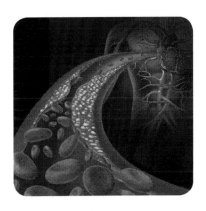

Heart and Vascular Health

One of the biggest myths about TOT is that it increases the risk of cardiovascular events and/or diseases. You may be aware of the many different advertisements (online, print and TV from 2014-2016) about TOT causing heart issues. Those ads claimed that if you've used TOT, you may be entitled to a financial recovery. This is because we live in a very lawyer-controlled society and the attorneys filing the lawsuits are opportunistic, not because of TOT causing heart issues.

Based on the most recent and relevant research on the matter[310] disputing the Testosterone in Older Men (TOM)[311] and Journal of

[310]   Patel P et al. Abstract 1195-376. Zuber A et al. Abstract 1126M-13. Both presented at: American College of Cardiology (ACC) 64th Annual Scientific Session & Expo; March 14-16, 2015; San Diego.

[311]   Basaria S, Davda MN, Travison TG, Ulloor J, Singh R, Bhasin S. Risk Factors Associated With Cardiovascular Events During Testosterone Administration in Older Men With Mobility Limitation. *The Journals of Gerontology Series A: Biological Sciences and Medical Sciences.* 2013;68(2):153-160. doi:10.1093/gerona/gls 138.

the American Medical Association (JAMA)[312] studies in question, there is no evidence to support the statement that 'TOT causes increased risk of heart attacks and strokes' in ***any man under the age of 65***. Both of those studies were inherently flawed as the patient population groups had previously existing heart and mobility issues. In other words, these were not normal, healthy aging men.

In randomized placebo-controlled trials, TOT *does not* increase the incidence of cardiovascular disease or events such as myocardial infarction, stroke, or angina[313]. In fact, most studies show improved survival in men treated with therapeutic testosterone (versus untreated men). Low levels of testosterone are predictive of an increase in coronary artery disease (CAD), cardiovascular disease (CVD), and cancer. Most of the data available provides clear evidence that supplemental testosterone reduces the risk of cardiovascular events in otherwise healthy and normal men[314,315].

---

[312] Vigen R, O'Donnell, Baron AE, et al. Association of testosterone therapy with mortality, myocardial infarction, and stroke in men with low testosterone levels. *JAMA* 2013; 310:1829-1835.Cappola AR. Testosterone therapy and risk of cardiovascular disease in men. *JAMA* 2013; 310:1805-1806.

[313] Testosterone and cardiovascular risk in men: a systematic review and meta-analysis of randomized placebo-controlled trials. Mayo Clin Proc. 2007;82(1):11-13. [PubMed]

[314] Oskui PM, French WJ, Herring MJ, Mayeda GS, Burstein S, Kloner RA. Testosterone and the Cardiovascular System: A Comprehensive Review of the Clinical Literature. Journal of the American Heart Association: Cardiovascular and Cerebrovascular Disease. 2013;2(6):e000272. doi:10.1161/JAHA.113.000272.

[315] Goodale, T., Sadhu, A., Petak, S., & Robbins, R. (2017). Testosterone and the Heart. Methodist DeBakey Cardiovascular Journal, 13(2), 68–72. http://doi.org/10.14797/mdcj-13-2-68.

Dr. Abraham Morgentaler, in his conclusion from the landmark 2015 Mayo Clinic study[316] *"Testosterone Therapy and Cardiovascular Risk: Advances and Controversies,"* couldn't have put it any more clearly (T = testosterone):

> *"In summary, we find no scientific basis for the suggestion that T therapy increases CV risk.*
>
> *In fact, as of this date, we are unaware of any compelling evidence that T therapy is associated with increased cardiovascular risk.*
>
> *On the contrary, the weight of evidence accumulated by researchers around the world over several decades clearly indicates that higher levels of T are associated with amelioration (improvement) of cardiovascular risk factors and reduced risk of mortality."*

One other biomarker to be aware of as a potential indicator of cardiovascular risk is **homocysteine**. Homocysteine is an amino acid that, when present in high concentrations, has been linked to an increased risk of heart attacks and strokes[317].

Observed normal levels of homocysteine are between 4.4 and 10.8 micromoles per liter of blood (mmol/L). Elevated **homocysteine levels** are thought to contribute to plaque formation by damaging arterial walls. If you have high levels of homocysteine, you may be at a greater risk for cardiovascular disease. For those faced with this issue, we recommend the complete

---

[316] Testosterone Therapy and Cardiovascular Risk: Advances and Controversies. Morgentaler, Abraham et al. Mayo Clinic Proceedings, Volume 90, Issue 2, 224 - 251.

[317] Correlation Between Hyperhomocysteinemia and Outcomes of Patients With Acute Myocardial Infarction.Am J Ther. 2014 Nov 17.

elimination of alcohol consumption, reduction of body fat and supplementation with *B Complex*[318] and *Folic Acid*[319] (all available over the counter) as excellent remedies to reduce elevated levels. The Life Extension Foundation has an excellent article on supplements to use to reduce homocysteine[320]. Additionally, an always prudent form of vascular protection (especially as we get older) is investing in regular and consistent endurance exercise. We discuss this much more in Chapter 16.

Lipids (Blood Fats) and Cholesterol Health

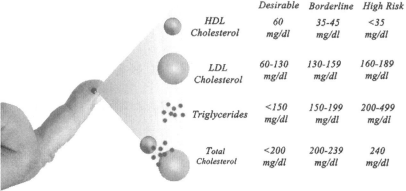

Lipid Profile

	Desirable	Borderline	High Risk
HDL Cholesterol	60 mg/dl	35-45 mg/dl	<35 mg/dl
LDL Cholesterol	60-130 mg/dl	130-159 mg/dl	160-189 mg/dl
Triglycerides	<150 mg/dl	150-199 mg/dl	200-499 mg/dl
Total Cholesterol	<200 mg/dl	200-239 mg/dl	240 mg/dl

TOT, in clinical dosages, has been shown to have little to no effect on plasma HDL (high-density lipoprotein, also known as

---

[318]   http://trtrev.com/b-complex

[319]   http://trtrev.com/folic-acid

[320]   http://www.lifeextension.com/Protocols/Heart-Circulatory/Homocysteine-Reduction/Page-03

the 'good' cholesterol) levels in multiple studies[321]. TOT has also been shown to decrease triglycerides and LDL (low-density lipoprotein, also known as the 'bad' cholesterol) levels[322]. For much more information on the roles that HDL and LDL cholesterol levels play in your health, read *HDL (Good), LDL (Bad) Cholesterol and Triglycerides*[323]. This is why it's important to have your LDL and HDL levels, along with your triglycerides, checked while in a fasted state (i.e. not having consumed any food for at least 10 hours prior) at least once a year as part of your general blood work.

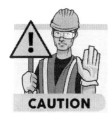

CAUTION

Some physicians believe that testosterone can negatively impact cholesterol levels, but there is no relevant data[324] to support this belief. The incorrect assumption often made is that excessively high (i.e. supraphysiologic) doses of testosterone and other synthetics (such as anabolic steroids) used by athletes and professional/recreational bodybuilders leads to reductions in **HDL** and increases in **LDL**. There is no conclusive peer-accepted research to support these beliefs—only the

321   Pharmacokinetics, efficacy, and safety of a permeation enhanced testosterone transdermal system in comparison with bi-weekly injections of testosterone enanthate for the treatment of hypogonadal men. J Clin Endocrinol Metab. 1999;84:3469–3478. [PubMed]

322   Chrysohoou C, Panagiotakos D, Pitsavos C, et al. Low Total Testosterone Levels are Associated With the Metabolic Syndrome in Elderly Men: The Role of Body Weight, Lipids, Insulin Resistance, and Inflammation; The Ikaria Study. The Review of Diabetic Studies : RDS 2013;10(1):27-38. doi:10.1900/RDS.2013.10.27.

323   http://bit.ly/2xpyO2k

324   Rubinow KB, Vaisar T, Tang C, Matsumoto AM, Heinecke JW, Page ST. Testosterone replacement in hypogonadal men alters the HDL proteome but not HDL cholesterol efflux capacity. *Journal of Lipid Research*. 2012;53(7):1376-1383. doi:10.1194/jlr.P026005.

perception that supraphysiologic dosages will elevate values in these population groups. Remember, this book talks about using THERAPEUTIC doses of testosterone to optimize your levels.

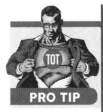

PRO TIP

Improving your cholesterol can be accomplished by modifying your diet and exercise. Proper eating and regular exercise should be the established foundation, prior to beginning any kind of statin medications. Chronically poor levels of cholesterol can increase your risk of cardiovascular disease, and sometimes medical intervention is needed to help restore a proper lipid balance.

Here are four OTC supplements which are known to improve your lipid profile, and each nutrient works differently: (1) Omega-3 Fish Oil[325] (2) Citrus Bergamot[326] (3) Red Yeast Rice[327] (4) Krill Oil[328].

---

[325] Yates A, Norwig J, Maroon JC, et al. Evaluation of Lipid Profiles and the Use of Omega-3 Essential Fatty Acid in Professional Football Players. *Sports Health*. 2009;1(1):21-30. doi:10.1177/1941738108326978.

[326] http://realcitrusbergamot.com/clinical-studies/

[327] Diane Peng; Amy Fong; Amanda van Pelt. The Effects of Red Yeast Rice Supplementation on Cholesterol Levels in Adults. AJN, American Journal of Nursing. 117(8):46–54, AUG 2017.

[328] Berge RK, Ramsvik MS, Bohov P, et al. Krill oil reduces plasma triacylglycerol level and improves related lipoprotein particle concentration, fatty acid composition and redox status in healthy young adults - a pilot study. *Lipids in Health and Disease*. 2015;14:163. doi:10.1186/s12944-015-0162-7.

Doctors sometimes prescribe Omega-3 as a blood thinner[329] for patients who have high RBC counts, as it has been found to be more effective than Aspirin for this purpose. This can be especially beneficial to men on TOT as testosterone can potentially thicken the blood via erythrocytosis (as previously discussed earlier in this chapter).

Statin drugs are commonly prescribed for patients who have high cholesterol levels. According to the CDC[330], 28% of men and women over the age of 40 are using statins in the United States. Statins have been found to significantly lower Co-Q10 levels, however, so it is essential for statin users to supplement with Co-Q10 to help restore depleted levels. We discuss the importance of supplementing with Co-Q10 in Chapter 13.

Pregnenolone

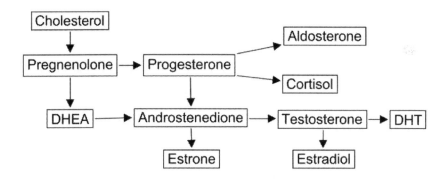

---

329 2017 Jan/Feb;24(1):15-18. doi: 10.1097/JTN. Omega-3 Fatty Acid Supplementation and Warfarin: A Lethal Combination in Traumatic Brain Injury.

330 https://www.nbcnews.com/health/heart-health/too-many-people-stop-their-lifesaving-statins-doctors-say-n789686

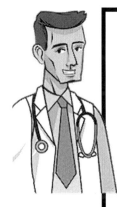

Pregnenolone is a hormone that very few doctors and their patients are familiar with. Restoring pregnenolone to optimal levels is critically important for overall hormonal health, especially for those undergoing TOT/HRT.

Pregnenolone sits at the pinnacle of 2 important hormone cascades, which have been found to influence neuronal functioning and the quality of aging. Pregnenolone plays an important role in memory, cognition, alertness, and mood. It is produced in three main organs (the brain, gonads and adrenal glands), which not only makes pregnenolone a neuroactive steroid, but a neurosteroid as well.

Notably, all other steroids including progesterone, cortisol, cortisone, aldosterone, DHEA, testosterone, dihydrotestosterone, estradiol, estrone, and allopregnenolone are all derived from this important hormone. Pregnenolone is the precursor to these other steroid hormones, and the main steroid hormone produced from cholesterol[331].

When you shut down **LH** and **FSH** because of therapeutic (i.e. exogenous) testosterone, you interfere with the initiation of steroidogenesis, the transport of cholesterol into the inner mitochondrial membrane, and the expression of the P450 cholesterol side chain cleavage

331 Neurosteroids and potential therapeutics: Focus on pregnenolone. Author links open overlay panel Monique Valléeab. INSERM U862, Neurocentre Magendie, Pathophysiology of Addiction, Bordeaux F33077, France Université de Bordeaux, Bordeaux F33077, France. Received 28 May 2015.

enzyme which catalyzes the conversion of cholesterol into pregnenolone. A word of caution: If you have a history of seizures, consult with your physician first as pregnenolone and its metabolite pregnenolone sulfate have been associated with increased seizure activity[332].

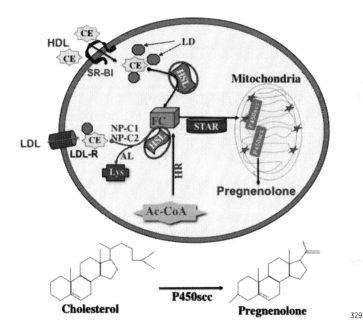

329

Pregnenolone is neuroprotective, enhances learning and memory[333] and increases the amount of deep sleep one gets[334]. Pregnenolone is also important for proper brain development,

---

[332] https://www.ncbi.nlm.nih.gov/pmc/articles/PMC4707056/figure/F1/

[333] Marx, C.E., Lee, J., Subramaniam, M. et al. Psychopharmacology (2014) 231: 3647. https://doi.org/10.1007/s00213-014-3673-4.

[334] Steiger A1, Trachsel L, Guldner J, Neurosteroid pregnenolone induces sleep-EEG changes in man compatible with inverse agonistic GABAA-receptor modulation.

cognition and mood. In fact, the most obvious sign of deficient pregnenolone levels is a loss of memory (or a decrease in cognition). These dramatic effects on the brain are why pregnenolone is known as a neurosteroid.

Our genetics can affect how pregnenolone works in our bodies. For example, a variation (rs6971) in the gene TSPO can influence internal production of pregnenolone (i.e. decrease production), meaning you may need to take a supplement to elevate pregnenolone levels to normal[335].

The **optimal serum levels for pregnenolone are between 80-180 ng/dL for men**[336]. If your pregnenolone is below those levels, speak to your doctor about potentially beginning a course of pregnenolone supplementation. If your levels are around that number, you may not need to take pregnenolone. **Dr. Rob Kominiarek** specifically states that in his practice, supplementing with pregnenolone is purely dependant on symptoms of a deficiency (loss of memory, decrease in cognition, etc.) rather than just lab measurement numbers. He also tests a patient's pregnenolone levels prior to starting TOT, 3 months after starting and also 12 months later.

The **typical dose of pregnenolone is between 30-60 mg per day**, usually taken at night along with DHEA. The pills are meant to be taken on an empty stomach, or you can use

---

[335] Barbara Costa, Stefano Pini, Pamela Gabelloni, Eleonora Da Pozzo, Marianna Abelli, Lisa Lari, Matteo Preve, Antonio Lucacchini, Giovanni B. Cassano, Claudia Martini; The Spontaneous Ala147Thr Amino Acid Substitution within the Translocator Protein Influences Pregnenolone Production in Lymphomonocytes of Healthy Individuals. *Endocrinology*, Volume 150, Issue 12, 1 December 2009, Pages 5438–5445.

[336] 1. Akwa Y, Young J, Kabbadj K, et al. Neurosteroids: biosynthesis, metabolism and function of pregnenolone and dehydroepiandrosterone in the brain. J Steroid Biochem Mol Biol. 1991;40(1-3):71-81.

a cream (i.e. transdermal application). Pregnenolone can be purchased over the counter (OTC) as a pill form (micronized slow release is the best for oral pills), or as a sublingual (under the tongue) treatment, in addition to transdermal applications. There is also the option of adding hCG to your TOT to help keep your pregnenolone, progesterone, and DHEA levels consistent. hCG activates the enzyme that turns cholesterol into pregnenolone. This ensures that your body gets the pregnenolone it needs to produce all the other important hormones.

Due to the potential of negative side effects (i.e. downstream conversion of pregnenolone to progesterone, and potentially estrogen), please ensure you test for pregnenolone before haphazardly supplementing with it. It is important (as with all forms of hormone supplements and medications) to assess whether there is a clinical need (i.e. a measured deficiency via lab work, and more importantly, the presence of SYMPTOMS) before one starts taking pregnenolone.

To find out much more about pregnenolone, we highly encourage you to read two thoroughly researched articles about pregnenolone: SelfHacked's "Top 11 Scientific Health Benefits of Pregnenolone (including side effects)"[337], and Nelson Vergel's "Pregnenolone - What You Need to Know"[338].

---

[337] https://selfhacked.com/blog/top-11-scientific-health-benefits-pregnenolone-including-drawbacks/

[338] https://www.discountedlabs.com/blog/post/pregnenolone-what-you-need-to-know/

Testicular Shrinkage, Low Sperm Count and HPTA/HPGA Dysfunction

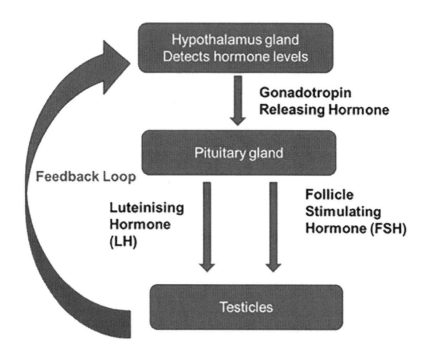

TOT inhibits the body's own (i.e. endogenous) testosterone production through negative feedback inhibition of **LH** levels. This results in suppression of **FSH** levels, which leads to suppression of sperm production (a.k.a. *azoospermia*).

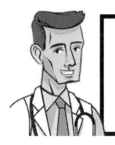

When exogenous (i.e. supplemental) testosterone is used, a cascade of biochemical actions take place. Your hypothalamus, the master gland in your brain, secretes **GnRH** (*Gonadotropin Releasing Hormone*) and this causes your pituitary gland to secrete **LH** and **FSH**. The increase in these hormones causes the testes to stimulate the Leydig cells to produce testosterone (via conversion of cholesterol). The produced testosterone then has the ability to undergo various metabolic processes that will inhibit **GnRH**, which in turn inhibits the secretion of **LH** and **FSH**, bringing a halt to endogenous (i.e. 'natural') testosterone production. This is referred to as the *negative feedback loop*. Once testosterone has stopped being produced, it no longer sends this negative signal, and GnRH eventually starts doing its job again (i.e. it returns to baseline levels). This is how homeostasis (balance) is maintained in the human body.

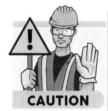

CAUTION

All men should be fully aware that using lifelong TOT protocols can (and most likely WILL) reduce the size of your testes, *potentially* interfere with your fertility, and suppress your **HPTA** (*Hypothalamic-Pituitary-Testicular Axis*). This means your natural testosterone production will be impaired, and potentially shut down altogether. While this might seem worrisome, especially to men who have little understanding of testosterone and fertility, we'll cover why this isn't something you need to worry about throughout this section (provided you work with a progressive and experienced TOT physician).

The question that might be racing through your mind right now will be answered: **Yes, you can still have kids while using therapeutic testosterone.** However, you MUST pay close attention to this chapter to best understand how to maintain your fertility through TOT.

To give you a deep insight into this subject, we interviewed **Dr. Merrill Matschke**, a Board Certified Urologist who is fellowship trained in Male Reproductive Medicine and Surgery. He is one of the most foremost and progressive physicians in his field.

Jay: How has the worldwide decline of testosterone and sperm levels affected the population of male patients who are using TOT?

Dr. Matschke: This has resulted in a huge increase in the use of exogenous testosterone replacement therapy (TRT), which I see you are now calling TOT. I really like that term. Between 2000 and 2011, there was a 12-fold increase in the sales of testosterone medications, with 12% of all therapeutic testosterone prescriptions being used by men less than 39 years of age.

The growing number of men of reproductive age drawn to TOT for relieving the associated symptoms of low testosterone levels (Types 1 and 2) has lead to a new appreciation for the negative impact that exogenous testosterone use has on a man's potential for fertility. Understanding the physiology of the hypothalamic-pituitary-gonadal (HPG) axis allows us to explain not only why this occurs, but also how to optimize and protect fertility while optimizing testosterone levels as well.

Jay: As you know, it gets tough trying to discuss the HPG/HPTA axis for those who aren't medically trained. I'm confident most readers have a good working knowledge of these acronyms, but let's be cognizant of this as we further discuss male fertility.

Dr. Matschke: Understood. Believe me, I have had these conversations daily for more than a decade now. Before diving into the HPG axis, we must recognize that the field of andrology and male infertility is relatively young, and there is still much we do not fully comprehend. All men are NOT created equal and no single cookie-cutter approach will work for everyone. Only an individualized approach will allow for the best outcomes possible. This requires finding a progressive physician with a deep working knowledge of both TOT and its impact on spermatogenesis (i.e. sperm production). Working together with the right physician can allow you to enjoy the many benefits of optimal testosterone levels while preserving fertility in all but a few instances.

Jay: Many readers should remember our discussion of the HPG Axis from Chapter 5. If not, this is a good review.

Dr. Matschke: The HPG axis (Figure 1) is the driving force for the production of testosterone (T), and is regulated via a negative feedback loop with both testosterone and estradiol (E2) acting as the mediators of that feedback control. Both T and E2 have an inhibitory effect at the hypothalamus and pituitary level. As T and E2 levels increase, there is a decrease in the release of GnRH, followed by a decrease in the release of LH and FSH and less drive through the system to stimulate T production from the Leydig cells. TOT obviously introduces increased levels of T into the system and the brain (the hypothalamus and pituitary in particular) sees this increase in T and shuts down the drive to produce T from the Leydig cells in the testes.

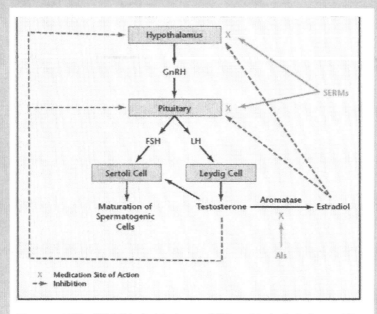

AI, aromatase inhibitor; FSH, follicle-stimulating hormone; GnRH, gonadotropin-releasing hormone; LH, luteinizing hormone; SERM, selective estrogen receptor modulator.

Figure 1[339]

---

[339] Rambhatla A, Mills J, Rajfer J. The Role of Estrogen Modulators in Male Hypogonadism and Infertility. Rev Urol. 2016; 18(2): 66-72.

With this knowledge of the HPG axis, it is easy to see how TOT will inevitably result in shutdown of natural T production at the level of the Leydig cells, and result in the plummeting of intratesticular testosterone (ITT) levels. Normally, ITT levels are 50-100x higher than serum T levels and these high ITT levels are required for normal sperm production. As ITT levels drop, a man's sperm count decreases rapidly.

Jay: This is fascinating intel, Dr. Matschke. It's rare to hear somebody explain the differences between ITT levels and serum T levels.

Dr. Matschke: No problem, Jay. I live to discuss this type of stuff with my patients. Multiple scientific trials using various forms of TOT have shown sperm counts drop below 1 million within 3.5 months of being on TOT, and many of these men end up being azoospermic. It is precisely this effect on ITT levels that drives the major negative effect of TOT on male fertility. All strategies to mitigate this negative effect work by attempting to maintain crucially high ITT levels.

We have two main players in our arsenal to preserve ITT, and thus normal sperm production in the face of using TOT. One is hCG (human chorionic gonadotropin), which literally replaces the Luteinizing Hormone (LH) that is normally produced by the pituitary. hCG is a near perfect mimic of LH, and by injecting it subcutaneously (i.e. into the skin), you can counteract the reduced LH secretion from the pituitary that occurs in response to

TOT. The hCG will directly stimulate the Leydig cells to continue testosterone production, thus maintaining high ITT levels and driving sperm production.

In many men (up to 70%), this is all that is required to maintain spermatogenesis. In others, however, hCG alone is not sufficient to recover or maintain normal spermatogenesis. In these men, Follicle Stimulating Hormone (FSH) and hCG are both needed to optimize the environment in the testis for quality sperm production.

This need for FSH can be met via SERMs (Selective Estrogen Receptor Modulators) or HMG (Human Menopausal Gonadotropin)/recombinant FSH. HMG and FSH can be difficult and expensive to obtain, whereas the SERMs are usually more readily available in oral formulations.

The more commonly used SERMs are Clomid and Tamoxifen. They act by inhibiting E2 feedback in both the hypothalamus and pituitary. Thus, their effect is to drive the release of GnRH from the hypothalamus and subsequently the release of BOTH LH and FSH from the pituitary. Therefore, the added benefit of SERMs over using HCG alone is that you also get the release of FSH. This will help men who need both LH and FSH to drive optimal sperm production.

Jay: What are your thoughts on Aromatase Inhibitor (AI) medications to maintain fertility in a similar vein?

Dr. Matschke: AIs can also serve an important role in some men. Recall that these medications will prevent the conversion of testosterone into estradiol within the peripheral tissues. This reduction in E2 will lead to less negative feedback inhibition of the HPG axis, and help to drive the production of both LH and FSH from the pituitary. By manipulating these various actors within the HPG axis, we can keep the drive within the system to maintain ITT levels. Keeping ITT levels high will maintain sperm production, even in the presence of TOT.

Jay: Again, it's fascinating to get this information into the book. Thanks, doctor!

Dr. Matschke: You and your readers are quite welcome. Honestly, the more men who read this book and become informed, the easier my job gets. So how do we put all this info together? First, it is absolutely essential to get a baseline evaluation of one's semen. We must know what the individual's starting point is with regard to both their HPG hormone profile and their semen analysis before we begin any kind of hormone manipulation.

One may have significant abnormalities at baseline that would require a different approach altogether. If TOT is to be contemplated, a thorough and thoughtful conversation must be had between the patient and provider regarding the potentially negative effect of TOT on fertility.

While we have avenues and tools to mitigate this risk (and many times completely remove it), there is always a small risk of experiencing a negative effect on fertility. By taking a proactive approach with an up-front evaluation, along with ongoing and regular follow-up studies for both hormones and semen analyses, it is certainly possible to watch for any signs of undesired changes early on and change course when necessary. This constant evaluation and re-evaluation is the key to optimization, given that each man's response is unique.

Once a man's baseline fertility status is established, if there exists a need for testosterone support, then the safest way of achieving that in a young man is to utilize either Clomid or hCG monotherapy. This can be done as long as his low testosterone levels are not due to primary hypogonadism (Type 1).

Jay: What would be the typical doses of monotherapy for both clomid and hCG?

Dr. Matschke: Typical doses would be Clomid 12.5 mg daily or 25-50 mg EOD (every other day). As for hCG, 500-1500 units taken 3 times a week works best. Many men will see good improvements in testosterone levels and a reduction of negative symptoms with either HCG or clomid, but some men will still complain of inadequate improvement in their hypogonadal symptoms.

Dr. Lipshultz and his colleagues at Baylor convincingly showed us that we can give exogenous TOT (delivered topically or intramuscularly) alongside 500 units of hCG taken 3 times a week (subcutaneously) and still maintain optimal semen parameters[340]. This same level

340 J Urol. 2013 Feb;189(2):647-50. doi: 10.1016/j.juro.2012.09.043. Epub 2012 Dec 20.

of spermatogenesis can also be achieved by using 25-50 mg of clomid EOD.

Again, these approaches cannot be applied in a cookie-cutter fashion, and it is strongly recommended to obtain a follow up semen analysis about 3 months after initiating TOT to confirm stability. Furthermore, it would be prudent to obtain periodic semen analyses 1-2 times per year, even if the initial 3-month semen analysis was stable. Lastly, the ultimate insurance policy would be to freeze a patient's sperm, prior to initiating any kind of TOT. This allows the physician and the patient to be prepared for the rare worst-case scenario of permanent azoospermia.

It cannot be stressed enough that a willing and enlightened medical provider can help carefully preserve, protect, and optimize fertility in a younger man who chooses to optimize his testosterone levels. Working together, along with having close and focused follow-ups, is essential for success.

There are highly effective medications one can use to maintain fertility while using TOT. The ones primarily used are *human chorionic gonadotropin* (**hCG**), *clomiphene citrate* (**clomid**) and *human menopausal gonadotrophin* (**hMG**). Each of these three, when administered by an experienced progressive physician, will restore natural testosterone production and ultimately lead to normal reproductive and sexual function[341].

---

[341] Preserving fertility in the hypogonadal patient: an update. Asian J Androl. 2014 Oct 3. doi: 10.4103/1008-682X.142772. [Epub ahead of print]

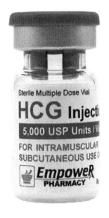

There are numerous accepted dosing protocols when using **hCG**. The protocol being used will vary, based on the experience of the prescribing doctor and their patients subjective responses to treatment. The physician also needs to take into consideration whether or not the patient's diagnosis is Type 1 or Type 2 Hypogonadism when contemplating hCG injection protocols. There are a number of hCG injection protocols that appear more commonly and are based on testosterone injection frequency and/or the use of a cream or gel.

hCG has been clinically proven to restore fertility in men when used concomitantly in men undergoing TOT[342,343]. This can be done intermittently (2-5 days in a row) or regularly (i.e. daily) at a dosage of ***100-500 IU per injection*** (***one injection per day***) by injecting subcutaneously into the fat tissue of your lower stomach, or the fat pad of your outer glute with an insulin syringe. This will provide your testicles with an increase in size, or fullness. We would like to point out that the dosage is purely dependent on the individual's tolerance of hCG. We believe it's always best to practice the minimum effective dose (MED) principle with regard to any medications that may interfere with the HPTA.

Some men psychologically need this cosmetic effect of 'full' testicles to feel normal. The "Dr. Crisler Method" of **hCG**

---

342   Ramasamy R, Stahl PJ, Schlegel PN. Medical therapy for spermatogenic failure. Asian Journal of Andrology 2012;14(1):57-60. doi:10.1038/aja.2011.63.

343   Ramasamy R, Armstrong JM, Lipshultz LI. Preserving fertility in the hypogonadal patient: an update. Asian Journal of Andrology. 2015;17(2):197-200. doi:10.4103/1008-682X.142772.

involves injecting **hCG** the last two days leading up to a once-a-week testosterone injection protocol (Example: If you inject your testosterone on Saturday, you would inject your hCG on Thursday and Friday). Alternatively, if you are injecting testosterone twice a week, inject hCG on the day before each testosterone injection[344]. There are numerous men who use hCG concomitantly with their testosterone delivery system as they believe it is necessary for overall health and wellbeing. For an excellent article covering much of the science as to why hCG can potentially improve health and wellbeing, read Gene Devine and Nelson Vergel's article *Human Chorionic Gonadotropin, Pregnenolone and DHEA*[345].

Monitor your blood work when you're on **hCG** because it *CAN* elevate estradiol (E2) levels, potentially causing estrogenic side effects in men with higher body fat percentages and higher genetic production of aromatase (acne, water retention, moodiness, sore nipples etc.). As previously discussed, aromatase is the enzyme responsible for converting testosterone into estrogen. We offer our personal usage insights on the usage of **hCG** later in the FAQ section of this book.

For those of you wishing to retain your fertility, we offer a very evidence-based protocol. **hMG** is a potent female fertility medication which also increases sperm count and stimulates sperm motility in men[346]. **hMG** is stronger than **hCG** because it

---

[344] Testosterone Replacement Therapy-A Recipe for Success-Dr. Crisler pg.73 Milestones Publishing (March 13, 2015).

[345] https://www.testosteronewisdom.com/hcg/human-chorionic-gonadotropin-pregnenolone-and-dhea/

[346] Hwang K, Walters RC, Lipshultz LI. Contemporary concepts in the evaluation and management of male infertility. Nature reviews. Urology 2011;8(2):86-94. doi:10.1038/nrurol.2010.230.

mimics the effects of both **LH** and **FSH**. It also binds to receptors in the testicles that **hCG** alone cannot bind to[347].

We have consulted with men who were on TOT for more than a decade without using any fertility medications at the same time, yet after starting a **protocol of hMG in combination with hCG**[348], they got their wives or girlfriends pregnant in under 90 days.

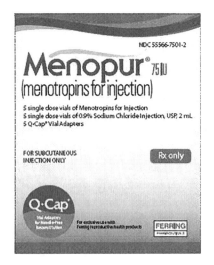

For any of you utilizing TOT and struggling to father children by using hCG or Clomid alone, bring this book to your physician as a starting place for a conversation. For an excellent and highly effective dosing strategy using *hCG* and *hMG* in combination with one another, read this article about understanding infertility treatment[349]. In combination with one another and due to hMG's stronger binding affinity to the receptors in the testicles, sperm motility

---

[347] Rate, extent, and modifiers of spermatogenic recovery after hormonal male contraception: an integrated analysis. Lancet. 2006 Apr 29;367(9520):1412-20.

[348] Ley SB, Leonard JM. Male hypogonadotropic hypogonadism: factors influencing response to human chorionic gonadotropin and human menopausal gonadotropin, including prior exogenous androgens. J Clin Endocrinol Metab. 1985 Oct;61(4):746-52. MID:3928676

[349] http://www.webmd.com/infertility-and-reproduction/gonadotropin-treatment-for-infertility

is enhanced and fertility improved[350]. Sometimes, men have trouble getting a prescription for fertility medications like hCG/hMG. If that's the situation you're in, we recommend consulting with an experienced doctor[351].

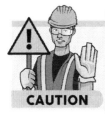

CAUTION

Some physicians will prescribe **hCG** and/or **clomid monotherapy** alone as a form of TOT (i.e. without using supplemental testosterone). The premise of this protocol is to stimulate the testicles with either **hCG** or **clomid** so they increase testosterone production. The success rate of this approach is highly dependant on how sensitive the Leydig cells are in the individual patient's testicles. This is the PREFERRED strategy for younger men (30-50 years old) desiring to maintain fertility and higher sperm count, while also *ATTEMPTING* to AVOID DISRUPTING their natural testosterone production.

---

[350] Mao J-F, Liu Z-X, Nie M, et al. Pulsatile gonadotropin-releasing hormone therapy is associated with earlier spermatogenesis compared to combined gonadotropin therapy in patients with congenital hypogonadotropic hypogonadism. *Asian Journal of Andrology.* 2017;19(6):680-685. doi:10.4103/1008-682X.193568.

[351] www.betterlifecarolinas.com

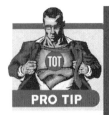

PRO TIP

For any man interested in guaranteeing the retention of their fertility when he has the means to afford it, consider getting a **measured sperm count** in order to understand your baseline values before undergoing TOT. It would also be prudent, as a precautionary measure, to have your sperm frozen to be used at a later date. The risks of becoming permanently infertile from TOT are supremely low when you take the precautionary measures of intermittently using **hCG** or **hMG**. However, freezing your sperm would be the ultimate preventative solution in a worst-case scenario.

The Myth of Penis Shrinking

It's also important to mention the societal myth about testosterone causing a man's penis to shrink. Quite honestly, it's nonsense. If anything, the penis can increase in size and/or girth because testosterone increases nitric oxide production, which stimulates nitrogen retention and enhances blood flow. All of this leads harder and thicker erections[352]. In fact, increasing nitric oxide is one of the things that Cialis does to give men stronger erections. We talk about Cialis in great depth in *Chapter 15: Agents of Change.*

---

[352] Recent insights into androgen action on the anatomical and physiological substrate of penile erection. Asian J Androl. 2006;8:3–9. [PubMed] Gooren LJ, Saad F.

Why Cycling Testosterone is a Myth

There is no such thing as 'cycling' testosterone when a person has a clinical need to optimize his blood testosterone levels. Once a person replaces his decreasing natural production with an external source of testosterone from any type of delivery system, this must be maintained for life due to the body shutting off its own natural production of testosterone. As already elegantly discussed, exogenous testosterone halts the HPT/HPG Axis (HPTA/HPGA) and as such the testicles are no longer receiving LH. This is known as inhibition (shut down) or HPTA suppression.

The benefits of ongoing, lifelong TOT are so strong that there would have to be a strongly compelling reason to stop therapy. Other than a very aggressive form of metastatic cancer appearing, the overwhelmingly positive biological benefits that exist for one's physical and mental health would make it illogical to even think of stopping. After all, men's natural testosterone levels decline by 1% (conservatively) every year after the age of 30[353].

We've already discussed the rampant environmental degradation that is placing your endocrine system under siege in this book. There doesn't appear to be any indication of this environmental situation improving in the near future. In our opinion, TOT is the only failsafe way to ensure you can control and maintain optimal levels of blood testosterone as you age.

---

[353] Morley JE, Perry HM 3rd: Androgen deficiency in aging men: role of testosterone replacement therapy. J Lab Clin Med. 2000;135:370-378.

CHAPTER 12 KEY TAKEAWAYS

- We discussed the importance of monitoring your TOT for optimum health by tracking key biomarkers on a regular basis. This allows you and your doctor to become intimately aware of your body's individual response to TOT.

- We reveal all of the blood biomarkers (values) you should be measuring, the specific tests to run, the ranges you should be within for each biomarker, how often to run each test and any exceptional circumstances to watch out for. Since TOT is a lifetime therapy, this means you'll be regularly running these tests and tracking the results for the rest of your life.

- We show you why salivary testing is an ineffective and inaccurate method for precisely measuring testosterone levels in your body. Drawing blood and pulling a serum testosterone panel are your only two reliable options for doing so.

- We talked about the differences between serum testosterone and free testosterone, and the ranges you should strive to be within. At the same time, it is imperative for progressive TOT physicians to treat the actual symptoms of their patients instead of solely relying on the findings of a lab report.

- The critical importance of sex hormone binding globulin (SHBG) in hormonal optimization (and therefore TOT) is discussed in an exclusive interview with Dr. Crisler.

- The importance of monitoring hemoglobin and hematocrit levels while on TOT, along with the reference ranges you should strive to stay within, is explored.

- Liver health is not compromised (i.e. no occurrence of liver toxicity, or development of tumors in the liver) by TOT, provided that one is not engaging in detrimental lifestyle habits.

- We debunk the myth that TOT leads to (or increases the risk of) prostate cancer, showing how low testosterone levels are actually the culprit. The long-held belief that raising total testosterone levels necessarily causes rapid and universal growth of existing prostate cancer has not been supported by the existing data.

- We show you how to maintain blood pressure and keep it in check while using TOT.

- We explain how TOT can be used without aggravating sleep apnea and other associated sleeping problems.

- Contrary to popular belief, TOT does not increase the risk of heart attacks, strokes and other cardiovascular diseases (hint: it actually reduces the risk or is cardioprotective). This myth was propagated by inherently flawed studies that did not use normal, healthy aging men. If anything, low testosterone levels are more predictive of an increase in cardiovascular disease.

- TOT has been demonstrated to lower 'bad' cholesterol levels while having next to no impact on 'good' cholesterol levels. We briefly discuss how you can improve and optimize your cholesterol levels.

- Pregnenolone is critically important for hormonal health and testosterone production. We show you how to maintain optimal serum levels of pregnenolone, and how you can supplement it alongside TOT (only if necessary).

- Through an extensive interview with Dr. Merrill Matschke, while drawing upon our own experience, we tell you everything you need to know about testicular shrinkage and decreased sperm count while on TOT. For those of you looking to maintain your fertility while on TOT, you don't want to miss this!

- Finally, we demonstrate the myths that lie behind 'penis shrinking' while using TOT, and 'cycling' testosterone.

CHAPTER 13
The Critical Role of Nutrition in TOT

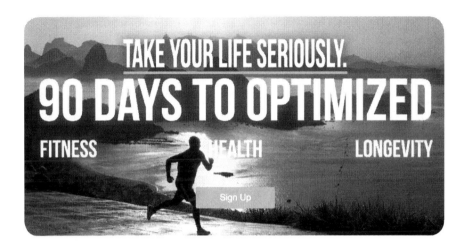

In Chapters 13 and 14, we will discuss maximizing your TOT through proper nutrition and living an Insulin Controlled Lifestyle (ICL). Understanding nutrition and harnessing the power of insulin (discussed in greater detail in Chapter 14) will play a critical role in getting the most out of your therapy. If you're lazy about your nutrition, you'll only reap a fraction of the rewards from TOT.

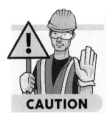

CAUTION

If you drink alcohol every night and your diet consists of nothing but processed food and soda, you will not experience the wonders of optimized testosterone levels. Testosterone isn't a magic bullet or wonder supplement that covers the damage done to your body from eating fast food and living a sedentary lifestyle.

But if you eat a clean diet and use an intelligently-designed resistance and endurance training program in combination with a sound TOT regimen, you will achieve outstanding results. We have created an excellent web-based video program that will teach you everything you need to know about nutrition. To find out more, visit 90Days2Optimized.com[354].

First, let's discuss how to best structure your diet and nutrition to maximize the benefits of TOT.

Your Caloric Intake is Dependent on Your Physical Goals

Your total food intake, which consists of the three primary macronutrients (protein, carbohydrates, and fats), is always dependant on your overall physical goals.

The chart on the next page shows the three specific types of physical goals, and the caloric intake needed to attain each of them.

---

[354] www.90days2optimized.com

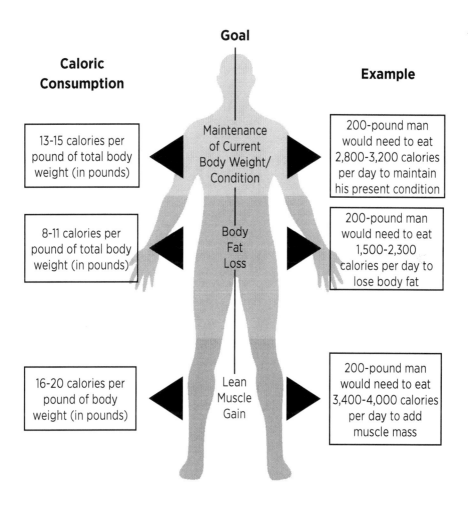

Goal

Caloric Consumption

Example

Caloric Consumption	Goal	Example
13-15 calories per pound of total body weight (in pounds)	Maintenance of Current Body Weight/ Condition	200-pound man would need to eat 2,800-3,200 calories per day to maintain his present condition
8-11 calories per pound of total body weight (in pounds)	Body Fat Loss	200-pound man would need to eat 1,500-2,300 calories per day to lose body fat
16-20 calories per pound of body weight (in pounds)	Lean Muscle Gain	200-pound man would need to eat 3,400-4,000 calories per day to add muscle mass

In order to calculate your exact consumption of macronutrients (relative to your goal), you need to understand the three somatotypes (i.e. body types) shown in the following chart:

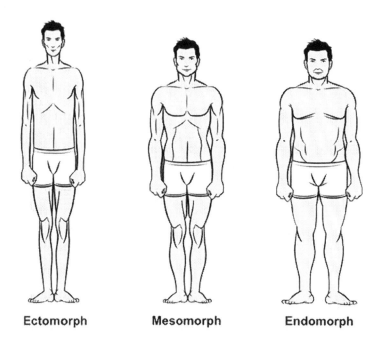

| Ectomorph | Mesomorph | Endomorph |

Ectomorphic body types are usually long, lean and skinny. **Mesomorphic** body types are normally muscular and look "naturally fit." **Endomorphic** body types are heavier and naturally possess higher body fat levels.

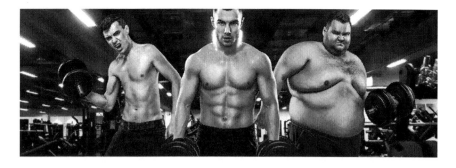

Most people are a combination of the 3 body types (for example, mix between ectomorphic and mesomorphic). Men who are less insulin-sensitive (i.e. have poor insulin sensitivity) will be naturally endomorphic (naturally heavy/fatter), and as a result will need to limit their carbohydrate intake more than the other two body types to avoid gaining fat.

There are biomarkers which can be measured (such as **HbA1c** and **fasted blood glucose**) to determine your insulin sensitivity. **HbA1c** stands for **glycated haemoglobin** (**A1c**), which identifies average plasma glucose concentration. By measuring the HbA1C it can tell you how high your blood glucose has been on average over the last 8-12 weeks. A normal non-diabetic **HbA1C is < 36 mmol/mol (5.5%).** For people without diabetes, the normal range for the hemoglobin A1c level is between 4% and 5.6%. Hemoglobin A1c levels between 5.7% and 6.4% mean you have a higher chance of getting diabetes. Levels of 6.5% or higher mean you have diabetes. To be truly healthy, 4.8% - 5.3% is where one should strive to maintain their HBA1c levels. Insulin is measured in "microunits per milliliter" (mcU/ml or mIU/ml). As a third alternative, you can also buy a glucometer[355] (glucose meter) and check your blood sugar from a pre and post meal pin prick (a drop of blood is taken from your finger).

NOTE: Naturally fatter people who are more insulin insensitive will have higher HbA1C levels on average. This is why they need to ALWAYS be mindful of carbohydrate intake to remain lean.

To figure out your own body type and insulin sensitivity, you'll need to experiment with your calorie (and carbohydrate) intake and keep close records to see what works best for you. The chart on page 257 has listed the estimated calorie intakes for each goal, but your body is unique and self experimentation is critical for achieving your fitness goals.

---

[355]   https://en.wikipedia.org/wiki/Glucose_meter

You should understand how your specific body type (i.e. somatotype) processes and responds to insulin when calculating your total calorie intake, regardless of your fitness goal. Insulin is the regulating hormone released by the pancreas when consuming food. How 'insulin-sensitive' you are ultimately determines the amount of carbohydrates you can consume without gaining fat. The role of insulin is intimately explained in *Chapter 14: What is Insulin Controlled Living and Why Is It Essential.*

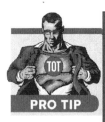

PRO TIP

If you're committed to looking your best, we recommend getting your body fat measured as precisely as possible. There are two specific ways to get your body fat measured with scientific accuracy: A DEXA scan[356], and a Bod Pod[357]. To understand the differences between the two testing procedures, read "Comparing Body Fat Test Methods" on BodySpec.com[358].

If you have higher body fat levels and are looking for a solution to burn fat as quickly and efficiently as possible, consider reading the best book ever written about optimizing **intermittent fasting (IF)**: *The Metabolic Blowtorch Diet*[359].

---

[356] https://www.bodyspec.com/what-is-dxa

[357] https://causenta.com/bodpod-body-fat-testing/

[358] https://www.bodyspec.com/blog/post/comparing_body_fat_testing_methods

[359] www.metabolicblowtorchdiet.com

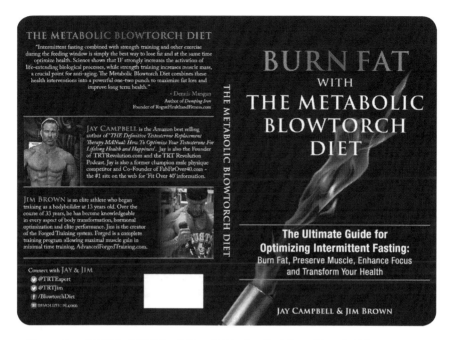

To get a FREE COPY of the Metabolic BlowTorch Diet, go to MetabolicBlowTorchDiet.com.

The Specific Macronutrients Needed on Your TOT Nutrition Plan

We believe it's important to briefly discuss the types of protein, carbs and fats you should focus on eating to maximize the results you get from TOT.

Protein

Protein is the most important macronutrient for performance and physique improvement. Without it, you cannot build or maintain muscle. Regardless of whether your goal is fat loss, maintenance or muscle gain, your diet needs to be rich in high-quality protein. **On top of needing protein to** build and maintain muscle, you need protein (in the form of amino acids) for proper brain function. Therefore, you need to get quality protein regularly throughout the day every 4-5 hours (when not fasting) and preferably at 20-50 grams per feeding.

Your daily protein requirements are based on one of your 3 physical goals, as previously discussed. Studies indicate that consuming *0.7 to 1 gram of protein per pound of total body weight daily* is required to support the anabolic (i.e. tissue-building) processes that build muscle[360]. When undergoing TOT, it is recommended to consume **at least 1 gram of protein per pound of LEAN body weight (not your total bodyweight)**. The exact amount you should eat is highly dependent on your age, as shown in the following chart:

Protein Requirements[361]

AGE GROUP (years)	MAINTENANCE (gram / lb of BW)	MUSCLE GAIN (gram / lb of BW)	FAT LOSS (gram / lb of BW)
15-19	1	1.5	1.25
20-49	0.85	1.25	1
50-65	.65	1	0.85
65+	0.55	0.75	0.65

BW = bodyweight

---

[360] Campbell B, Kreider RB et al. International Society of Sports Nutrition position stand: protein and exercise. J Int Soc Sports Nutr. 2007; 4:8.

[361] Please refer to this link for a detailed explanation on our recommended guidelines for daily protein requirements: http://fabfitover40.com/2014/06/02/know-daily-protein-requirements/

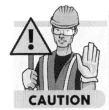

CAUTION

If you're worried that consuming high levels of protein might be detrimental to your kidneys, worry no more! The myth that high-protein diets impair kidney function is based on studies on individuals with renal (kidney) disease. In otherwise healthy individuals, protein intakes well over 1 gram per pound of bodyweight show no adverse effects on kidney function[362,363]. As long as you don't have any pre-existing kidney disease(s), a higher protein diet does not pose any issues to your health.

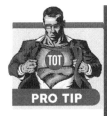

PRO TIP

All proteins are not made equal, as our bodies absorb some proteins better than others. For each protein source listed in the table on the next page, their bio-availability refers to the amount the body typically absorbs. by looking at the table on the next page, you can see that whey and eggs are some of the best protein sources you can consume from an absorption standpoint.

---

[362] Martin WF, Armstrong LE, Rodriguez NR, Dietary protein intake and rental function. Nutr Metab(Lond) 2005; 2:25.

[363] Poortmans JR, Dellalieux O. Do regular high protein diets have potential health risks on kidney function in athletes? Int J Sport Nutr & Exerc Metab. 2000; 10(1):28-38.

Protein Source	Bio-Availability Index
Whey Protein Isolate Blends	100-159
Whey Concentrate	104
Whole Egg	100
Cow's Milk	91
Egg White	88
Fish	83
Beef	80
Chicken	79
Casein	77
Rice	74
Soy	59
Wheat	54
Beans	49
Peanuts	43

(Chart taken from "Protein Availability & Bioabsorption" on Dioxyme.com[364])

There are five basic types of protein you need to focus on if you want to meet your target protein intake every day:

Animal Protein

Lean cuts of red meat, fish, turkey, chicken should be organic and wild-caught. They will have fewer toxins (pesticides, antibiotics, etc.), most of which will accumulate in the animal's fat. Cows and fish should not be raised eating corn, because in some cases this will lower or get rid of all omega 3's that would be found in a wild-caught or grass-fed animal. For the same reason, eggs should be organic and free-range if possible.

These are 'complete' proteins because they contain all of the essential amino acids your body needs to build and maintain muscle. Aim to consume meat a couple of times a day, no

---

[364]   https://dioxyme.com/protein-absorption/

matter your goal. If you are a vegan (or somebody who avoids meat), no problem!

For those of you who are consuming vegan protein, stay as far away from soy-based products as possible! Concentrated soy products have high levels of estrogen that can lead to undesired effects in the body such as lowered libido, decreased sperm count and breast enlargement[365].

Fortunately, you do not need to rely on this inferior choice as there are many healthy plant-based options for getting your protein. Don't be fooled by meat-substitute products either because they might contain soy. Read the labels carefully! The only exception to this rule is FERMENTED soy protein, and even then it has to be organic and properly fermented.

An example of a reliable vegan protein source is concentrated pea protein powder[366], which has a great amino acid profile. TrueNutrition.com offers many great vegan alternatives in several delicious flavors.

Long story short: Eliminate all soy additives, soy proteins, and soy bi-products from your diet AND NEVER LOOK BACK!

Whey Protein

This is the cheapest, most efficient way to add supplemental protein into your diet. It is also the most common ingredient in protein powder formulations seen in supplement stores and magazine advertisements. It can be used in multiple ways: mixed with oatmeal, in shakes by itself, combined with other

---

[365]   https://www.newscientist.com/article/dn12792-eating-soya-could-slash-mens-sperm-count/

[366]   https://truenutrition.com/p-1115-pea-protein-isolate-non-gmo-1lb.aspx

foods when cooking, and so on. Due to its rapid absorption by the body, you should use it immediately before, during and after training as part of your post-training shake. The rapid influx of amino acids into your bloodstream from whey protein has been shown to increase protein synthesis (i.e. muscle gain)[367]. The best form to use is Whey Protein Isolate Cold-Filtration, as it is the most highly filtered whey. The filtration is done at a cold temperature that leaves you with a undenatured, virtually fat- and lactose-free, protein source.

Casein Protein

Technically known as 'micellar casein,' it is a natural and undenatured milk protein that is separated from milk through ultrafiltration. Unlike whey protein, it provides a much slower and steady release of amino acids into the bloodstream upon consumption. It is used by people who want to prevent muscle tissue breakdown during situations where a large caloric deficit is needed (ex. Fitness competitions). It is best consumed at night so that your body can use the slow-digesting amino acids while in an overnight fasted state.

Egg Albumin

This is the protein you can find in egg whites. Minimal in fat and rich in protein, it is one of the easiest protein sources to use for busy people who are always on the go. You can buy egg white formulations, or eat whole eggs. Combined with meats and veggies, it is a very satiating option you will often find yourself going back to.

---

[367]   Tipton KD, Elliott TA, Cree MG, Wolf SE, Sanford AP, Wolfe RR. Ingestion of casein and whey proteins result in muscle anabolism after resistance exercise. Med Sci Sports Exerc. 2004;36(12):2073-81.

Carbohydrates

Some people still believe that eating carbs is *inherently* detrimental to body composition. As such, many have developed 'carbophobia' and do not consume enough carbohydrates. This causes great confusion around carbohydrates, from a nutritional perspective. Carb consumption is always *time-specific* and *goal-dependent*. More specifically, as long as you *consume the* **proper amount of carbs (relative to your insulin sensitivity)**[368] **and the right TYPES of carbs at specific times**, you will remain lean and energetic.

In regards to your carbohydrate intake and your goal of *losing body fat, maintaining body composition* or *increasing muscle mass,* harnessing the power of your body's insulin production is critical. You need excess insulin from higher carb intakes to build muscle, and you need to reduce insulin by reducing your carb intake to lose body fat. For a much greater understanding of insulin's role in the human body with respect to building muscle and losing fat, read *Chapter 14 - What is Insulin Controlled Living and Why it is Essential.*

To keep things simple, let's use the charts on the next page to determine your carb consumption based on the goals of *muscle gain, maintenance* or *fat loss,* relative to your individual body type:

---

[368]   http://www.ironmanmagazine.com/dont-be-so-sensitive/

Carbohydrate Requirements for Muscle Gain:	
Somatotype (Body Type)	Total Carbohydrate Consumption (grams)
Ectomorph (naturally skinny and lean)	250
Mesomorph (naturally muscular and athletic)	200
Endomorph (naturally chunky, 'heavy set')	75 or less (no more than 100)

Carbohydrate Requirements for Fat Loss	
Somatotype (Body Type)	Total Carbohydrate Consumption (grams)
Ectomorph	75
Mesomorph	50
Endomorph	Zero (no more than trace except vegetables

Carbohydrate Requirements for Maintenance	
Somatotype	*Total Carbohydrate Consumption (grams)*
Ectomorph	175
Mesomorph	150
Endomorph	50 or Less

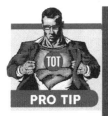

PRO TIP

To gain muscle, most ectomorphic and mesomorphic men generally do best when consuming the amounts shown in the chart. For endomorphic men who are usually less insulin sensitive, you'll likely have to consume fewer carbs. Remember: It is critical to establish baselines and self experiment to figure out how your body type individually responds to your carbohydrate intake.

Here are the 'right' (i.e. clean) carbs to eat, along with some guiding principles of when to eat them depending on your goals.

Complex Carbs

Eat these earlier in the day to provide a slow and steady release of insulin throughout the day. If you want to 'eyeball' it, add a fist full of these complex carbs alongside a high-quality lean protein for your dinner:

- Brown Rice
- Oatmeal
- Sweet Potatoes / Yams
- Oatbran
- Couscous
- Matza
- Ezekiel Bread
- Quinoa

Additionally, we recommend you consume high glycemic index carbs[369] (ex. cyclic dextrin[370]) within 30 minutes after finishing your workout. You can also consume them before and during your workout for fast absorption and replenishment of your muscle glycogen stores. This is especially important if you are trying to gain lean muscle.

Vegetables / Legumes

Anything that is green can be eaten in huge amounts, but avoid adding high-calorie dressings or additives to them. If you are hardcore dieting to drop a lot of body fat, lean protein + tons of green veggies are a tried-and-true combination:

[369] https://www.livestrong.com/article/279222-a-list-of-high-glycemic-carbs/

[370] http://truenutrition.com/blog/highly-branched-cyclic-dextrin-hbcd/

- Any vegetables that are green and leafy
- Asparagus
- Broccoli
- Green Beans
- Spinach
- Cauliflower
- Mushrooms
- Artichokes
- Lima Beans
- Okra

Fruits

The best time to consume fruits is right before your workout as a snack for some simple, quick-release sugars. You can also consume them with protein right after your workout. With that said, it's best to minimize fruit consumption altogether[371] if you want to get super lean.

This is because fructose digestion is rate limited by a specific enzymatic process. If you eat too much fruit over this rate limitation (usually 50 grams of fructose in a day, i.e. two apples), the body's liver glycogen over fills during digestion, which can lead to fat gain. This is not optimal for maximum leanness.

The more fiber a fruit has, the more readily it will be digested and the less likely the body will be subject to the rate limiting digestion effect mentioned above. The following fruits are fibrous and excellent choices to consume for maintenance and muscle gain programs:

---

[371] http://fabfitover40.com/2014/01/22/truth-fructose/

- Apples
- Blueberries
- Cherries
- Pineapple
- Fresh Melon / Cantaloupe
- Papaya
- Grapefruit
- Pears

As a bonus, we offer you Alexander Juan Antonio Cortes' "10 'Almost' Rules of Carbohydrate Consumption":

1. **Minimize sugar intake -** Sugar, which is made up of monosaccharides and disaccharides (carbohydrates are trisaccharides), are 'generally' not good for you.

   Bluntly, it is not satiating (i.e. leaves you feeling full). Not only does it interfere with the brain's pleasure centers for eating, but it also tampers with the hormones responsible for your appetite. This makes you want to eat more, which naturally leads to overeating and eventually becoming overweight. It also lowers your testosterone and creates an unwanted inflammatory state in the body.

   From a mostly objective standpoint, you are not 'missing out' on anything by not eating sugar. If needed (i.e taken post-workout or pre-workout for energy and glycogen replenishment), get your sugar from fruit and honey.

2. You probably need fewer carbohydrates than you think - People who are less physically active should consume fewer carbs.

While there isn't an 'exact' amount of carbs to consume, there are general ranges to consider depending on your level of physical activity. If you are physically inactive and barely do any walking, 50-100 grams of carbohydrates per day is probably all you need (the rest of your calories come from fats and proteins). When in doubt, less is more! Despite the bad rap they sometimes get, lower carb diets improve metabolic health and lead to better long-term adherence to your diet.

If you are physically active and move around often, you can consume 100 grams of carbs or more. The range to follow here is anywhere from 1-4 grams of carbs per pound of total bodyweight. The more active you are and the more muscle you have, the more carbs you can consume on a daily basis.

3. Your body needs 3-4 grams of water for every 1 gram of carbohydrate stored[372].

Carbohydrates are hydrophilic (i.e. 'water-loving'). Therefore, water is necessary to store them and burn them for energy when needed. This is why carbs can make some people bloat, while leading to the common mistake of confusing carb consumption (and water retention) for fat gain.

---

[372] https://www.deanza.edu/faculty/ackergigi/n62carbs.pdf

The weight you have gained is 'water weight', and indicates that you are not feeding yourself properly. Furthermore, your body is more likely to retain water if you are chronically dehydrated.

4. **The more muscular you are, the more carbs you can consume -** As previously stated, people who are close to achieving their natural muscular potential (i.e. being lean while having a decent amount of muscle) can tolerate higher carbohydrate intakes.

   Why? Because muscular people have the following qualities[373]:

   - Better insulin sensitivity
   - Better glucose management
   - Better nutrient partitioning

   It's also worth noting that people who are more muscular are also more metabolically active. This means they do not store carbohydrates as fat (or create an inflammatory reaction) in the same way that an overweight and inactive person would. Additionally, they can consume more sugar for this same reason.

   NOTE: This is not implying that sugar should be a primary source of carbohydrates, as explained in Rule #1.

---

[373] Cartee GD. Mechanisms for greater insulin-stimulated glucose uptake in normal and insulin-resistant skeletal muscle after acute exercise. American Journal of Physiology - Endocrinology and Metabolism. 2015;309(12):E949-E959. doi:10.1152/ajpendo.00416.2015.

5. **If you are overweight or obese, a low-carb diet is your best option -** Many individuals with excess body fat got to where they are by over-consuming sugars and processed foods. Ultimately, this leads to metabolic syndrome, increased blood pressure, high blood sugar, excess body fat around the waist, abnormal cholesterol levels and type 2 diabetes.

    Not only can a low-carb diet help these individuals lose fat, but it can also improve metabolic health through the control of insulin. This is discussed in greater detail in *Chapter 14: What is Insulin-Controlled Living and Why Is It Essential.*

6. **Most people should avoid processed carbs -** First and foremost, processed carbs are designed to make you WANT to overeat them without thinking about it. You are not going to feel 'full' after eating them.

    When in doubt, you should opt for leaving them out of your diet, especially if you are lethargic and/or overweight. Lean individuals are an exception to this rule and can eat processed carbs in moderation.

7. **Front-loading carbohydrates is a great strategy for any kind of fitness goal (fat loss / maintenance / muscle gain) -** In plain English, this means you eat carbohydrates right before your workout. This ensures the carbs you consume will be used by your muscles for your workout performance and your post-workout recovery. It also ensures your energy levels will be high during your training session, which is especially useful for those eating a low-carb diet.

NOTE: Lean and muscular people should consume carbs before, during AND after working out (a total of 3 times) for maximum performance and recovery.

8. **Eat fast-digesting carbs**[374] **right before AND immediately after intense physical activity (ex. resistance training). Otherwise, stick to slow-digesting carbs**[375] - Fast-digesting carbs (i.e. processed carbs and sugar) will be used as fuel before your workout, and as glycogen replenishment for your muscles after your workout. For those of you who are not working out on a regular basis, stick with slow-digesting carbohydrates.

9. **The faster you can consume it, the worse it is for your health** - In my experience, this is a general rule of thumb that works well for most people.

I once ate an entire bag of gummy worms in less than 5 minutes before I trained legs. It contained 120 grams of carbs that almost all came from sugar, and I did NOT feel full at all. I would have to eat 5 apples in a row just to eat the SAME amount of carbohydrates!

Obviously, the apples are the healthier carb source and they take a lot longer to eat. Complex carb sources should almost always be chosen over processed, sugar-heavy carbs. As previously discussed, they are designed to make you want to eat more of them without feeling satiated.

---

[374] https://www.livestrong.com/article/319828-list-of-fast-digesting-carbs/

[375] https://www.livestrong.com/article/84650-list-slow-digestible-carbs/

10. When in doubt, stick to vegetables, whole grains, rice, and fruit - Follow this rule and you will likely end up eating a healthy diet. You could even do what I do, and simplify this rule down to vegetables and rice alone. This is my quick and easy way of avoiding overconsumption of carbs, and it's really hard to screw up.

Not only do you end up getting a lot of fiber, but you also find yourself feeling full on a regular basis. Add in some fruit on occasion for a quick energy boost before lifting, and you have a way of eating that is sustainable for a very long time.

Fats (Essential Fatty Acids)

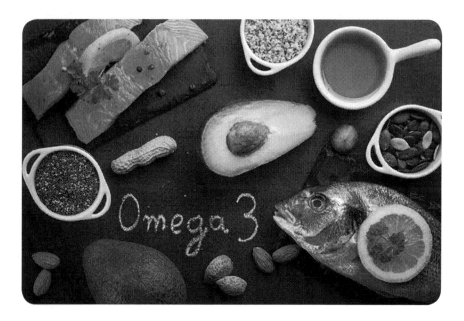

Essential Fatty Acids (EFAs) are the most critical macronutrient for your overall health.

Humans need EFAs to control important cellular processes, while maintaining optimal health & fitness. Without them, your skin would dry out, your brain would cease to function and your nervous system would shut down completely. Ironically, 90% of people in the world are deficient in EFAs from eating an average 'everyday' diet.

Supplementing with EFAs will result in significant improvements in muscular and neural coordination, along with improvements in memory, metabolism and skin elasticity[376].

---

[376] http://doktori.bibl.u-szeged.hu/34/1/tz_eredeti927.pdf

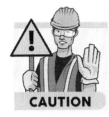

CAUTION

EFA consumption greatly impacts your testosterone levels. A diet high in EFA's will help keep your body in a state of positive nitrogen retention (i.e. a muscle-building state) and ensures the positive benefits of your TOT are fully maximized. For those of you who embrace an intermittent fasting[377] lifestyle, a diet rich in EFA's will allow you to remain satiated (feeling 'full') and improve your mental focus during long fast windows.

Understanding this, it is important to focus on eating the right EFA's. Here are a few recommend sources of EFA's.

- Udo's Oil[378]: Add it to protein shakes and salads, 2-4 tablespoons a day

- Deep Marine Fish Oil[379] (High in Omega 3): 4-6 grams of Omega-3 minimum per day

- Coconut Oil[380]: You can cook your meals with 2-3 tablespoons

- Avocado Oil[381]: 2-4 tablespoons per day (in addition to, or instead of Coconut Oil)

- Olive Oil[382]: 2-4 tablespoons to be used on salads or with cooking

---

[377]   www.metabolicblowtorchdiet.com

[378]   https://www.amazon.com/exec/obidos/ASIN/B0010ED3DQ/fabfitove40-20

[379]   http://www.amazon.com/exec/obidos/ASIN/B00CAZAU62/fabfitove40-20

[380]   http://www.amazon.com/exec/obidos/ASIN/B00CXA0AKA/fabfitove40-20

[381]   http://www.amazon.com/exec/obidos/ASIN/B007XA49O8/fabfitove40-20

[382]   http://www.amazon.com/exec/obidos/ASIN/B01IR6KI3M/fabfitove40-20

- Red Palm Oil[383]: 2-4 tablespoons per day
- Nut Butters: Almond, Peanut, Cashew
- Nuts: Almonds, Sunflower Seeds, Macadamia Nuts
- Medium Chain Triglycerides (MCTs)[384]: Supplemental capsule form, or liquid form added to protein shakes

Vitamin & Mineral Supplementation to Maximize TOT

It is important to realize that highly active people who train intensely on a frequent basis need adequate vitamin and mineral replenishment, and this may require additional supplementation. This section is a quick hit list of essential things that men on TOT should add to their nutritional regimen.

Eating broccoli, cauliflower, and cabbage will help rid your body of excess estrogen.

Cruciferous vegetables are high in **indole-3-carbinol**, which is an estrogen-lowering food compound[385]. These veggies are also high in fiber[386], which help with weight control and losing body fat[387]. Because we recommend you only use AI medications when there is a measured clinical need, the usage of natural remedies & foods that minimize estrogen production is a great failsafe to ensure your body maintains a healthy amount of estrogen.

---

[383]   http://www.amazon.com/exec/obidos/ASIN/B00IMQC78C/fabfitove40-20

[384]   http://www.amazon.com/exec/obidos/ASIN/B0019LRY8A/fabfitove40-20

[385]   Indole-3-carbinol, a vegetable phytochemical, inhibits adipogenesis by regulating cell cycle and AMPKα signaling. Biochimie. 2014 Sep;104:127-36. Epub 2014 Jun 18.

[386]   http://fabfitover40.com/2014/05/12/the-importance-of-fiber-in-your-diet-2/

[387]   www.metabolicblowtorchdiet.com

The body uses **magnesium** and **zinc** to maintain normal nerve function and muscle function. Both minerals support a healthy immune system, keep the heartbeat steady and help bones remain strong. Proper levels of **magnesium** and **zinc** can also increase free testosterone levels significantly in men[388]. **Dr. Robert Kominiarek** has seen TOT deplete intracellular magnesium stores in many of his patients, leading to hand tremors and tics. He recommends supplementing **200-400 mg of magnesium glycinate per day** as a good failsafe to prevent any potential testosterone-induced magnesium depletion.

Calcium hydroxyapatite improves bone mineral density while strengthening ligaments and tendons at the same time. Calcium hydroxyapatite, magnesium and zinc are all found in the supplement "Ultra Bone-Up"[389]. Take 3 capsules twice a day (6 capsules total) with meals if you're doing intense, heavy resistance training.

Curcumin (the active ingredient of Tumeric)[390] is a potent antioxidant that decreases oxidative stress responsible for suppressing testosterone production in aging males[391]. It is known as one of nature's 'super nutrients', and a powerful ally in the protection against cancer. Curcumin also protects and strengthens your joints and soft tissues during bouts of

---

[388] Effects of magnesium supplementation on testosterone levels of athletes and sedentary subjects at rest and after exhaustion. Biol Trace Elem Res. 2011 Apr. Epub 2010 Mar 30.

[389] http://www.amazon.com/exec/obidos/ASIN/B0013OUJIU/trtrevbook-20

[390] http://www.amazon.com/exec/obidos/ASIN/B00JA4TLTI/trtrevbook-20

[391] Abarikwu SO, Akiri OF et al. Combined administration of curcumin and gallic acid inhibits gallic acid-induced suppression of steroidogenesis, sperm output, antioxidant defenses and inflammatory responsive genes. J Steroid Biochem Mol Biol. 2014;143, 49060.

heavy resistance training, while helping fight arthritis[392]. We recommend anyone who is training intensely with weights to take **500 mg, 3-5x a day (1500-2500 mg total)** with food. For those who have suffered a joint, tendon or soft tissue injury, dosages of up to **5-6 grams a day** have shown to be effective at significantly reducing inflammation[393]. Very recently, curcumin was found[394] to be useful in the treatment of several neurological diseases. Specifically, the research found that curcumin reduces the effects of neurotoxicity induced by fluoride. Clearly, this is a powerful antioxidant that has a wide range of beneficial uses. We strongly recommend you supplement with it.

Ubiquinol Kaneka QH Coenzyme Q-10[395] **(CoQ-10)** is a vitamin-like substance found throughout the body, especially in the heart, liver, kidney, and pancreas. Coenzyme Q10 may protect against many age-related disorders including cancer, heart disease, diabetes, and various neurological disorders[396]. Taking **200-300 mg a day** has been clinically proven to offer powerful disease-resistant benefits[397]. If you are using statin medications to control blood cholesterol levels, it is critically important to

[392] Curcumin: A Review of Its' Effects on Human Health. Foods. 2017 Oct 22;6(10). pii: E92. doi: 10.3390/foods6100092.

[393] Sun Yufeng, Liu Wei, Zhang Hao, Li Hongtao, Liu Jiakun, Zhang Fayao, Jiang Tao, and Jiang Shan. Journal of Interferon & Cytokine Research. October 2017, 37(10): 449-455. https://doi.org/10.1089/jir.2017.0069

[394] Sharma C, Suhalka P, Sukhwal P, Jaiswal N, Bhatnagar M. Curcumin attenuates neurotoxicity induced by fluoride: An *in vivo* evidence. *Pharmacognosy Magazine*. 2014;10(37):61-65. doi:10.4103/0973-1296.126663.

[395] http://www.amazon.com/exec/obidos/ASIN/B00EFVQ3BA/trtrevbook-20

[396] Effects of Coenzyme Q10 on Markers of Inflammation: A Systematic Review and Meta-Analysis. *Zhai J, Bo Y, Lu Y, Liu C, Zhang L.PLoS One. 2017;* 12(1):e0170172. Epub 2017 Jan 26.

[397] Dhanasekaran M, Ren J. The emerging role of coenzyme Q-10 in aging, neurodegeneration, cardiovascular disease, cancer and diabetes mellitus. Curr Neurovasc Res. 2005 Dec;2(5):447-59.

supplement with CoQ-10 as well, due to the fact that statins will reduce your natural levels of CoQ-10.

Betaine TMG and Alpha GPC are 2 other supplements we recommend TOT users consider adding to their supplement regime. *Alpha glycerylphosphorylcholine (Alpha GPC)* is a naturally occurring choline-containing compound found in a variety of sources. It's been on our radar because it can get choline to the brain by passing the blood-brain barrier. It's also a precursor of acetylcholine. Acetylcholine is a neurotransmitter that is needed for proper function of the motor, autonomic, sympathetic and parasympathetic nervous systems[398]. Put simply, it helps your brain and skeletal muscle systems function more effectively.

Alpha GPC has shown promise in three areas: Cognitive decline, power output and nootropic qualities. In relation to cognitive decline, Alpha GPC has been shown to have protective and/ or reparative qualities for recent stroke victims[399]. It also improves symptoms of dementia in Alzheimer's patients[400], and significantly enhances power output during exercise while effecting peak serum growth hormone secretions after exercising[401]. If one is deficient in consuming choline-containing

---

[398] Tiwari P, Dwivedi S, Singh MP, Mishra R, Chandy A. Basic and modern concepts on cholinergic receptor: A review. *Asian Pacific Journal of Tropical Disease.* 2013;3(5):413-420. doi:10.1016/S2222-1808(13)60094-8.

[399] alpha-Glycerophosphocholine in the mental recovery of cerebral ischemic attacks. An Italian multicenter clinical trial. Ann N Y Acad Sci. 1994 Jun 30;717:253-69.

[400] Cognitive improvement in mild to moderate Alzheimer's dementia after treatment with the acetylcholine precursor choline alfoscerate: a multicenter, double-blind, randomized, placebo-controlled trial. Clin Ther. 2003 Jan;25(1):178-93.

[401] Acute supplementation with alpha-glycerylphosphorylcholine augments growth hormone response to, and peak force production during, resistance exercise. Journal of the International Society of Sports Nutrition 20085 (Suppl 1):P15.

foods (like most American diets), supplementation with Alpha GPC may show a significant improvement in learning, memory, focus and motor skills. All of these are influenced by acetylcholine and will function more effectively with adequate amounts. We recommend a **dosage of anywhere between 400 and 1200 mg per day** in either capsule or powder form.

We typically recommend Betaine HCL for someone who is having digestive issues. As we age, we oftentimes release less HCL (hydrochloric acid) in the stomach to breakdown foods and our food digestion becomes less optimal. Supplementing with Betaine HCL will increase the amount of HCL in the gut biome, which may help improve digestive issues. The other way we find betaine is through betaine anhydrous, also known as trimethylglycine (TMG). Betaine anhydrous, made from choline, offers the key benefit of lowering homocysteine levels[402]. As already mentioned in Chapter 12, homocysteine is an amino acid that is thought to be a measurement of inflammation related to cardiovascular disease. The higher your level of homocysteine, the greater your risk for cardio-vascular disease[403]. The data supports both sides of this argument, but most agree that high levels of this amino acid are not good for endothelial lining and function[404].

One of the main things betaine does in the body is act as a methyl donor. Basically, it's a compound that will take a methyl group from one compound and donate it to another. There are

---

[402] Dietary and supplementary betaine: acute effects on plasma betaine and homocysteine concentrations under standard and postmethionine load conditions in healthy male subjectsAm J Clin Nutr March 2008 87: 3 577-585.

[403] Ganguly P, Alam SF. Role of homocysteine in the development of cardiovascular disease. *Nutrition Journal*. 2015;14:6. doi:10.1186/1475-2891-14-6.

[404] Homocysteine and endothelial dysfunction: a link with cardiovascular disease. J Nutr. 2000 Feb;130(2S Suppl):369S-372S.

a lot of processes in the body that are found to be rate limited by the available methyl group, with creatine synthesis being one of them. Protein synthesis is another, and betaine may influence that positively as well (i.e. increase the rate of protein synthesis)[405].

Betaine supplementation has been shown to increase physical performance[406-407], and is typically found in combination with creatine and compounds that affect nitric oxide. Most of the studies cited show a clinical benefit when **supplementing with at least 2.5 mg daily**. This is also our recommended dose.

Most men over the age of 40 can benefit from the regular use of a **prostate supplement** to support the prostate and prevent potential prostate problems. Optimally, one should choose a formulation that contains Saw palmetto berry (*Serenoa repens*) and Pygeum (*Pygeum africanum*), along with other herbs like nettle, pumpkin seed extract/oil and beta-sitosterol. All of these herbs have been shown to support proper prostate function[408]. One of the strongest over-the-counter (OTC) prostate supplements on the market today is **New Chapter Prostate 5LX**[409].

---

[405] Betaine supplementation enhances anabolic endocrine and Akt signaling in response to acute bouts of exercise. Eur J Appl Physiol. 2013 Mar;113(3):793-802. doi: 10.1007/s00421-012-2492-8. Epub 2012 Sep 14.

[406] Effects of betaine on body composition, performance, and homocysteine thiolactone. Journal of the International Society of Sports Nutrition 2013;10:39.

[407] Effect of betaine supplementation on cycling sprint performance J Luke Pryor, Stuart AS Craig and Thomas Swensen. Journal of the International Society of Sports Nutrition 2012;9:12.

[408] Cole C, Burgoyne T, Lee A, Stehno-Bittel L, Zaid G. Arum Palaestinum with isovanillin, linolenic acid and β-sitosterol inhibits prostate cancer spheroids and reduces the growth rate of prostate tumors in mice. *BMC Complementary and Alternative Medicine.* 2015;15:264. doi:10.1186/s12906-015-0774-5.

[409] http://www.amazon.com/exec/obidos/ASIN/B0009F3RTW/trtrevbook-20

Glutathione is produced by every single cell in the human body, and has an impressive list of scientifically-proven health effects. By scavenging free oxy radicals from the body, glutathione protects most biological systems from disease and deterioration[410]. Glutathione has been described as a defensive agent against the action of toxic xenobiotics (drugs, pollutants, carcinogens, etc.)[411]. Because of its many uses in the body, it is important to prevent glutathione levels from becoming too low.

Glutathione deficiency leads to an increased susceptibility to the many diseases of aging, such as cancer and Alzheimer's disease[412]. Men using TOT and subjecting themselves to intense weight lifting and cardiovascular training should consider supplementing with it. Regulating your glutathione metabolism is critical to ensure optimal health. Taken orally, glutathione is absorbed very poor by the body. The **optimal dosage of glutathione is 200 mg once a day, injected subcutaneously** with an insulin needle. To learn much more about glutathione, read Self Hacked's "27 Proven Health Benefits of Glutathione"[413].

---

[410]   Chen J, Wu F, Long Y, Yu W. Glutathione Supplementation Attenuates Oxidative Stress and Improves Vascular Hyporesponsiveness in Experimental Obstructive Jaundice. Oxidative Medicine and Cellular Longevity. 2015;2015:486148. doi:10.1155/2015/486148

[411]   Pompella A, Corti A. Editorial: the changing faces of glutathione, a cellular protagonist. Frontiers in Pharmacology. 2015;6:98. doi:10.3389/fphar.2015.00098.

[412]   Identification of cytotoxic, glutathione-reactive moieties inducing accumulation of reactive oxygen species via glutathione depletion. Bioorg Med Chem. 2017 Nov 4. pii: S0968-0896(17)31533-X. doi: 10.1016/j.bmc.2017.11.009. [Epub ahead of print]

[413]   https://selfhacked.com/blog/glutathione-30-scientifically-proven-health-benefits-glutathione/

What to Minimize and Avoid While on TOT

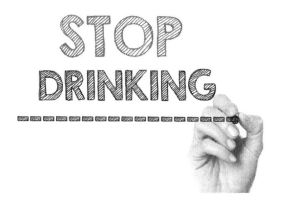

Alcohol

Alcohol, even in moderation[414], lessens the beneficial effects of TOT. It increases estrogen conversion, leading to excess body fat and the atypical 'dad bod'. On top of that, overconsumption puts an unnecessary amount of stress on the liver. Alcohol also has toxic effects on the testes and decreases your overall testosterone levels[415].

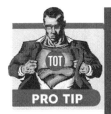

PRO TIP

Alcohol is a subject that elicits strong feelings from users because of the popular mainstream opinion which states that moderate alcohol consumption offers positive health benefits. Additionally, there are an overwhelming number of studies that contradict each other regarding the benefits and downfalls of regular alcohol consumption. ***The best data we've***

---

[414] http://suppversity.blogspot.de/2014/06/true-or-false-occasional-weekend.html

[415] Rachdaoui N, Sarkar DK. Effects of Alcohol on the Endocrine System. Endocrinology and metabolism clinics of North America 2013;42(3):593-615. doi:10.1016/j.ecl.2013.05.008.

> *found shows that ONLY 4 ounces of red wine per day (due to the presence of pycnogenol, resveratrol and other flavonoids) is good for reducing blood sugar*[416] *in otherwise normal and healthy aging adults.* 4 ounces isn't very much when you think about it! If you justify your alcohol consumption as 'much more' than 4 ounces of red wine per night, you have a drinking problem and TOT isn't going to do much for you or your health.
>
> We understand that telling men to give up alcohol will be met with great resistance, but if you want the best results while on TOT, you must minimize or eliminate your alcohol consumption altogether.

Even if you just drink alcohol once in a while[417], detoxifying your metabolic system with a powerful liver protectant is a good protective policy. We recommend **N-Acetyl-Cysteine (NAC)** as an excellent detoxification supplement. Typical dosages are between **300-2000 mg daily**. NAC works by providing a source of cysteine that acts to recycle glutathione in the liver[418].

NAC has also been shown to treat liver failure caused by excessive alcohol consumption and environmental pollutants[419].

[416] http://time.com/4070762/red-wine-resveratrol-diabetes/

[417] http://fabfitover40.com/2014/01/14/is-alcohol-in-moderation-really-good-for-you-2/

[418] Lai IK, Dhakal K, Gadupudi GS, et al. N-acetylcysteine (NAC) diminishes the severity of PCB 126 – induced fatty liver in male rodents. Toxicology. 2012;302(1):25-33. doi:10.1016/j.tox.2012.07.007.

[419] De Andrade KQ, Moura FA, dos Santos JM, de Araújo ORP, de Farias Santos JC, Goulart MOF. Oxidative Stress and Inflammation in Hepatic Diseases: Therapeutic Possibilities of N-Acetylcysteine. Haenen G, ed. International Journal of Molecular Sciences. 2015;16(12):30269-30308. doi:10.3390/ijms161226225.

Glutathione also plays an essential role as an antioxidant in the liver, and when taken together with **NAC** it ensures a more powerful antioxidant effect[420]. Along with reducing oxidative damage in the liver, NAC also decreases bodily inflammation[421].

Sugar and HFC's

Consumption of **refined sugar** and **high fructose corn syrup (HFC)** should also be minimized. After consuming refined sugar, testosterone levels decrease due to the release of insulin[422]. Despite all the refined sugar that exists in our modern diets, the human body rarely needs it. The obvious exception to this rule is consuming high glycemic index sugars immediately before, after or during an intense weight training session or long endurance event. Otherwise (and especially if you're trying to reduce body fat levels), strive to minimize your simple sugars, including refined and processed carbs, as much as possible.

Soy Protein and Soy Bi-Products

Consuming soy protein and its variants[423] are absolutely counter productive to maximizing TOT. Soy products are part of the the many environmental, endocrine-disrupting toxins causing breast enlargement (gynecomastia), decreased facial and

---

[420] Kaplowitz N. The importance and regulation of hepatic glutathione. *The Yale Journal of Biology and Medicine.* 1981;54(6):497-502.

[421] Regulation of cyclooxygenase-2 expression in human osteoblastic cells by N-acetylcysteine. Origuchi, Tomoki et al. Translational Research, Volume 136, Issue 5, 390 - 394.

[422] Aromatase, adiposity, aging and disease. The hypogonadal-metabolic-atherogenic-disease and aging connection. Cohen, P.G. Medical Hypotheses, Volume 56, Issue 6, 702 - 708.

[423] http://fabfitover40.com/2014/06/06/soy-protein-friend-foe/

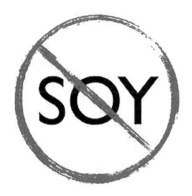

body hair growth, lowered libido, wild mood swings, higher body fat storage, erectile dysfunction and lowered sperm count. It has also recently fostered a popular internet meme of "soy boys" to describe soft, weak and effeminate men who got that way from overeating soy and its various by-products[424].

Next time you go grocery shopping, check the nutritional labels of food you normally buy and look for soy in the list of ingredients. There's a good chance you'll see soy or one of its various by-products. Unfortunately, most processed and refined foods are laced with soy by-products. The more of these foods you can remove from your diet, the healthier you'll be. Read this excellent article[425] summarizing the dangers of soy.

Proper Hydration - How Much Water is Enough?

Water is the principal component of plasma, which aids the body in the transportation of nutrients through the bloodstream. Drinking enough water also ensures proper metabolic function. Additionally, it helps regulate body temperature, moisten the air used for breathing and keep our mucous membranes hydrated.

Water is crucially important to our body's two organ systems: the kidneys and the lower gastrointestinal tract. Both systems function almost exclusively to ensure that excess water is not lost. You need to constantly replace water in your body due

---

[424] https://youtu.be/QtOJIR8KwMY

[425] https://paleoleap.com/dangers-soy/

to losing it through breathing, sweating and normal digestion. Honestly, how hard is it to drink 6-8 small water bottles a day? Apparently much harder than it seems for most folks. DRINK WATER. A LOT of it!

Part of staying hydrated also means avoiding (or at least minimizing) your consumption of carbonated beverages. The carbonic and phosphoric acids in sodas are terrible for your digestive tract and are a chief component of metabolic syndrome[426]. These acids also wreak havoc on your gums and tooth enamel[427]. Carbonated mineral water is not as bad, provided it doesn't have sugar sweeteners or other additives.

The Importance of Vitamin D from Sunlight and Supplementation

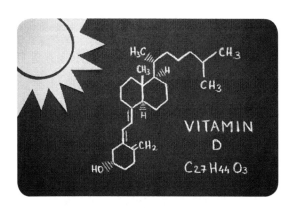

Get out in the sun for a bare minimum of 10-20 minutes a day for at least 3-4 days per week. If you live in a place where sunlight is hard to come by, visit a tanning salon that offers beds which minimize / avoid the use of harmful ultraviolet (UV) spectrum rays. In most cities, tanning bed companies offer the usage of

---

426 The Oslo health study: soft drink intake is associated with the metabolic syndrome. Appl Physiol Nutr Metab. 2010 Oct;35(5):635-42. doi:10.1139/H10-059.

427 Effect of soft drinks on the release of calcium from enamel surfaces. Southeast Asian J Trop Med Public Health. 2013 Sep;44(5):927-30.

beds that prevent UV burning within a specified time frame. Additionally, some people have found that using SAD lamps helps them experience the positive benefits of sunlight if they live in dark, cold areas that rarely get any sunlight at all[428].

We're not advocating that people sit in a tanning bed for too long and get a sunburn. We are simply saying this: You need sunlight, and where sunlight is hard to come by, you need a workaround solution. Sunlight exposure increases the body's production of melanin. Melanin is a very powerful hormone you'll read more about in *Chapter 15: Agents of Change* when we discuss the peptide hormones Melanotan I and II.

Vitamin D isn't technically a vitamin, despite its name. The name actually encompasses a vitally important group of micronutrients. It is a potent steroid hormone responsible for switching our genes on or off. It is structurally similar to steroids like testosterone, cholesterol, and cortisol. In other words, it's more of a hormone than it is a vitamin, and that's why we highly recommend having your Vitamin D levels checked with a simple blood test.

Vitamin D's effects are varied and profound. It is essential to the formation of male sperm cells[429] and the production of natural and free testosterone[430]. Supplementation with Vitamin D has also been associated with higher levels of testosterone

---

[428]   https://selfhacked.com/blog/blue-light-therapy-benefits/

[429]   Vitamin D and male reproduction. Nat Rev Endocrinol. 2014 Mar;10(3) Epub 2014 Jan 14.

[430]   Vitamin D levels and bone mineral density: are LH levels involved in the pathogenesis of bone impairment in hypogonadal men? J Endocrinol Invest. 2014 Oct 17.

and Sex Hormone Binding Globulin[431]. On top of its positive testosterone-boosting effects, Vitamin D is essential for cell-to-cell communication.

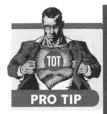

PRO TIP

To make sure you get enough sunlight, despite being unable to fully control how much sunlight exposure you'll receive, have your physician test your blood levels of **Vitamin D, 25-Hydroxy** to make sure you fall into the upper end of the accepted value range **(30-100 ng/mL or 75-250 nmol/L)**. To ensure your score is *70 ng/mL (or 175 nmol/L)* or above[432], we recommend supplementing with **5,000-10,000 IU's of Vitamin D daily.**

---

[431] Vitamin D is significantly associated with total testosterone and sex hormone-binding globulin in Malaysian men. Kok-Yong Chin, Soelaiman Ima-Nirwana, Wan Zurinah Wan Ngah (doi: 10.3109/13685538.2015.1034686).

[432] Andrology. 2014 Sep;2(5):748-54. doi: 10.1111/j.2047-2927.2014.00247.x. Epub 2014 Jul 16.

CHAPTER 13 KEY TAKEAWAYS

- We discuss the three specific types of physical fitness goals (fat loss / maintenance / muscle gain), and the amount of calories you need to eat in order to achieve each of them.

- We talked about the importance of figuring out your own body type and its unique insulin sensitivity.

- For each of the three primary macronutrients (Protein, carbohydrates, fats), the following items were explained in great detail: The importance of each macronutrient in relation to your health and success with TOT, the exact amounts of each to eat depending on your fitness goals (and body type), the 'right' types of each macronutrient to eat, and when you should be eating them.

- We reveal our list of supplements we highly recommend you take to replenish your body's vitamins and minerals, thereby maximizing the benefits you get from TOT.

- We show you what you should be minimizing and avoiding altogether while on TOT (Alcohol, refined sugars, soy products).

- Lastly, we remind you why it's important to stay properly hydrated with adequate water intake, while getting enough vitamin D from sunlight and supplementation (regardless of whether you are on TOT or not).

What is Insulin-Controlled Living, and Why Is it Essential?

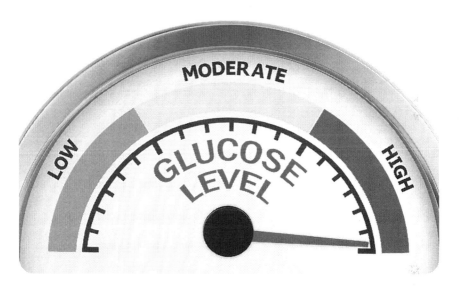

Insulin is a hormone that regulates how your body uses carbohydrates, fat, and protein. More specifically, it helps your muscles, liver, and fat cells process and utilize glucose (i.e. blood sugar). This chapter will teach you why an insulin-controlled lifestyle is critical for optimal health, and how you can live this way.

An insulin-controlled lifestyle is a way of living that will maximize your long-term health by properly controlling your body's insulin response to the foods you consume. By minimizing your insulin response and improving your body's usage of glucose, you will avoid the detrimental health effects of aging that are associated with excess insulin and insulin resistance, such as increased vascular inflammation and/or type 2 diabetes. In turn, you will significantly lower your risk for age related diseases.

The typical American diet is high in processed foods, grains, and sugar. Combined with poor meal frequency (i.e. irregular eating habits), these foods cause the body to release massive amounts of insulin when they are consumed. The excess insulin release and overconsumption of calories both lead to fat gain, which desensitizes the body to insulin and starts a vicious health-damaging cycle.

The fat gain also leads to several negative downstream effects, such as increased body inflammation (via cellular degradation) and increased blood glucose levels. The average American is either overweight or obese, and likely suffers from some level of insulin resistance (ex. prediabetes, or type 2 diabetes) due to their diet and overall lifestyle.

Obesity among all US adults reaches all-time high

By Victoria Larned, CNN
Updated 11:00 AM ET, Fri October 13, 2017

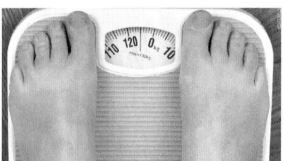

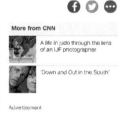

More from CNN

A life in judo through the lens of an IJF photographer

'Down and Out in the South'

Advertisement

The most recent statistics from the Center for Disease Control (CDC)[433] regarding the overall health of adults in the USA states that 40% of people are obese. Let's state that number again.

4 out of 10 adults in America are obese.

The cost of being overweight and obese is HUNDREDS OF BILLIONS of dollars for the US healthcare system. But more importantly, obesity-related health risks exponentially increase the chances of mortality (death).

How Insulin Works

Insulin is a peptide chain hormone (i.e. made up of proteins) created by beta cells in your pancreas. Beta cells are simply a type of cell in the pancreas that makes insulin. The pancreas is a glandular organ that is specifically evolved to produce insulin. Your pancreas works with your cardiovascular system 24/7 to produce insulin. There are cells called chemoreceptors in your vascular system (i.e. your blood vessels and veins) that constantly monitor glucose levels within the body. When you have excess blood glucose, your body produces insulin to bring the glucose level back to homeostasis (i.e. normal balance).

What does all of this mean? It means that your body tries to keep blood sugar stable, and within a certain healthy range. Anytime blood sugar goes up, insulin gets released to bring it back down.

Why does blood sugar go up? It goes up because you ate FOOD, some of which gets converted into glucose. Different foods cause different increases in blood sugar and insulin - some

---

[433]   https://www.cdc.gov/nchs/products/databriefs/db288.htm

higher, some lower. Carbohydrates, especially processed sugar and carbs, will make glucose go up the most. Foods that have zero sugar, such a sirloin steak, will cause an insulin response but there is little to no increase in blood sugar.

You now understand that insulin is released in response to blood sugar levels increasing, which happens whenever you eat food that contains carbohydrates. But how exactly does insulin lower blood sugar?

HOW DOES INSULIN WORK?

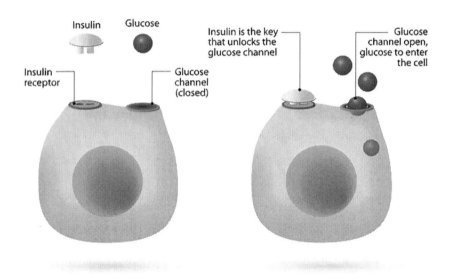

Insulin and Glucose Utilization

To answer that question, insulin lowers blood sugar by sending a signal to muscle cells, fat cells, and liver cells which tells them to absorb glucose from the blood. In essence, insulin tells these cells that there is way too much sugar floating around and it has to go somewhere, and so they are going to store the excess sugar.

In short, your body has three options for deciding WHERE the stored glucose goes: fat tissue, muscle tissue, and the liver.

Where it goes, however, depends on a few factors:

- Your muscle mass
- Your fat mass
- Your glycogen (stored glucose) stores in your liver
- Your resting blood sugar levels

Muscles use glycogen when they contract and extend during exercise. If you are about to exercise, are in the process of exercising, or have already exercised, then the glucose is going to go to the muscles first. This is a good thing, as it means that very little of the glucose will be stored as fat. When you have muscle and you regularly do resistance training with proper intensity, your body is far less likely to store glucose in fat cells. This is why building muscle tissue is so critical for overall health.

If your liver is depleted of glucose, which happens when you fast (i.e. don't eat for an extended period of time, or follow an insulin-controlled diet where carb intake is controlled), then your body will replenish the depleted glucose in the liver. When liver glycogen is depleted, your body is more likely to use stored body fat for fuel. When liver glycogen is full, however, fat storage is more likely. The liver can store anywhere between 100-200 grams of glucose in the form of glycogen[434].

---

[434] http://main.poliquingroup.com/ArticlesMultimedia/Articles/PrinterFriendly.aspx?ID=1122&lang=en

Fat cells can store glucose by converting it into fat. You do NOT want this to happen for the most part, as adding stored fat is never as good thing. Unfortunately, this is what happens for around 75% of Americans: They over-consume carbs, sugar and calories, which eventually get stored as excess body fat.

Insulin Resistance

With all of the above information taken into consideration, why is it therefore important to have stable blood sugar levels?

Your body stores blood sugar because too much sugar in the blood becomes TOXIC. Hyperglycemia (excess blood sugar) causes the following[435]:

- Vascular inflammation
- Long-term organ damage
- Cognitive decline (which contributes to Alzheimer's and dementia)
- Neurological dysfunction
- Immune system decline
- Damaged vision

Long story short: Your body does not want excess sugar in the blood, EVER. This is why being overweight or obese, along with overeating, is so damaging to your overall health. All of this damage eventually leads to insulin resistance and ultimately some level of diabetes.

---

[435] [Diabetes Mellitus, a prothrombotic disease]. Ann Cardiol Angeiol (Paris). 2017 Dec;66(6):385-392. doi: 10.1016/j.ancard.2017.10.011. Epub 2017 Oct 27.

Insulin resistance refers to a cascade effect that happens in the following manner:

- You eat too much, which leads to excess fat storage.
- Overeating, combined with poor diet choices, constantly spikes your insulin levels. As a result, your body's tissues STOP responding to elevated insulin levels.
- This lowered insulin response means that EVEN MORE insulin has to be produced in order to have the same effect.
- You store EVEN MORE fat. And now, you literally have a metabolism that is constantly in "store fat" mode.
- With worsened insulin sensitivity, you eventually develop type 2 diabetes if this excessive insulin environment persists long enough.
- On top of vascular inflammation, your cardiovascular system is being damaged daily due to your diet and body composition.

By now, it should be plainly obvious why you MUST live an insulin-controlled lifestyle!

The Major Myth of "Insulin Hypothesis"

One might think that insulin is the secret to losing fat, or that insulin by itself causes fat storage. WRONG!

While insulin plays a huge role in fat storage, insulin ALONE does NOT cause anyone to become overweight or obese. High insulin levels are a symptom of EXCESS CALORIE INTAKE. Remember how your body responds to insulin, as previously discussed: You overeat, and insulin levels increase as a result. This increase in insulin makes you more likely to overeat, among other factors. Following that, insulin increases from overeating, and so on and so forth.

Keep in mind that insulin is SUPPOSED to go up whenever you eat food. The major issue is when it goes up too high on a regular basis. This only happens when you are overeating, and/or eating lots of processed carbs and sugar.

Insulin is not the problem: YOUR LIFESTYLE IS! Insulin does not make you fat, and while controlling insulin IS a vital component of a healthy lifestyle, understand that CALORIE RESTRICTION is the ONLY thing that has been proven 10,000 times over to generate fat loss. LIkewise, consuming calories in excess is the ONLY thing that makes someone gain excess fat.

The science on this is extremely clear. Research has been done on all kinds of diets that have been heavy in sugar, potatoes, McDonald's, sodas and more. Over and over again, it is observed that regardless of food choice, weight loss will ALWAYS happen if calorie intake is controlled and kept below maintenance levels (i.e. the number of calories your body requires to sustain its current weight[436]). This is really the law of thermodynamics here.

Every study that has ever attempted to "prove" that calories don't matter, and that insulin alone makes you fat, have all failed. Every single one. There is no evidence that supports the idea.

---

[436] http://junkfoodscience.blogspot.com/2008/10/first-law-of-thermodynamics-in-real.html

How Do You Manage Your Insulin?

The fast and easy answer is DIET, followed by exercise. But diet always comes first. By making better choices with what you eat and when you eat it, you can begin altering your body's biochemistry almost immediately.

An insulin-controlled diet is one that is based upon whole, nutrient-rich foods. You can tailor this list to suit your preferences, but a good diet should consist of the following:

- Meat, fish, poultry, eggs
- Dairy products (greek yogurt, cottage cheese, etc.)
- Vegetables and tubers
- Fruit
- Legumes
- Nuts
- Healthy fat sources (ex. olive oil, walnut oil, macadamia nut oil, coconut oil, avocado oil)

With an insulin-controlled diet, the majority of your carbohydrate consumption should revolve around "low glycemic index (GI) carbs" (i.e. carbs that do not dramatically raise blood sugar levels or insulin levels).

The truth about carbohydrates is this: Not all carbs are equal, as different carbs affect the body in different ways. In fact, you can divide carbs into 'good' carbs and 'bad' carbs.

Good Carbs vs Bad Carbs

GOOD carbs are complex in structure, higher in fiber content, lower in sugar content and are digested slower by the body. They raise blood sugar the least, resulting in a lower insulin response. They are also known as low GI carbs, and are considered to be the healthiest carb sources.

Examples of good carbohydrates would be vegetables, rice, tubers, legumes (if your body digests them well), and fruit.

BAD carbs are simple in structure (comprised of simple sugars like monosaccharides and disaccharides), low in nutrients and fiber, higher in sugar content and are digested faster by the body. They sharply elevate blood sugar, causing a heightened insulin response. They are known as high GI carbs, and unsurprisingly they are also less satiating.

Examples of bad carbohydrates would be sugar, processed sugars, and processed grains.

If you want to learn more about the specific effects of individual foods, you can look them up on a glycemic load chart[437,438]. However, simply following the above heuristic should be enough to dramatically improve your food choices and therefore your health.

Optimal Versus Suboptimal Carbohydrate Consumption

In an optimal scenario, you strategically consume carbohydrates before, during, and after resistance training. You consume little to no sugar-heavy carbs, thereby avoiding excess glucose spikes

---

[437] https://www.health.harvard.edu/diseases-and-conditions/glycemic-index-and-glycemic-load-for-100-foods

[438] Atkinson FS, Foster-Powell K, Brand-Miller JC. International Tables of Glycemic Index and Glycemic Load Values: 2008. *Diabetes Care*. 2008;31(12):2281-2283. doi:10.2337/dc08-1239.

and insulin spikes. Your body stores the carbs you consume in the muscles as muscle glycogen. If you increase your muscle mass, your metabolism can better tolerate carbohydrates as your muscles use them for energy. You are also more physically active, which further increases the odds of your body using carbohydrates for energy instead of storing them as fat.

In a suboptimal situation, you have carbohydrates and sugar whenever you feel like it. You have excess body fat, are physically inactive, and do not have much lean body mass. The ongoing consumption of processed carbs and sugars means your body is often storing fat. The increased body fat leads to excessive levels of insulin and elevated blood sugar, and as a result you develop insulin resistance over time.

Overall Plan of Attack

With the dietary change established, an insulin-controlled lifestyle would consist of the following lifestyle habits:

1. **Lift weights to build muscle**[439]. 4 days a week is the sweet spot for optimal results. This will almost immediately begin to improve your insulin sensitivity.

2. **Eat low GI carbs and TIME your carb intake.** This means all your carbohydrates should come from veggies, rice, possibly some fruit. You should also eat your carbs around your training sessions, or minimally on the days you don't train. Essentially, this is a 'meat and veggies' diet.

---

[439] www.advancedforgedtraining.com

3. **Manage your SLEEP.** Sleep affects EVERY hormone in your body, including insulin. 6-8 hours of deep, uninterrupted sleep a night will improve your insulin sensitivity.

4. **Do CARDIO.** Start with aerobic cardio if you are deconditioned. If you are in better shape, do interval cardio 2-4 times a week. The effects of cardio done properly and frequently are powerful, especially on your insulin sensitivity.

5. **Use Metformin.** This will require a conversation with your doctor and a prescription. Metformin is a diabetes drug that not only improves insulin sensitivity, but also possesses profound anti-aging and life-extension properties. If you can get your doctor to prescribe it, it can be used to augment your health. If not, Berberine is an alternative that can be obtained over the counter.

Summary

Practicing a controlled insulin lifestyle will lead to a leaner & more muscular physique, lower incidence of disease, improved energy and better overall health.

CHAPTER 14 KEY TAKEAWAYS

- We tell you about the importance of living an insulin-controlled lifestyle and why the typical American diet has led to an all-time high in obesity and diabetes.

- We present a high-level overview of how insulin works in your body and when it is released.

- We provide much more detail about how insulin lowers blood sugar, and how exactly the body decides where it will store blood sugar. From this, you learn how fat storage becomes possible.

- We discuss why it is important to have stable blood sugar levels, and how one develops insulin resistance. We also outline the negative health effects of insulin resistance.

- We debunk the myth that insulin alone causes fat storage, and why losing fat all boils down to calorie restriction.

- We explain how to manage your insulin through an insulin-controlled diet. Specifically, we make the distinction between 'good' and 'bad' carbs while examining optimal and suboptimal strategies for carbohydrate consumption.

- With all of the above information taken into consideration, an overall plan of attack that gets you started on living a controlled insulin lifestyle is presented to you.

CHAPTER 15
Agents of Change

This chapter details the supplements, medications, and exotic substances we've personally used that have the ability to completely and radically alter human physiques while enhancing performance at the same time.

Both Jim and Jay have successfully used these "agents of change" on themselves, and have also recommended them to male and female professional athletes, bodybuilders, actors, Olympic athletes, high-level fitness competitors, and regular everyday people.

Each of the agents, listed in this chapter in alphabetical order, are worth the time and attention of any man or woman who truly wants to take their body to the ultimate level. These agents are safe and can be considered ultimate tools for a healthy optimized lifestyle. Think of this chapter as our biohacking guide to building the best YOU ever!

Albuterol

Albuterol is used for the treat-ment and management of asth-ma, bronchospasm and COPD (Chronic Obstructive Pulmonary Disease) to a lesser extent. Most of you have seen, or have direct experience with an Albuterol inhaler. However, you may not

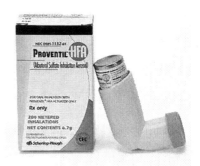

realize that Albuterol has been used as a safe and effective fat loss agent in select fitness and bodybuilding circles.

How Does It Work?

Albuterol is known as a beta-2 receptor adrenergic agonist. Beta-2 receptor agonists are known to accelerate fat burning[440], especially when they are in a low insulin environment (typically produced during the end of a long fasting window). Because Albuterol is a beta-2 receptor agonist, it will slowly downregulate the beta-2 receptors over time[441]. This means that its fat loss effects are lessened, and eventually fat loss from Albuterol will stall. Our real-world experience with using Albuterol for fat loss has shown us that dosing for two weeks "on" (taking it once a day), followed by two weeks "off" (not taking it at all) is optimal for maximum fat loss.

Side Effects

When dosed as recommended, side effects are rare. Some people may experience nervousness, or involuntary shaking of the hands or feet. Headaches and nausea is also listed on the insert packaging as a potential side effect. It is our opinion that these side effects would only appear with an over dosage (i.e. taking too much Albuterol).

---

[440] Molecular insights into the dynamics of pharmacogenetically important N-terminal variants of the human β2-adrenergic receptor. Shahane G, Parsania C, Sengupta D, Joshi M.PLoS Comput Biol. 2014 Dec; 10(12):e1004006. Epub 2014 Dec 11.

[441] Schiavone A, Tarantola M, Perona G, Pagliasso S, Badino P, Odore R, Cuniberti B, Lussiana C. Effect of dietary clenbuterol and cimaterol on muscle composition, beta-adrenergic and androgen receptor concentrations in broiler chickens. J Anim Physiol Anim Nutr (Berl). 2004;88(3-4):94-100.

Our Recommended Dosage and Usage

A peak fat-burning Albuterol dose is 3-6 mg per day, depending on body size (over 200 pounds would be 5-6 mg, below 200 pounds would be 3-4 mg). Albuterol can be found in pill form, research chemical liquid form, or as the image indicates, inhaler form. Because Albuterol possesses a half-life of only 4 – 6 hours, it is recommended that you use it early in the morning before doing fasted cardio. This recommendation stems from Albuterol's ability to mobilize stubborn fat tissue when combined with a low insulin environment. As we've already stated, it is best used for two weeks on, followed by two weeks off when fat loss is your primary goal.

Ashwagandha

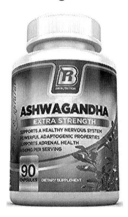

Ashwagandha is one of the most vital herbs in Ayurvedic (traditional Indian) healing. It's been known to provide several positive health benefits:

- Reduces anxiety and depression without causing fatigue[442].

- Stabilizes blood sugar and lowers LDL cholesterol levels[443].

---

[442] Andrade C1, Aswath A, Chaturvedi SK, Srinivasa M, Raguram R. A double-blind, placebo-controlled evaluation of the anxiolytic efficacy of an ethanolic extract of withania somnifera. Indian J Psychiatry. 2000 Jul;42(3):295-301.

[443] Andallu B1, Radhika B. Hypoglycemic, diuretic and hypocholesterolemic effect of winter cherry (Withania somnifera, Dunal) root. Indian J Exp Biol. 2000 Jun;38(6):607-9.

- Stimulates libido and enhance fertility in some men[444].

How Does It Work?

Ashwagandha is an adaptogen, which means it helps the body deal with stress by normalizing cortisol levels. Through lowering blood levels of cortisol, it reduces anxiety and increases relaxation at the same time[445]. Additionally, it's been used successfully with depressed people to enhance mood and improve overall well-being[446].

Side Effects

Ashwagandha should not be used by pregnant women as it may cause premature delivery. If you have an ulcer, Ashwagandha may aggravate your digestive tract. In diabetics, it can lower blood glucose levels. Finally, Ashwagandha may cause drowsiness as it slows down the nervous system. For that reason, you should stop using it 2 weeks before any medical procedure where an anesthetic is given because the anesthetic may accelerate the effects of Ashwagandha.

---

[444] Evid Based Complement Alternat Med. 2009 Sep 29. [Epub ahead of print] Withania somnifera Improves Semen Quality in Stress-Related Male Fertility. Mahdi AA1, Shukla KK, Ahmad MK, Rajender S, Shankhwar SN, Singh V, Dalela D.

[445] Indian J Psychol Med. 2012 Jul;34(3):255-62. doi: 10.4103/0253-7176.106022. A prospective, randomized double-blind, placebo-controlled study of safety and efficacy of a high-concentration full-spectrum extract of ashwagandha root in reducing stress and anxiety in adults.

[446] Anxiolytic-antidepressant activity of Withania somnifera glycowithanolides: an experimental study. Bhattacharya SK, Bhattacharya A, Sairam K, Ghosal S.Phytomedicine. 2000 Dec; 7(6):463-9.

Our Recommended Dosage and Usage

The minimum effective dose (and arguably the most cost-effective dose) is 300-500 mg taken on an empty stomach every day. However, it also can be taken with food.

The optimal dose for cortisol suppression is 6,000 mg a day, usually divided into three doses of 2,000 mg spread out evenly. While 300-500 mg taken daily is effective for most situations, a lower dose of 50-100 mg per day is effective in reducing the immunosuppression seen with high levels of stress. Jim and Jay have noticed that taking 2-4 grams right before bed promotes deeper sleep and increased relaxation.

Astaxanthin

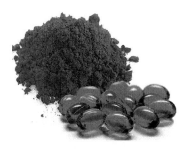

Astaxanthin is a powerful, naturally occurring carotenoid pigment that's found in certain marine plants and animals. Often called "the king of the carotenoids," astaxanthin is recognized as being one of the most powerful antioxidants found in nature. Unlike some other types of antioxidants, astaxanthin never becomes a pro-oxidant in the body, and therefore it can never cause harmful oxidation[447].

---

[447] https://www.amazon.com/Spirulina-Natures-Superfood-Helen-Morgan/dp/0963751131

How Does it Work

Astaxanthin is a carotenoid closely resembling beta-carotene in molecular structure. Naturally occurring in foods such as salmon, trout, lobster and shrimp, it is responsible for the reddish color found within these food sources. In fact, the microalgae known as *Haematococcus pluvialis* is the best source for finding this molecule at high concentrations[448]. Because of astaxanthin's unique molecular structure, this red-colored pigment is an extremely powerful antioxidant. Astaxanthin is the most powerful antioxidant in the carotenoid class (consisting of compounds such as zeaxanthin, tunaxanthin, lutein, etc.). It has been called "Super Vitamin E" due to its strength as an antioxidant in comparison to Vitamin E's tocopherol antioxidant activity.

While astaxanthin was initially introduced as a "super antioxidant" to the world at large, it has also been found to benefit a number of bodily functions. There have been at least eight clinical studies conducted in over 180 humans using astaxanthin to assess its safety, bioavailability and health benefits in relation to oxidative stress, inflammation and the cardiovascular system[449].

Eye Health – The chemical structure of astaxanthin is similar to lutein and zeaxanthin, two antioxidants that have been shown to reduce the risk of nuclear cataracts. However, astaxanthin has stronger antioxidant activity, along with a UV-light protection effect, both of which point to it being an excellent supplement for maintaining eye health.

---

[448] Shah MMR, Liang Y, Cheng JJ, Daroch M. Astaxanthin-Producing Green Microalga *Haematococcus pluvialis:* From Single Cell to High Value Commercial Products. *Frontiers in Plant Science.* 2016;7:531. doi:10.3389/fpls.2016.00531.

[449] Fassett RG, Coombes JS. Astaxanthin: A Potential Therapeutic Agent in Cardiovascular Disease. *Marine Drugs.* 2011;9(3):447-465. doi:10.3390/md9030447.

Cardiovascular – Astaxanthin has been shown to lower lipid levels, increase HDL levels and improve cognition and visual acuity[450]. In vivo studies of astaxanthin showed promise in protecting mitochondria from oxidative stress, allowing them to operate more efficiently[451]. Astaxanthin has also shown promise in potentially lowering blood pressure, as it may improve elastin levels and arterial wall thickness[452].

Fertility – There was a small study that showed improvements in sperm count, motility and overall fertility[453]. Would the benefit of improving fertility be compromised by TOT? A study would have to be designed to look more closely at the mechanisms of these findings.

Skin Health – Astaxanthin has been shown to help improve skin moisture levels, elasticity, and smoothness while reducing wrinkles, freckles, and spots[454].

Side Effects

Very few side effects are known and/or have been reported, and we don't know if it's safe to use astaxanthin during pregnancy

---

[450] Ambati RR, Siew Moi P, Ravi S, Aswathanarayana RG. Astaxanthin: Sources, Extraction, Stability, Biological Activities and Its Commercial Applications—A Review. *Marine Drugs*. 2014;12(1):128-152. doi:10.3390/md12010128.

[451] Ambati RR, Siew Moi P, Ravi S, Aswathanarayana RG. Astaxanthin: Sources, Extraction, Stability, Biological Activities and Its Commercial Applications—A Review. *Marine Drugs*. 2014;12(1):128-152. doi:10.3390/md12010128.

[452] Kumi Tominaga, Nobuko Hongo, Mariko Karato and Eiji Yamashita. Cosmetic benefits of astaxanthin on humans subjects*Fuji Chemical Industry Co. Ltd., Kamiichi, Toyama, Japan.

[453] Donà G, Kožuh I, Brunati AM, et al. Effect of Astaxanthin on Human Sperm Capacitation. *Marine Drugs*. 2013;11(6):1909-1919. doi:10.3390/md11061909.

[454] Kumi Tominaga, Nobuko Hongo, Mariko Karato and Eiji Yamashita. Cosmetic benefits of astaxanthin on humans subjects*Fuji Chemical Industry Co. Ltd., Kamiichi, Toyama, Japan.

and breastfeeding. If you're pregnant, stay on the safe side and avoid using it.

Our Recommended Dosage and Usage

If you are taking astaxanthin as part of your daily health maintenance regimen, **4 to 6 mg of BioAstin per day is recommended**. However, if you are taking astaxanthin for serious joint or tendon health problems, or if you're someone who does a lot of physical work or exercise, **12 mg per day is generally recommended**. It is important to note that since astaxanthin is a fat-soluble carotenoid, it works best when taking it with food as fat aids in the absorption of the antioxidant.

Cialis

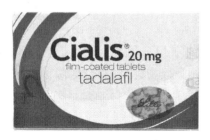

When men think of the drug Cialis, they think about older men enhancing erectile strength for better sex. We're here to tell you that this medication does much more than fix erectile dysfunction.

In fact, it has massive benefits for the aging male who is into TOT and life optimization as a whole! In fact, we rank Cialis just a shade below Metformin as the most effective anti-aging medication.

Cialis (**Tadalifil**) is a PDE5 inhibitor (i.e. a vasodilator, which describes a drug that 'opens' your blood vessels for increased blood flow). It is an FDA-approved medication in the USA for benign prostate hyperplasia[455] (BPH), a condition where the prostate constantly grows in size as a man ages. Cialis can also treat high blood pressure, but it is marketed under the brand name Adcirca for this specific purpose. Additionally, it will help individuals with normal blood pressure who are looking to improve their current numbers[456].

What if we told you that Cialis can also reduce inflammation in the body? It has been proven to reduce C-reactive protein levels (one important biomarker of body inflammation), and in doing so, it drastically lowers the buildup of plaque in your arteries[457]. This also makes Cialis a cardioprotective drug. Unsurprisingly, there are breakthrough studies[458] showing that Cialis has powerful protective effects against several clinical scenarios including myocardial ischemia/reperfusion injury, doxorubicin and post-MI, heart failure, cardiac hypertrophy and heart transplantation. In plain English, Cialis is clinically proven to help prevent heart disease and reduce the probability of heart attacks.

On top of all that, Cialis has been proven to increase lean muscle tissue in healthy aging males[459], while improving their

---

[455] Hatzimouratidis K. A review of the use of tadalafil in the treatment of benign prostatic hyperplasia in men with and without erectile dysfunction. *Therapeutic Advances in Urology.* 2014;6(4):135-147. doi:10.1177/1756287214531639.

[456] Safety and effectiveness of tadalafil in patients with pulmonary arterial hypertension: Japanese post-marketing surveillance data. Hiroyoshi Yamazaki, Noriko Kobayashi, Masanori Taketsuna, Koyuki Tajima & Masahiro Murakami.

[457] Lee JW, et al. Serum High-Sensitivity C-Reactive Protein Levels and Response to 5 mg Tadalafil Once Daily in Patients With Erectile Dysfunction and Diabetes. Korean J Urol. 2013 Dec;54(12):858-64.

[458] Kukreja RC. Sildenafil and cardioprotection. Curr Pharm Des. 2013;19(39):6842-7.

[459] Aversa A, et al. Tadalafil improves lean mass and endothelial function in nonobese men with mild ED/LUTS: in vivo and in vitro characterization. Endocrine. 2017 Jun;56(3):639-648.

testosterone-to-estrogen ratios[460]. Because of these benefits, some men may be able to use a lower dosage of an AI medication if Cialis is also being taken at daily low doses. The less you have to rely on AI medications, the better results you will see with your HDL cholesterol levels and your bone mineral density as you get older.

Finally, a big fear of prescribing testosterone to patients is the fear of prostate enlargement (even though this is a myth, as already proven in Chapter 12). Cialis is proven to relax the smooth muscles of the prostate, ultimately reducing any symptoms of BPH[461].

How Does It Work

When a man is sexually stimulated, nitric oxide is released into the penis. Nitric oxide enables the production of cGMP (Cyclic guanosine monophosphate), which controls the dilation (opening) and contraction (closing) of the blood vessels that carry blood to and from the penis. Another substance, PDE5 (phosphodiesterase type 5 inhibitor), destroys cGMP. When this occurs, the blood vessels return to their normal size and the erection ends. Cialis stops PDE5 from destroying cGMP, thereby causing the erection to last longer.

---

[460] Aversa, A., Fittipaldi, S., Bimonte, V.M. et al. Tadalafil modulates aromatase activity and androgen receptor expression in a human osteoblastic cell in vitro model. J Endocrinol Invest. (2016) 39: 199. https://doi.org/10.1007/s40618-015-0344-1.

[461] Effectiveness of tadalafil 5 mg once daily in the treatment of men with lower urinary tract symptoms suggestive to benign prostatic hyperplasia with or without erectile dysfunction: results from naturalistic observational TadaLutsEd study. Bechara A, Casabe A, Rodriguez Baigorri G, Cobreros C.J. *Sex Med.* 2014 Feb; 11(2):498-505. Epub 2013.

Cialis also works by increasing nitric oxide formation throughout the entire body. This causes vasodilation (opening of blood vessels) and improved blood flow to many tissues, including the brain. The improved blood flow also provides a better 'pump' in the gym[462]. In short, dosing Cialis at low levels will not only strengthen erections and protect the brain, but it will also improve exercise performance through vasodilation of the muscle cells.

Side Effects

Cialis, when used daily at low dosages, causes very few side effects. The reported side effects from taking too much Cialis include nausea, headache, flushing, dizziness, runny nose, indigestion, and muscle aches. Most of these side effects make sense, as dilating your blood vessels may cause your blood pressure to change. Therefore, a man who is already prescribed a nitrate drug for heart problems or chest pain should not use Cialis. Like any new drug you introduce into your daily regimen, consult with your physician and start at very low doses. It is highly unlikely that you will suffer any of the mentioned side effects if you follow our recommended dosages.

Our Recommended Dosage and Usage

To experience the numerous long-term health benefits of Cialis and avoid potential side effects, we recommend a minimum daily dosage of 2.5 to 7 mg. This is enough to get all of the

---

[462] Jacqueline K. Limberg, Katherine R. Malterer, J. Mikhail Kellawan, William G. Schrage, Brad W. Wilkins, Wayne T. Nicholson, John H. Eisenach, Michael J. Joyner, Timothy B. Curry. Phosphodiesterase-5 inhibition preserves exercise onset vasodilator kinetics when NOS activity is reduced. J Appl Physiol (1985). 2017 Oct 5:jap.00483.2017.

benefits previously discussed, while providing stronger erections. If you want to use this medication for a sexual 'boost' over the weekend, dosages up to 30 mg daily for the event are effective, with a return (following the event) to your smaller daily dose. Used correctly, a daily microdose of Cialis might be one of the most important life-enhancing medications an aging male can take.

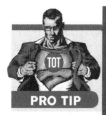

PRO TIP

It is unfortunate that the pharmaceutical industry charges such exorbitant rates for Cialis (Tadalafil) tablets. A very real and effective option to acquire Cialis for much cheaper is buying it from Research Chemical Companies. One can purchase 30 mg/mL, 30 mL vials for around $30[463]. We can not vouch for any specific company, but if you do purchase Cialis from any source, we recommend you have your product's efficacy tested first before using it. Bunk Police will test any research chemical. Their analyses are conducted at a government-sanctioned harm reduction facility in Europe that has access to the finest analytical technology available (GCMS, HPLC, and HPLC/UV, etc.)[464]. There are also off-shore pharmacy options with generic pill and tablet formulations cheaper than most US pharmacies. Just let Google be your friend.

---

[463] http://www.maximpeptide.com/tadalafil-30mg/

[464] http://bunkpolice.com/

Citrulline Malate

Citrulline is a nonessential amino acid that is isolated and extracted from watermelon rind. Commonly sold as L-Citrulline or Citrulline Malate (CM), it was identified as an essential catalyst in the body's urea cycle for proper kidney filtration and function[465]. Citrulline will also aid in nitric oxide (NO) production by raising arginine levels. As previously explained when discussing Cialis, NO is considered a potent vasodilator for the vascular system. Vasodilators improve blood flow.

How Does It Work

Citrulline is converted into arginine by the kidneys, which results in a greater rise in arginine blood levels than taking supplemental arginine at the same dosage[466]. However, it is believed that increasing arginine may not increase NO production as it isn't the rate limiting factor (i.e. the raw material needed in the synthesis of NO that runs out first) in NO synthesis. This is assuming that you have normal blood levels of arginine.

Certain disease processes, such as high blood pressure and/or adult onset diabetes, will lower arginine levels. In those cases, citrulline is effective at raising arginine levels back to normal levels while increasing NO production.

---

[465] Acute citrulline-malate supplementation improves maximal strength and anaerobic power in female, masters athletes tennis players. Glenn JM, Gray M, Jensen A, Stone MS, Vincenzo JL. Eur J Sport Sci. 2016 Nov; 16(8):1095-103. Epub 2016 Mar 28.

[466] L-citrulline-malate influence over branched chain amino acid utilization during exercise. Sureda A, Córdova A, Ferrer MD, Pérez G, Tur JA, Pons A. Eur J Appl Physiol. 2010 Sep; 110(2):341-51. Epub 2010 May 25.

There is scientific data[467] suggesting that CM reduces lactic acid, aids in removing ammonia during exercise, increases nitrogen retention, and plays a role in increasing ATP (a vital factor in the creation of cellular energy). The study in question said this: "This increase was positively correlated with the number of sets, achieving 52.92% more repetitions and the 100% of response in the last set. A significant decrease of 40% in muscle soreness at 24 hours and 48 hours after the pectoral training session and a higher percentage response than 90% was achieved with CM supplementation."

Going by the results of the study, it can be concluded that CM might be useful for increasing athletic performance in high-intensity anaerobic exercise with short rest times, while relieving post-exercise muscle soreness. Thus, athletes undergoing intensive preparation that involves a high level of training (or a competitive event) may benefit from using CM.

Side effects

Citrulline supplementation is considered to be safe and well tolerated. No common side effects have been found to date.

Our Recommended Dosage and Usage

We use CM around workouts, normally in a pre-workout or peri-workout drink combined with creatine monohydrate. The typical dosage is 3-12 grams per day, but we personally use 8 grams and experience noticeable effects such as better muscle pumps and an increased ability to train at a higher intensity.

---

467   Pérez-Guisado J1, Jakeman PM.Citrulline malate enhances athletic anaerobic performance and relieves muscle soreness. J Strength Cond Res. 2010 May;24(5):1215-22.

You can also add L-Arginine to the mix as a way to optimize NO levels. However, we recommend you start with low doses and gradually work your way up, especially if you are using CM alongside other NO-enhancing agents such as Cialis.

Creatine

Creatine is a naturally occurring compound in the body that is made up of three amino acids: Glycine, methionine and arginine. It can also be found in foods such as beef, chicken, and fish. It is mostly produced in the liver, but it may also be produced in the kidneys or pancreas. No matter where it is produced, it ultimately gets stored in muscle cells as creatine phosphate. Most readers of this book are likely familiar with creatine's use in fitness and weightlifting, but not nearly as many people understand its role in improving memory and cholesterol profiles.

How Does it Work?

Creatine is essential in regulating adenosine triphosphate (ATP) levels. It removes a phosphate group from ATP, resulting in the creation of creatine phosphate and adenosine diphosphate (ADP). Later on, creatine phosphate can return the phosphate to ADP and form ATP. Having an abundant supply of creatine phosphate is beneficial during short periods of intensive activity involving high energy demands (i.e. anaerobic activities such as sprinting or lifting weights, especially in the last few seconds).

Study after study has shown that creatine has multiple benefits. Here are a few:

- Significant improvements in repetitive high-power exercises (i.e. more total reps and less perceived fatigue)[468].

- Significant improvements in increasing bench press volume and total weight lifted, along with improvement in sprint performance[469].

- Significant increases in lean body mass[470].

- One study showed that creatine supplementation has positive effects on total cholesterol by lowering low density lipoproteins (LDL's) and triglycerides[471].

- Creatine reduces memory decline[472], while improving memory span and working memory[473,474].

Side Effects

If you have high blood pressure, or any kind of liver or kidney disease, you should consult your physician before supplementing with creatine. When starting to supplement with creatine, some

---

[468] Bird SP. Creatine supplementation and exercise performance: a brief review. *J Sports Sci Med.* 2003;2(4):123-32.

[469] Kreider RB, Ferreira M, Wilson M, Grindstaff P, Plisk S, Reinardy J, Cantler E, Almada AL. Effects of creatine supplementation on body composition, strength, and sprint performance. *Med Sci Sports Exerc.* 1998;30(1):73-82.

[470] http://thesportjournal.org/article/effects-of-creatine-supplementation

[471] Earnest CP, Almada AL, Mitchell TL. High-performance capillary electrophoresis-pure creatine monohydrate reduces blood lipids in men and women. *Clin Sci (Lond).* 1996;91(1):113-8.

[472] McMorris T, Mielcarz G, Harris RC, Swain JP, Howard A. Creatine supplementation and cognitive performance in elderly individuals. *Neuropsychol Dev Cogn B Aging Neuropsychol Cogn.* 2007;14(5):517-28.

[473] Rae C, Digney AL, McEwan SR, Bates TC. Oral creatine monohydrate supplementation improves brain performance: a double-blind, placebo-controlled, cross-over trial. *Proc Biol Sci.* 2003;270(1529):2147-50.

[474] Benton D, Donohoe R. The influence of creatine supplementation on the cognitive functioning of vegetarians and omnivores. *Br J Nutr.* 2011;105(7):1100-5.

people will experience water retention, but it tends to subside quickly. A few people may experience an upset stomach and loose bowels. While this typically subsides with frequent use, some people simply can't tolerate it well. Overall, creatine has been heavily studied and the consensus amongst experts is that it's a safe and effective supplement.

Our Recommended Dosage and Usage

If you naturally have a high amount of creatine in your body, you won't experience the same benefits as a person who naturally has a lower amount of creatine in their body. Your body can only hold so much creatine at one time, as some of it is circulating in your blood as pure creatine and the rest is stored in your muscles as creatine phosphate. You can take 50 grams a day (which is overkill), but you will only be able to retain and use a certain amount (the rest will be removed and excreted in your urine). If you are a regular meat eater, you will have a higher level of creatine in your body than someone who only consumes vegetables.

Most supplement companies recommend you use 'loading periods', where you will take a larger-than-normal dose of creatine for a short period of time before dropping down to a maintenance-level dose. This is unneeded. Instead, we recommend a maintenance dose of 3-6 grams a day.

You can take it in coffee, tea, or water. Some recommend taking creatine with carbs to increase absorption. However, the truth is that you don't need anything special to help absorption. In fact, you absorb it just fine when you eat meat!

There are a few different types of creatine sold on the market. We like creatine monohydrate. Some companies will try and sell you more expensive forms of creatine. In our experience, we have found a high-quality creatine monohydrate works very well. We tend to look for Creapure® Creatine Monohydrate, as it's a patented form that is easily affordable and ensures you are getting the best form of creatine available.

Desiccated Thyroid

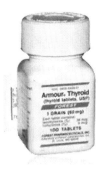
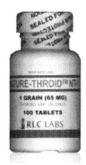

NatureThroid, Armour Thyroid and WP Thyroid (among others) are natural, dessicated thyroid hormone medications containing the active thyroid hormone constituents T_4, T_3, T_2 and T_1. Using any of these medications can slightly increase your basal metabolic rate (BMR) without the risk that comes with using harsh thyroid medications like Synthroid or Cytomel. Both Synthroid and Cytomel have well-understood side effects of permanently altering natural thyroid output when used inappropriately.

In plain English, using these medications in combination with a calorie-restricted diet can improve fat loss. Using them in combination with a muscle-building diet (i.e. your caloric intake is above your maintenance level caloric intake) can also improve caloric processing and burning. In essence, you will burn more calories while building muscle, leading to more lean muscle gain and less fat gain.

How Does it Work

Your physician must prescribe this for you. Your ability to qualify for a prescription is based on your TSH (Thyroid Stimulating Hormone) levels and whether there is an observed clinical need. If you do not qualify, there are over-the-counter (OTC) desiccated thyroid supplements available in a pill or capsule form. Dr. Robert Komininarek discusses subclinical hypothyroidism in clear detail in *Chapter 17 - The State of the Science in Male Hormonal Optimization.*

Side Effects

Negative bodily reactions due to a therapeutic overdose are rare (excluding those attributable to hyperthyroidism, where your thyroid is overactive). Side effects include changes in appetite, a fast (or irregular) heartbeat, nervousness and headaches.

Our Recommended Dosage and Usage

We recommend following the dosing instructions provided by your physician, or the manufacturer in countries where it's legal to purchase desiccated thyroid without a prescription. In either case, you want to consistently monitor your blood work. The end goal is to move your thyroid levels from the low range to the high range of what is considered optimal.

Energy Memory Focus (EMF) (OTC Nootropic)

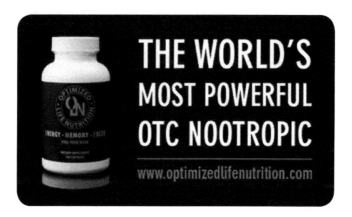

EMF by Optimized Life Nutrition (OLN)[475] is the strongest OTC (over the counter) nootropic we know of on the planet. It is an excellent nootropic to improve focus due to its unique formula. All of the ingredients within the formulation have been proven to improve cognition, drive and focus. It also has a mild appetite-suppressing ability, making it an excellent choice to use while on a fat loss diet. It's especially helpful during long fasting windows for improved fat loss and enhanced cognition.

How Does it Work?

By providing the breakdown of ingredients that are used in Energy Memory Focus, you will understand how it works.

Magnesium L-Threonate (MgT)

The typical American diet will lead to magnesium deficiency throughout the body. Among other roles within the brain, magnesium is involved in the activation of nerve canals responsible

---

[475] www.optimizedlifenutrition.com

for the plasticity of synaptic pathways. It is vital to the biological processes needed for learning and memory.

MgT is unique in that it can cross the blood brain barrier and activate these processes. Studies have clearly shown that MgT can increase long-term and short-term processes that are critical to learning[476]. The optimal human dose per serving has been widely accepted at 144 mg. This is why we put that exact amount in our formula.

Bacopa Monnieri (BM)

BM has been used since the 6th century to sharpen mental processes. It has been shown to improve attention, cognitive processing, and working memory. This is partly due to the suppression of acetylcholinesterase (AChE) and monoamine oxidase (MAO) activity[477].

AChE and MAO are enzymes that break down neurotrans-mitters such as dopamine and choline. Certain kinds of antidepressants can block the action of these enzymes, such as selective serotonin uptake inhibitors (SSRIs) and MAO inhibitors. This is also why BM has been reported to give users a better positive feeling after taking it. Additionally, drug cocktails made for treating Alzheimer's will typically include an AChE inhibitor.

---

[476] Slutsky I, Abumaria N, Wu LJ, Huang C, Zhang L, Li B, Zhao X, Govindarajan A, Zhao MG, Zhuo M, Tonegawa S, Liu G. Enhancement of learning and memory by elevating brain magnesium. Neuron. 2010;65(2):165-77.

[477] Peth-Nui T, Wattanathorn J, Muchimapura S, Tong-Un T, Piyavhatkul N, Rangseekajee P, Ingkaninan K, Vittaya-Areekul S. Effects of 12-week Bacopa monnieri consumption on attention, cognitive processing, working memory, and functions of both cholinergic and monoaminergic systems in healthy elderly volunteers. Evid Based Complement Alternat Med. 2012;2012:606424.

You will find BM in many formulas, but the research studies we based our dosage on averaged 500 mg per day from STANDARDIZED sources[478-479].

Rhodiola Rosea (RR)

RR is another herb with a very long use in human history, dating back to several centuries ago when it was first used to deal with extremely harsh living conditions and high levels of stress. Like BM, RR is an effective MAO inhibitor[480].

Recent studies have shown a significant reduction in self-reported anxiety, stress, anger, confusion and depression at 14 days, with major improvements in total mood when taking RR[481]. So, why did we specifically include it in our formula if it just makes you 'feel better'?

More research has concluded that RR will result in a reduction of mental fatigue and an improvement in mental processes involving complex perceptive and cognitive cerebral functions, such as associative thinking, short-term memory, mathematical

---

[478] Aguiar S, Borowski T. Neuropharmacological review of the nootropic herb Bacopa monnieri. Rejuvenation Research. 2013;16(4):313-26.

[479] Kumar N, Abichandani LG, Thawani V, Gharpure KJ, Naidu MUR, Venkat Ramana G. Efficacy of standardized extract of Bacopa monnieri (Bacognize®) on cognitive functions of medical Students: A six-week, randomized placebo-controlled trial. Evidence-based complementary and alternative medicine : eCAM. 2016;2016:4103423.

[480] van Diermen D, Marston A, Bravo J, Reist M, Carrupt PA, Hostettmann K. Monoamine oxidase inhibition by Rhodiola rosea L. roots. J Ethnopharmacol. 2009;122(2):397-401.

[481] Cropley M, Banks AP, Boyle J. The effects of Rhodiola rosea L. extract on anxiety, stress, cognition and other mood symptoms. Phytother Res. 2015;29(12):1934-9.

calculation, mental concentration, and speed of audio-visual perception[482].

What better addition to a nootropic than a compound that will help your brain deal with stress so it can be focused on the task at hand? Again, we included a CLINICAL RR dosage of 500 mg in our formulation.

TeaCrine®

TeaCrine® is the trademarked version of theacrine. TeaCrine® inhibits adenosine, which decreases feelings of fatigue. It also enhances neural drive, providing better focus while also supporting a positive mood and heightened motivation. TeaCrine is such a revolutionary supplement that it does all of the following[483]:

- Boosts mental + physical energy
- Increases mental energy without jitters, irritability, or habituation
- Supports a positive mood
- Increases one's motivation to exercise
- Improves perceived focus + concentration

---

[482] Darbinyan V, Kteyan A, Panossian A, Gabrielian E, Wikman G, Wagner H. Rhodiola rosea in stress induced fatigue—a double blind cross-over study of a standardized extract SHR-5 with a repeated low-dose regimen on the mental performance of healthy physicians during night duty. Phytomedicine. 2000;7(5):365-71.

[483] Please refer to this page for more information: http://www.compoundsolutions.com/benefits.html

L-Tyrosine

L-Tyrosine is a supplement that is also known as a building block of various neurotransmitters. It has been clinically shown to help during periods of stress and sleep deprivation by replenishing neurotransmitters[484]. Research data has shown that L-Tyrosine may also increase working memory while performing multiple tasks at once[485]. Once again, we have a REAL dose of 500 mg.

Although studies show mixed results, empirical evidence suggests that L-Tyrosine is useful as a pre-workout stimulant when combined with other substances such as caffeine. It seems to enhance the effect of other stimulatory substances, which we have both experienced.

L-Tyrosine has also shown promise in alleviating the decrease in cognitive performance associated with stress and fatigue. For this reason, it might be useful for keeping your mind sharp during intense stints of dieting, such as what is found in *The Metabolic Blowtorch Diet*[486].

Our Recommended Dosage and Usage

EMF can be used for many applications! It can be used for improved focus during intense work tasks, blunting appetite during long fast windows and improving your energy levels before cardio or weight training. We have found that using

---

[484] Magill RA, Waters WF, Bray GA, Volaufova J, Smith SR, Lieberman HR, McNevin N, Ryan DH. Effects of tyrosine, phentermine, caffeine D-amphetamine, and placebo on cognitive and motor performance deficits during sleep deprivation. Nutr Neurosci. 2003;6(4):237-46.

[485] Thomas JR, Lockwood PA, Singh A, Deuster PA. Tyrosine improves working memory in a multitasking environment. Pharmacol Biochem Behav. 1999;64(3):495-500.

[486] www.metabolicblowtorchdiet.com

it on fasting days before early morning cardio and early/mid afternoon will help suppress appetite while increasing energy and focus. Many people have also found that using EMF before training sessions improves neural drive during the workout.

The optimal dosage really depends on one's body size and whether a person is sensitive to stimulants or not. We have found that 2-3 capsules on an empty stomach in the early morning to be a good starting point for most people. If you are a heavy stimulant user, a full dosage (5 capsules) will provide the best response.

For a concise explanation on how to best use EMF, read "How to Use the World's Strongest Nootropic - Energy Memory Focus" on TRTRevolution.com[487]. Make sure you also watch the video Jay did discussing how to use it on YouTube[488].

EMF is sold exclusively at: www.OptimizedLifeNutrition.com

Human Growth Hormone (HGH)

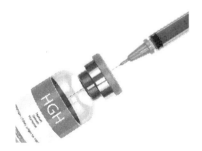

HGH is a peptide hormone (i.e. protein molecule), also medically known as 'somatropin', that is secreted and regulated by the pituitary gland. It plays many vital roles in the body, such as cellular regeneration, reproduction and growth.

One of the most pronounced roles of HGH is to stimulate IGF-1 (insulin-like growth factor 1) synthesis by binding to the growth

---

[487] http://www.trtrevolution.com/how-to-use-energy-memory-focus/

[488] https://youtu.be/IhX4edxPdKs

hormone receptors found in various muscle tissues. IGF-1 is responsible for growth of almost every cell in the body, thereby highlighting the importance of HGH.

HGH generally counteracts the effects of insulin on glucose and lipid metabolism[489]. Specifically, it acutely decreases glucose oxidation (secondary to an increase in lipid oxidation) and suppresses muscle uptake of glucose, suggesting that HGH redistributes glucose through a buildup of glycogen (via gluconeogenesis). Since HGH secretion is blocked in the fed state (i.e. when you have eaten food), these actions are mainly important in the fasting state. Under pathological conditions of excess HGH levels (e.g. acromegaly, or high dose HGH treatment) the diabetogenic (i.e. diabetes-promoting) actions of HGH become apparent.

We're briefly mentioning HGH, only because it is legal to use in the USA with a highly specific medical diagnosis of growth hormone deficiency (GHD). The best way for a clinician to obtain this diagnosis is through Glucagon Stimulation Testing[490]. For most healthy aging patients, this diagnosis normally comes from a head trauma, even though the cause is likely idiopathic (i.e. it is presently unknown). There are also certain genetic mutations that can arise in HGH receptors and result in a pituitary hormone deficiency. In our opinion, for the average male or female looking to optimize their health and combat the effects of aging, the cost of using a medically prescribed dose of HGH (when there is measured and legal clinical need) far outweighs the potential benefits, especially in comparison to peptide hormones.

---

489   Møller N1, Jørgensen JO. Effects of growth hormone on glucose metabolism. Horm Res. 1991;36 Suppl 1:32-5.

490   Cesar L. Boguszewski. Glucagon stimulation test: has its time come? Endocrine (2017) 57: 361. https://doi.org/10.1007/s12020-017-1356-8.

How Does It Work?

It functions by binding to the growth hormone receptor found on the cell surface of many different organs and tissues within the body. The binding of HGH to the receptors will trigger biochemical signalling cascades that stimulate an anabolic environment, which supports greater muscle growth while also promoting fat loss. One of the primary ways that HGH triggers muscle growth is by binding to HGH receptors on liver cells, stimulating the production of insulin-like growth factor 1 (IGF-1). This stimulates the muscle satellite cells to increase muscle cell protein synthesis levels, ultimately leading to muscle growth[491]. In our experience, if you want a cost-effective way to improve your IGF-1 levels while on TOT, using a **G**rowth **H**ormone **R**eleasing **P**eptide like Ipamorelin (discussed later in this chapter) is the best option.

Side Effects

There are no systematic research studies on the adverse effects of HGH usage. Much of the information regarding negative side effects comes from the studies of patients with acromegaly. This is a disease caused by excessive HGH production, resulting in abnormal growth of the hands, feet and face. High HGH levels in these patients often leads to hypertension, congestive heart failure, cardiomyopathy, insulin resistance, diabetes and even increased mortality[492].

In the competitive bodybuilding community, known side effects from supraphysiologic dosages (i.e. excessively high dosages)

---

[491] Schiaffino S, Mammucari C. Regulation of skeletal muscle growth by the IGF1-Akt/PKB pathway: insights from genetic models. Skeletal Muscle. 2011;1:4.

[492] Wass J, Trainer P and Korbonits M. Oxford Textbook on Endocrinology and Diabetes. 1994 (2nd ed): p. 197-209

are carpal tunnel, water retention, edema, insulin resistance, type 2 diabetes and accelerated cancer growth in individuals who are predisposed to it.

Our Recommended Dosage and Usage

When one has a legal prescription to use HGH, physiologic dosages of 1-3 IU's (international units) injected daily are reasonably safe and will enhance fat loss and nutrient partitioning (uptake) via a slight increase in BMR (Basal Metabolic Rate). HGH will also improve sleep, recovery and skin elasticity in aging men and women. Long-term therapy with adults deficient in HGH has shown no increase in the incidence of cardiovascular disease or cancer[493] (although pre-existing cancers can arise more often).

Some clinicians recommend dosing schedules of every other day (EOD) or even a "5-2" schedule (i.e. you take a dose each day on Monday through Friday, but don't take a dose on Saturday or Sunday). A patient's response to HGH dosing is monitored by measuring IGF-1 levels, which should not exceed the normal range[494] (i.e. levels should not go above 1.96 µg/L). As we've already stated, using 3 IU's of pharmaceutical-grade HGH (with a prescription) 5 days a week will cost around $3000-$4500 per month. For the average person, the cost does not equal the

[493] Christa C. van Bunderen, I. Caroline van Nieuwpoort, Lucia I. Arwert, Martijn W. Heymans, Anton A. M. Franken, Hans P. F. Koppeschaar, Aart J. van der Lely, Madeleine L. Drent; Does Growth Hormone Replacement Therapy Reduce Mortality in Adults with Growth Hormone Deficiency? Data from the Dutch National Registry of Growth Hormone Treatment in Adults, *The Journal of Clinical Endocrinology & Metabolism,* Volume 96, Issue 10, 1 October 2011, Pages 3151–3159. https://doi.org/10.1210/jc.2011-1215.

[494] Rosario, Pedro Weslley. (2010). Normal values of serum IGF-1 in adults: results from a Brazilian population. *Arquivos Brasileiros de Endocrinologia & Metabologia,* 54(5), 477-481.

reward, especially when there are *growth hormone releasing peptides* (GHRP's) that provide a similar beneficial effect for far less money.

Ipamorelin

In the last 10 years, a class of drugs known as growth hormone

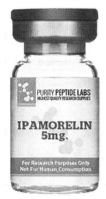

releasing peptides (GHRPs)[495] have come into the marketplace. GHRPs are synthetic forms of the natural hormone ghrelin. They are known for their ability to increase insulin-like growth factor (IGF-1) and natural Human Growth Hormone (HGH) production, all while being affordable.

As already mentioned earlier in this chapter, HGH is naturally produced in the pituitary gland and plays a vital role in cell regeneration, cell growth and maintaining healthy human tissues in the brain and various vital organs. Once secreted, HGH remains active in the bloodstream for a few minutes, allowing just enough time for the liver to convert it into various growth factors. Out of all the growth factors, the most crucial one is IGF-1[496], which has growth-promoting properties for every cell in the body.

Peptides are chains of amino acids that serve as the building blocks of proteins. There are numerous forms of these peptides that are sold as drugs on the market. Many of them are not FDA-approved, and are sold online by research chemical

---

[495] Ghigo E1, Arvat E, Muccioli G, Camanni F. Growth hormone-releasing peptides. Eur J Endocrinol. 1997 May;136(5):445-60.

[496] https://en.wikipedia.org/wiki/Insulin-like_growth_factor_1

manufacturers[497]. The most prescribed FDA-approved growth hormone secretagogue is **Sermorelin**, which many anti-aging practices provide to their patients. Sermorelin is a 29-amino acid polypeptide containing the 1st through 29th amino acids found in endogenous growth hormone releasing hormone (GHRH). It is the most widely used member of the GHRH analogue drug class. It can significantly promote the release of growth hormone (GH), improving the serum concentrations of GH and subsequently insulin-like growth factor 1 (IGF-1)[498,499].

Due to the short biological half-life (15 minutes) of Sermorelin, administration must occur periodically several times a day in multiple subcutaneous injections[500]. The best time to inject Sermorelin is right before sleeping as it will help increase the amplitude of the largest natural GH pulse, which occurs during your first REM cycle. Sermorelin has also been shown to be a regulator of sleep patterns and hormone secretion[501]. It elicits an increase in the amount of slow wave sleep (SWS) while augmenting GH secretion and reducing cortisol secretion. Many users report better sleep and feeling more refreshed in the morning after taking Sermorelin[502].

[497] http://www.maximpeptide.com/peptides/

[498] Chen, R.G., et al., A comparative study of growth hormone (GH) and GH-releasing hormone(1-29)-NH2 for stimulation of growth in children with GH deficiency. Acta Paediatr Suppl, 1993. 388: p. 32-5; discussion 36.

[499] Perez-Romero, A., et al., Effect of long-term GHRH and somatostatin administration on GH release and body weight in prepubertal female rats. J Physiol Biochem, 1999. 55(4): p. 315-24.

[500] Walker, R.F., Sermorelin: a better approach to management of adult-onset growth hormone insufficiency? Clin Interv Aging, 2006. 1(4): p. 307-8.

[501] Walker RF. Sermorelin: A better approach to management of adult-onset growth hormone insufficiency? *Clinical Interventions in Aging.* 2006;1(4):307-308.

[502] Steiger, A., et al., Growth hormone-releasing hormone (GHRH)-induced effects on sleep EEG and nocturnal secretion of growth hormone, cortisol and ACTH in patients with major depression. J Psychiatr Res, 1994. 28(3): p. 225-38.

Another FDA-approved secretagogue is **Tesamorelin** (sold as Egrifta), which we briefly mention as 'on our radar' later in this chapter.

Jim and Jay have experimented with all of the various GHRP's, and in our opinion the best one is **Ipamorelin**. Why? Put simply, it allows users to experience the positive benefits of increased natural HGH production with next to no side effects. Due to its ability to increase natural HGH production without stimulating the release of both cortisol and prolactin[503], it is the most strategically effective GHRP on the market. Increased levels of cortisol and prolactin often lead to potential negative side effects such as increased breast tenderness and discharge (i.e. gynecomastia and lactation), a suppressed immune system, hypertension (high blood pressure), high blood sugar (hyperglycemia), insulin resistance, metabolic syndrome and type 2 diabetes.

Other GHRPs (GHRP-6, GHRP-2, Hexarelin, etc.), some of which are stronger in their ability to increase growth hormone release than Ipamorelin, have noticeable negative side effects that normally come from increased cortisol and prolactin production. GHRP-6 and GHRP-2 also elevate hunger levels, which is terrible for people trying to lose body fat while reducing their insulin signal and ultimately their risk of inflammation. These side effects do not exist with Ipamorelin, even with high doses administered at a higher frequency. This makes it a much more versatile peptide for usage at night before bed, and if you choose to dose it throughout the day. If you want to know more about the various GHRP's available and how to best use them, read Ben Greenfield's excellent article titled '*How To Use Growth*

---

[503] Ipamorelin, the first selective growth hormone secretagogue. Eur J Endocrinol. 1998 Nov;139(5):552-61.

Hormone Stacks For A Better Body: Everything You Need To Know About IGF-LR3, GHRP, and GHRH Peptide Stacks[504].'

Ipamorelin is the mildest GHRP, but it's not the weakest. It can be used at 1,200 mg a day without stopping your body from producing HGH naturally. Studies have even shown[505] that large saturation (i.e. extremely high) doses of Ipamorelin have almost no effect on the body's natural production of growth hormone (GH). As a GHRP, it has the longest half life[506] and at higher doses it is even more potent. For all the reasons described thus far, we recommend Ipamorelin as the first and primary GHRP for people to use.

How does it Work?

After injecting Ipamorelin subcutaneously (i.e. under the skin), a selective pulse that lasts for roughly 3 hours stimulates the pituitary to release HGH. Once the HGH pulse is sent, it goes directly to the muscle to support development (i.e. lean muscle growth) while staying clear of any possible bone or cartilage growth. This is especially important as accidental growth in either of the two areas can lead to deformities later down the road.

For long-term Ipamorelin users, consistent usage will increase cell synthesis, elevate secretion levels of insulin from pancreatic

---

504 https://bengreenfieldfitness.com/article/supplements-articles/how-to-use-growth-hormone-stacks/

505 Histol Histopathol. 2002;17(3):707-14. Influence of chronic treatment with the growth hormone secretagogue Ipamorelin, in young female rats: somatotroph response in vitro. Jiménez-Reina L1, Cañete R, de la Torre MJ, Bernal.

506 Pharm Res. 1999 Sep;16(9):1412-6. Pharmacokinetic-pharmacodynamic modeling of ipamorelin, a growth hormone releasing peptide, in human volunteers. Gobburu JV1, Agersø H, Jusko WJ, Ynddal L.

tissue, and increase ghrelin in the stomach (which helps release HGH and control hunger). All of these functions work together to promote fat loss, improve the shuttling and absorption of nutrients, and potentially build skeletal muscle mass. This improves overall body composition and also minimizes, if not entirely suppresses unwanted side effects.

The pituitary gland releases HGH due to the action of chemicals that attach to two receptors: the Growth Hormone Releasing Hormone Receptor (GHRH-R) and the Growth Hormone Secretagogue Receptor (GHS-R).

The graph shows how combining a GHRH (Sermorelin, CJC-1295) with a GHS (Ipamorelin, GHRP-2, GHRP-6) causes synergistic release (i.e. their positive effects are combined to create one larger positive effect). GHS requires endogenous hypothalamic GHRH for maximal GH stimulation[507].

Using Ipamorelin with a **GHRH** like Sermorelin or CJC-1295 without DAC, also known as DAC:GRF (short for drug affinity complex:growth hormone-releasing factor), will give users the biggest increase in GH and IGF-1. CJC-1295 without DAC is a 30-amino acid peptide hormone that will release a series of pulses over a long period of time.

GHRHs are paired specifically with GHRPs in order to create a synergy between the peptides that will unlock the body's own stores of HGH, ultimately improving the benefits of Ipamorelin over time. Again, for a detailed discussion about why you would want to stack a GHRP with a GHRH, read Ben Greenfield's excellent article, 'How To Use Growth Hormone Stacks For A

---

[507]   Naushira Pandya, Roberta Demott-Friberg, Cyril Y. Bowers, Ariel L. Barkan, And Craig A. Jaffe, Journal of Clinical Endocrinology and Metabolism 1998 Vol. 83, No. 4.

Better Body: Everything You Need To Know About IGF-LR3, GHRP, and GHRH Peptide Stacks'[508].

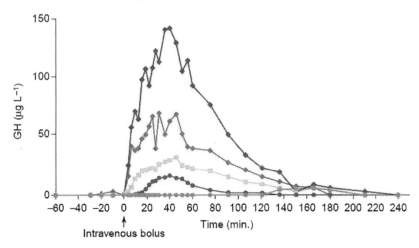

Comparative growth hormone (GH) responses in individual subjects. GH responses, together with the area-under-the-curve (in µg L⁻¹ after 4 h treatment) is as follows: placebo (orange, 540); 0.1 µg kg⁻¹ growth hormone-releasing peptide (GHRP; blue, 916); 1 µg kg⁻¹ GHRP (green, 5319); 1 µg kg⁻¹ growth hormone-releasing hormone (GHRH; yellow, 2590); 0.1 µg kg⁻¹ GHRP plus 1 µg kg⁻¹ GHRH (red, 10,065) in two normal men J. Clin. Endocrinol. Metab. 70, 975-982*

Side Effects

Even though Ipamorelin is the mildest and safest GHRP, it still comes with the possibility of some minor side effects. Theoretically, Ipamorelin at high doses could lead to higher cortisol levels. But in practice, when Ipamorelin is the only GHRP used as part of a nightly (before bed) dosing regimen, there is very little increase in cortisol levels (if at all).

---

[508] https://bengreenfieldfitness.com/article/supplements-articles/how-to-use-growth-hormone-stacks/

Some users will experience a "head rush" and get slight headaches. Therefore, start supplementation at a lower dose and gradually work your way up. GHRPs can also cause slight water retention (most noticeable in the lower abdominal region). However, it will disappear when you stop using it. Specifically, we have observed that water retention stops within 10 days of consistent usage.

Our Recommended Dosage and Usage

Ipamorelin, like other peptides, comes as a delicate freeze-dried powder. You can store it in the refrigerator, or at room temperature before reconstituting it (i.e. preparing it for injection). Once reconstituted with bacteriostatic water, the vials must be stored in a cool and dry place like your refrigerator. Bacteriostatic (i.e. stops bacteria from reproducing without necessarily killing them) water[509] is a sterile, non-pyrogenic (non-flammable) preparation of water used for injection. It contains 0.9% (9 mg/mL) of benzyl alcohol, which is used as a bacteriostatic preservative. Insulin syringes are the best way to administer Ipamorelin after reconstitution, usually via subcutaneous injection (lower abdominal region or gluteal fat pocket).

The average dose for Ipamorelin is **200-300mcg, injected subcutaneously one to three times daily**. Some users inject Ipamorelin **30-45 minutes before training** to take advantage of the HGH pulse and maximize both training intensity and fat loss. Most users will see body composition changes with 300 mg, once or twice per day, over a 3 month period (or longer).

---

[509]   https://westendmedicalsupplies.com/products/bacteriostatic-water-30ml

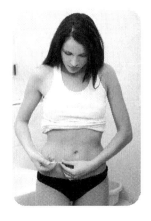

Ipamorelin for Women

Ipamorelin is an amazing agent for women who want to improve their body composition. An **injection of 200-300mcg immediately before bed** can produce dramatic fat loss and improved body composition in less than 3 months (when combined with resistance training[510], cardiovascular training and insulin-controlled living).

It also significantly improves REM sleep, skin quality and (often times) libido. Most of the women we've consulted with who have used Ipamorelin (3-6 months or longer) experienced dramatic transformations in their physique. In fact, when used at the minimum effective dose (MED), it actually works much better in women than men.

Melanotan I and Melanotan II

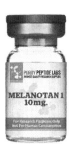

Melanotan I (**M1**), also known as Afamelanotide, and **Melanotan II** (**M2**) are both analogs of the peptide hormone called "alpha-melanocyte stimulating hormone" (a-MSH). Both **M1** and **M2** are naturally occurring melanocortin peptide hormones that research and clinical trials have shown to induce skin pigmentation (tanning) via melanogenesis (i.e. the formation of melanin).

---

[510] www.advancedforgedtraining.com

The more melanin you have, the more protection your skin has against the sun[511]. This subsequently reduces ultraviolet damage done to your skin. Both of these peptide hormones increase production of the hormone melanin, allowing for the skin to naturally darken when exposed to the sun's UV rays.

Melanotan I and II are primarily used by people who want to achieve a tanned skin color (i.e. a darker complexion) without having to sit in the sun for long hours and expose themselves to UV radiation (and hence increase the risk of getting sunburn). Based on our combined 20 years of experience in using Melanotan, it is our belief that increasing one's production of melanin (thereby darkening the skin) also improves or enhances conscious awareness. It's hard to explain in words.

Dr. Frank Barr, pioneering discoverer of melanin's overall organizing ability in living systems and other fascinating properties, proposes the following theory in his technical work *Melanin: The Organizing Molecule*[512]:

> *"The hypothesis is advanced that (neuro)melanin (in con-junction with other pigment molecules such as the isopen-tenoids) functions as the major organizational molecule in living systems. Melanin is depicted as an organizational "trigger" capable of using established properties such as photon-(electron)-photon conversions, free radical-redox mechanism, ion exchange mechanisms, and semi-conduc-tive switching capabilities to direct energy to strategic mo-lecular systems and sensitive hierarchies of protein enzyme*

---

[511]   The protective role of melanin against UV damage in human skin. *Brenner M, Hearing VJ.Photochem Photobiol.* 2008 May-Jun; 84(3):539-4.

[512]   Melanin: the organizing molecule. Med Hypotheses. 1983 May;11(1):1-139.

cascades. Melanin is held capable of regulating a wide range of molecular interactions and metabolic processes..."

Dr Barr's work is so profound that he summarized the role of melanin in his obscured research study from 1983:

> **Melanin's role in embryological organization and tissue repair /regeneration via sustained or direct current is considered in addition to its possible control of the major homeostatic regulatory systems—autonomic, neuroendocrine, and immunological.**

Another fascinating study titled *The self-organizing fractal theory as a universal discovery method: the phenomenon of life*[513] makes the following incredible statements about Melanin:

> *Consider melanin, an ancient pigment found in all biological kingdoms. In humans, melanin is present in skin, hair, the brain, the nervous system, the eye, the adrenal gland, and the inner ear.*

> *Melanin acts as an amorphous semiconductor. Melanin can quench radical species as well as produce them. Melanin dissipates all sorts of absorbed radiation in a non-radiative manner **through an efficient but rather mysterious process.***

> *Melanin participates in electron transfer reactions, reducing and oxidizing other molecules. A key monomer of melanin has been reported to perform photon-driven proton transfer cycles. Melanin exhibits strong electron-phonon coupling and is one of the best sound-absorbing materials known.*

---

[513]   Kurakin A. The self-organizing fractal theory as a universal discovery method: the phenomenon of life. Theoretical Biology & Medical Modelling. 2011;8:4. doi:10.1186/1742-4682-8-4.

Consequently, it has been proposed that melanin may function as a broad-band radiation energy harvester, in a manner similar to chlorophyll.

How Does It Work?

First let's discuss the differences between Melanotan I (M1) and Melanotan II (M2).

M1 *emulates the action* of the melanocyte-stimulating hormone (MSH), while also emulating the effect of naturally produced melanocyte. In other words, it tans you more naturally (relative to your maximum allowable tan). In the experience of most users, M1 gradually tans you and provides a more uniform color based on your skin tone (while working in unity alongside your body's natural melanocytes).

M2 *emulates the effect* of naturally produced melanocyte, and is a shorter version of the peptide called afamelanotide. M2 also has the unique ability to stimulate erections[514]. Most users notice a reddish brown tint to their skin with it, and their skin darkens much faster than when using M1.

M2 acts as a non-selective agonist of the melanocortin receptors MC_1, MC_3, MC_4, M[515]. To the extent that M2 produces melanin, this is thought to be caused by activation of the MC1 receptor. Its observed sexual effects, on the other hand, are thought to be related to its ability to activate the MC_4 receptor (though

---

[514] Synthetic melanotropic peptide initiates erections in men with psychogenic erectile dysfunction: double-blind, placebo controlled crossover study. Wessells H, Fuciarelli K, Hansen J, Hadley ME, Hruby VJ, Dorr R, Levine N.J Urol. 1998 Aug; 160(2):389-93.

[515] Wikberg, Jarl ES (2001). "Melanocortin receptors: new opportunities in drug discovery." *Expert Opinion on Therapeutic Patents.* 11 (1): 61–76. ISSN 1354-3776. doi:10.1517/13543776.11.1.61.

the MC$_3$ is thought to possibly be involved as well)[516]. In plain English, M2 works to darken skin tone faster that M1 does (and in a more pronounced way) while also stimulating erections.

Side Effects

In our experience with using M1, noticeable side effects are next to none. Some people have reported a slight flushing sensation at the point of injection. Others report a temporary head rush, similar to what people feel when taking the supplement niacin.

Potential side effects of M2 are sometimes more pronounced, including flushing, nausea, vomiting, yawning, and loss of appetite[517]. The other known issue with M2 are the potential side effects of uneven skin pigmentation, new nevi development (i.e. moles) and the darkening or enlargement of existing moles. These side effects are essentially why the medical community discourages the use of M2[518].

Our Recommended Dosage and Usage

Jim and Jay have both been using Melanotan on and off for close to 10 years. Jay has been using it in a minimum effective dose (MED) fashion at one to two sub-q (subcutaneous) injections per week, dosing 0.25 mg per injection. This has

---

[516] King SH, Mayorov AV, Balse-Srinivasan P, Hruby VJ, Vanderah TW, Wessells H (2007). "Melanocortin receptors, melanotropic peptides and penile erection." Curr Top Med Chem. 7 (11): 1098–1106. PMC 2694735 . PMID 17584130. doi:10.21 74/156802661070701111.

[517] Alan J. Wein; Louis R. Kavoussi; Andrew C. Novick; Alan W. Partin; Craig A. Peters (28 September 2011). Campbell-Walsh Urology. Elsevier Health Sciences. pp. 743. ISBN 1-4557-2298-7.

[518] Brennan R, Wells JS, Van Hout MC. The injecting use of image and performance-enhancing drugs (IPED) in the general population: a systematic review. Health Soc Care Community. 2016 Jan 25

produced a complete change in his complexion (a darker skin tone year-round with minimum sun exposure), while elevating his consciousness. This has manifested itself in his overall productivity, and an improved ability to read voraciously and recall vast quantities of information. We don't recommend M2 as strongly as M1 (based on documented research studies and the empirical observation of peers) due to its ability to increase mole formation and darken EXISTING ONES. At the same time, there are many members of the fitness community who use M2 in microdose fashion, and report few (if any) side effects. As always, experiment for yourself to see what works best for you.

We've already written about how melatonin and melanin have the ability to stimulate the pineal gland (via increasing production by using M1 or M2). The pineal gland secretes the hormone melatonin (primarily during the hours of 2 a.m. to 6 a.m.), which literally bathes the brain and creates the chemical condition necessary for "inner vision" to take place. It is Jay's belief (based on empirical observation of his own life) that using M1 has helped significantly in his spiritual evolution and connection to "WHAT IS" (a.k.a. his inner knowing or the soul).

Metformin

We strongly believe that Metformin is one of the most effective 'wonder drugs' available for optimizing human life. Metformin originates from the French Iliac, a plant that has been used for centuries in traditional folk medicine. In the last year, the media has paid significant attention to Metformin, using phrases such as "anti-aging" and "life-extension."

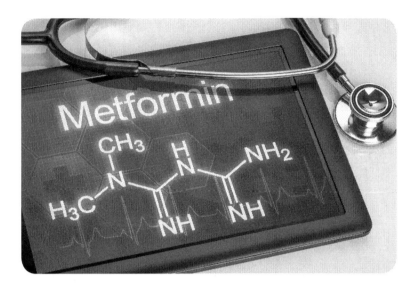

Recently, a long term study (Targeting Aging with Metformin, or "TAME") started looking at Metformin as an anti-aging drug[519]. TAME is a novel clinical trial aimed at testing whether Metformin can delay the onset of age-related diseases and conditions including cancer, cardiovascular disease and Alzheimer's disease.

Metformin has been the primary treatment for diabetes for over 60 years, and as such it's one of the most studied drugs in existence. There is also ample research data suggesting that Metformin has anti-aging and life-extending properties[520]. If you're in doubt, Google "Metformin + Life Extension" and see for yourself. The number of citations touting the amazing

---

[519] Nir Barzilai, Jill P. Crandall, Stephen B. Kritchevsky, Mark A. Espeland. Metformin as a Tool to Target Aging. Institute for Aging Research, Albert Einstein College of Medicine, Bronx, NY 10461, USA.

[520] C.A. Bannister, S.E. Holden, S. Jenkins-Jones, C.L. Morgan, J.P. Halcox, G. Schernthaner, J. Mukherjee, C.J. Currie. Can people with type 2 diabetes live longer than those without? A comparison of mortality in people initiated with Metformin or sulphonylurea monotherapy and matched, non-diabetic controls. Diabetes Obes. Metab., 16 (2014), pp. 1165-1173.

effects of the drug is astounding. We would also encourage you to watch this fascinating live stream Jay did with Nelson Vergel, where they examined all of the relevant research data on Metformin[521].

NOTE Unfortunately there is a contingent of people (including physicians) who claim that long-term usage of Metformin causes mitochondrial dysfunction. This leads to the increased risk of neurological disease, such as dementia and/or Alzheimer's. Jay has spent a great deal of time countering the research[522] supporting this group's argument. The research in support of their argument is inherently flawed, and it involves a patient population group (obese diabetics) who are not using Metformin in the way we recommend, nor in the way the research documents the use of Metformin to support life extension.

[521]   https://youtu.be/GbeKDYz-RTw - Is Metformin a Miracle Drug?

[522]   Metformin directly acts on mitochondria to alter cellular bioenergetics. Cancer Metab. 2014 Aug 28;2:12. doi: 10.1186/2049-3002-2-12. eCollection 2014.

How Does it Work

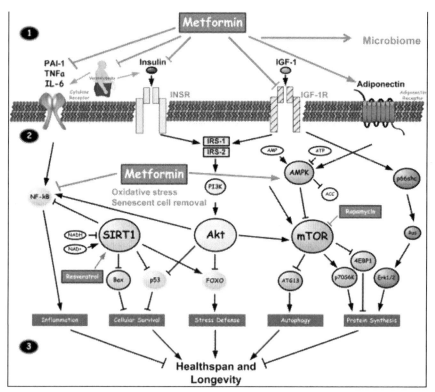

523

Metformin's mechanism of action (in relation to aging at the cellular level) is depicted in the picture above.

Here is a summary from the study *Metformin As a Tool to Target Aging*[524], which shows how Metformin targets multiple aging pathways in the chart shown:

---

523   Nir Barzilai, Jill P. Crandall, Stephen B. Kritchevsky, Mark A. Espeland. Metformin as a Tool to Target Aging. Institute for Aging Research, Albert Einstein College of Medicine, Bronx, NY 10461, USA.

524   NirBarzilai Jill P.Crandall Stephen B.Kritchevsky Mark A.Espeland. Metformin as a Tool to Target Aging. Institute for Aging Research, Albert Einstein College of Medicine, Bronx, NY 10461, USA.

The figure depicts schematically the current consensus within the biology of aging community as to pathways that are important in order to target aging and indicates at which points Metformin has been shown to have effects. Key take-away: outside of the cell (1, top), Metformin has been shown to affect the receptors for cytokines[525], insulin[526], IGF-1[527], and adiponectin[528], all pathways that are activated with aging and, when modulated, are associated with longevity. (1) Intracellular (2, middle) Metformin inhibits the inflammatory pathway and activates AMPK, increasing inhibition of mTOR, which seems to be a major target to modulate aging. Through some of these mechanisms, it also modulates oxidative stress[529] and removes senescent cells (the mitochondrial pathways are not shown, and the mechanisms by which Metformin induces senescent cell removal remain unclear). (2) These processes jointly (3, bottom) affect inflammation, cellular survival, stress defense, autophagy[530], and protein synthesis[531], which are major biological outcomes associated with aging/longevity.

Metformin enhances insulin sensitivity and lowers blood levels of insulin, but it also reduces the formation of AGEs (advanced glycation end-products) that dramatically accelerate the process of heart disease. Cardiovascular diseases, such as heart

---

[525] http://www.sciencedirect.com/topics/medicine-and-dentistry/cytokines

[526] http://www.sciencedirect.com/topics/medicine-and-dentistry/insulin-medication

[527] http://www.sciencedirect.com/topics/biochemistry-genetics-and-molecular-biology/insulin-like-growth-factor-1

[528] http://www.sciencedirect.com/topics/medicine-and-dentistry/adiponectin

[529] http://www.sciencedirect.com/topics/medicine-and-dentistry/oxidative-stress

[530] http://www.sciencedirect.com/topics/medicine-and-dentistry/autophagy

[531] http://www.sciencedirect.com/topics/biochemistry-genetics-and-molecular-biology/protein-biosynthesis

attacks and strokes, kill more Americans per year than any other forms of disease[532]. Metformin is so effective in extending one's lifespan that there is data showing people with type 2 diabetes living longer than those without diabetes when the former group (people with type 2 diabetes) is using Metformin[533].

This is a major discovery, considering that diabetics easily succumb to the effects of accelerated aging (i.e. increased whole body inflammation that is manifested as a development of cancer, heart disease, Alzheimer's, dementia, or any number of age-related diseases). Therefore, Metformin's life-extension effects comes from negating the unwanted metabolic effects of elevated glucose levels and insulin. Less insulin exposure over time will help make you more sensitive to it, leading to less inflammation and a longer lifespan.

Secondly, by reducing the **mTOR** (**m**amalian **T**arget **O**f **R**apamycin) signaling pathway, Metformin integrates both intracellular and extracellular signals, thereby serving as a central regulator of cell metabolism, growth, proliferation and survival. Metformin also reduces blood levels of "growth factors" that accelerate both the heart disease and cancer-forming processes[534].

---

[532] CDC, NCHS. Underlying Cause of Death 1999-2013 on CDC WONDER Online Database, released 2015. Data are from the Multiple Cause of Death Files, 1999-2013, as compiled from data provided by the 57 vital statistics jurisdictions through the Vital Statistics Cooperative Program. Accessed Feb. 3, 2015.

[533] C.A. Bannister, S.E. Holden, S. Jenkins-Jones, C.L. Morgan, J.P. Halcox, G. Schernthaner, J. Mukherjee, C.J. Currie. Can people with type 2 diabetes live longer than those without? A comparison of mortality in people initiated with Metformin or sulphonylurea monotherapy and matched, non-diabetic controls. Diabetes Obes. Metab., 16 (2014), pp. 1165-1173.

[534] Repurposing Metformin for cancer treatment: current clinical studies. Chae YK, Arya A, Malecek MK, Shin DS, Carneiro B, Chandra S, Kaplan J, Kalyan A, Altman JK, Platanias L, et al.Oncotarget. 2016 Jun 28; 7(26):40767-40780.

Thirdly, Metformin inhibits the liver's ability to release glucose into the bloodstream[535]. When taken with the ingestion of carbs, it may inhibit the absorption of carbs into your bloodstream.

In addition to its capacity to prevent the release of glucose from the liver, Metformin helps turn on adenosine monophosphate kinase (AMPK), an enzymatic "master switch" that is crucial for regulation of cellular energy, proper hormone expression and protein synthesis. Metformin upregulates AMPK[536] and increases lipolysis (i.e. fat-burning), similar to how lipolysis increases while fasting[537]. From a bio-evolutionary standpoint, the presence of famine induces a metabolic shift, where we call upon our fat stores for energy production. By increasing the expression of AMPK, Metformin mimics the effects of caloric restriction (a.k.a. the only proven life-extension strategy in mammalian models).

We know that Metformin has life-extending benefits for diabetics, but can it exert similar effects in people with normal insulin levels? From personal experience, most physicians shudder at the thought of using Metformin for an off-label purpose such as life extension. However, all of the recent research data on Metformin cannot be ignored.

Pharmaceutical companies have zero interest in sponsoring trials such as TAME for medicines that potentially play a major role in disease prevention. Furthermore, there is no money in research for a product that has an expired patent. This is why Big Pharma is developing a new class of diabetic drugs that

---

[535]   Gong L, Goswami S, Giacomini KM, Altman RB, Klein TE. Metformin pathways: pharmacokinetics and pharmacodynamics. Pharmacogenetics and genomics. 2012;22(11):820-827. doi:10.1097/FPC.0b013e3283559b22.

[536]   Ibid.

[537]   www.metabolicblowtorchdiet.com

are combinations of Metformin and something else — that way, they can patent these combinations and make large sums of money off of them.

Side Effects

Metformin has a fairly mild side effect profile and is usually well tolerated. In fact, one of the often-noted "side effects" is fat loss from lowered blood levels of insulin. Most of the side effects are experienced by people who possess an unhealthy and infected gut biome, which is caused by a diet high in refined carbs, sugar and alcohol. This often produces gastric distress in the form of nausea, flatulence or a stomach discomfort. These effects are usually short-lived, and will disappear over time with improved gut health and a cleaner diet.

Our Recommended Dosage and Usage

Jim and Jay are extremely passionate in their advice about using Metformin, and they can't promote its use more strongly. Almost everyone can (and should) start using Metformin ASAP.

Discuss this book's information with your doctor and don't wait for the data from the TAME trial either. Inform your doctor of the available study data, as there's a good chance they'll be unaware of it.

Go into their office and tell them the following:

> **You want to use Metformin because it is cardioprotective, prevents cancer, and it is believed to stop the progress of neurodegenerative diseases such as Alzheimer's and dementia. It's also affordable and easily provided by your local pharmacist.**

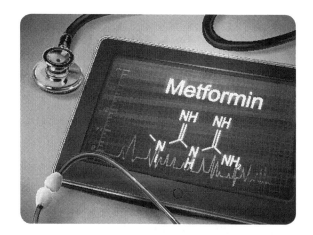

We recommend that **men start with 500 mg twice a day (once in morning and once at night) on an empty stomach** to reduce their insulin production even further. Women should be taking half that dosage (250 mg, twice a day). For those of you with an inflamed gut biome, make sure to use the "XR" (extended release) form and be prepared for short-term side effects that may last a couple of weeks.

With that said, there are people in the Life Extension Foundation (LEF) who are using dosages as high as 3 grams a day. Jim and Jay have been using Metformin for more than a decade, and have found that 1 gram taken twice a day (AM and PM) is highly effective in reducing insulin levels. This ultimately reduces their body fat levels and improves their inflammatory biomarkers.

Modafinil

Modafinil[538] is generally thought of as a wakefulness medication. In the U.S., it is normally prescribed to treat conditions such as

---

[538] http://fabfitover40.com/2014/01/06/do-you-know-the-benefits-of-modafinil/

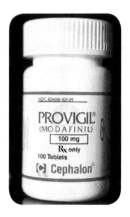

narcolepsy and shift work sleep disorder. It is also used off-label to battle the fatigue that arises from conditions such as fibromyalgia, cerebral palsy, and Parkinson's.

Also known as a nootropic (i.e. a drug that enhances cognitive performance and health), its use is notoriously widespread. From surgical personnel and soldiers in combat to super-focused entrepreneurs and business leaders, high-profile people are using Modafinil as the ultimate drug for hacking sleep.

While amphetamine-based agents such as Dexadrine and Adderall are popularly used to achieve optimal cognitive performance, we believe Modafinil should be the preferred drug of choice because it does not affect the beta adrenergic pathways. In plain English, it will make you much more focused without speeding up your heart rate, nor will you become addicted to it with repeated use[539].

Modafinil is classified as a Schedule IV controlled substance under United States federal law, which means you need a doctor's prescription to legally obtain it or import it into the U.S. You will also find that various athletic organizations have Modafinil listed as a banned substance.

There are two common analogs of Modafinil you should be aware of. Adrafinil is a precursor to Modafinil (i.e. it produces Modafinil when metabolized in the body). This analog is easier to obtain than Modafinil in some areas. The effects are lighter,

---

[539] Dopamine D1 and D2 Receptor Family Contributions to Modafinil-Induced Wakefulness. Jared W. Young. Journal of Neuroscience, 4 March 2009, 29 (9) 2663-2665; DOI:10.

and only last a short period of time. Adrafinil can be useful for situations where you only need 1-2 hours of laser focus.

FLmodafinil (FLmoda) is a newer analog of Modafinil, with a double flouro group added to the molecule. This version will enter the bloodstream faster and seems to be stronger than the original version. There is no legal way to obtain this version yet, and can only be found on the grey market (it's classified as a research chemical). We personally found that it works faster than Modafinil does. The dosing is much different, so if you are going to experiment with FLmoda, start conservatively at low doses. FLmoda doesn't last as long as Modafinil, which may or may not fit your needs. In our minds, the regular version (Modafinil) is still the best option for 3-6 hours of mental enhancement.

How Does It Work

Modafinil is a relatively low-risk drug with respect to side effects, or becoming overly dependent on it. Contraindications are few (i.e. it won't negatively interact with other drugs you are taking), and there are no allergies and or hypersensitivities associated with the drug. It is sold under several brand names, such as Provigil, Modafinil, and Alertec. Modafinil is a dopamine reuptake inhibitor (DRI), a class of drugs which increase dopamine production while slowing down the breakdown of dopamine (i.e.more dopamine is available for cellular usage).

Dopamine is a neurotransmitter that mainly influences reward-motivated behavior. It is part of the main mechanism behind motivation, cravings, and desire in animals. Although this explains a possible mechanism of action by which Modafinil works, some people also suspect that there are other unknown mechanisms of action which are specifically tied to its ability to induce wakefulness.

Side Effects

We find it to be as effective as promised, with relatively low side effects. Anybody who has taken Modafinil before will have noticed that their mood was elevated, while feeling an enhanced sense of well-being. The most commonly reported side effects include nausea, anxiety, feelings of nervousness, headaches and insomnia.

Our Recommended Dosage and Usage

Clinical dosages are listed anywhere from 50 to 400 mg daily, and sometimes as high as 1200 mg per day. Jim has used Modafinil, on and off, for 9 years. He originally started using it to stay awake at a late-night job after working a full 8-hour day. This job required him to stay focused for long periods of time, and Modafinil worked great for this. His only complaints were that Modafinil lasts for a long time, sometimes dries out the eyes, and affects the quality of your sleep after a few days of consistent dosing at 200 mg or more. Jay had similar observations, except that he experienced headaches late in the day instead of dry eyes.

After using Modafinil for 10 days straight at 100 mg per day (or more), both Jim and Jay noticed a higher frequency of side effects and the dose becoming less effective over time.

Aside from that, it's one of the best nootropics you can get your hands on and we highly recommend it. We suggest you limit the dosage to 100 mg a day, and use it sparingly for highly specific purposes (ex. While preparing research, writing a book like the *TOT Bible* or before taking challenging exams). This means you will have to cycle off Modafinil to avoid any side effects, while ensuring it does not lose its efficacy. Jay often uses 50 mg (¼ of 200 mg tab) in the morning before cardio for an energy boost, and to dull his appetite on long fasting days.

Nicotine

The supplemental form of nicotine[540] has been used as a cognitive enhancer[541] with great results. It improves attention in a wide variety of cognitive tasks, while also improving immediate and long-term memory. Additionally, nicotine has been shown to improve attention span in patients with probable Alzheimer's disease[542].

IMPORTANT While one can become addicted to nicotine in any form, is it likely when you are using 1-2 mg daily for a short period of time? NO, it isn't. We have done this time and time again, never experiencing any dependence or negative symptoms when we stopped using it[543].

When you use nicotine in a nasal spray, gum or lozenge, it is much different than using a tobacco product. Tobacco is a known carcinogen, whereas nicotine is not. Tobacco products have a multitude of other ingredients to make you want to use them more. Nicotine, on the other hand, is just one of the chemicals

[540] http://www.amazon.com/exec/obidos/ASIN/B0039ZAF44/fabfitove40-20

[541] Warburton DM. Nicotine as a cognitive enhancer. Prog Neuropsychopharmacol Biol Psychiatry. 1992;16(2):181-91.

[542] Jones GM, Sahakian BJ, Levy R, Warburton DM, Gray JA. Effects of acute subcutaneous nicotine on attention, information processing and short-term memory in Alzheimer's disease. Psychopharmacology (Berl). 1992;108(4):485-94.

[543] Besson M, Forget B. Cognitive dysfunction, affective states, and vulnerability to nicotine addiction: A multifactorial perspective. Front Psychiatry. 2016;7:160.

found in tobacco products. Nicotine, by itself in its pure form, has shown no adverse health effects. This is particularly true at the dosages we are talking about.

When used in conjunction with a fat loss diet, such as The Metabolic Blowtorch Diet[544], supplemental nicotine gum has been shown to suppress appetite. If it is combined with caffeine, these actions are enhanced[545]. Lastly, nicotine can also help your body convert stored fat into energy that is used by your muscle tissues[546].

How Does it Work?

When your body is in a state of low insulin/glucose (i.e. during the last few hours of a fasting window), using nicotine will help get stored fat out of cells and make it ready to be used as energy. However, if you have a sufficient amount of glucose and insulin in your system (i.e. when eating carbs), these fats will NOT be used as energy. This is why you don't want to use nicotine outside of your fasting windows.

Side Effects

When dosed correctly (i.e. according to our recommendations), side effects are rare. Dizziness, upset stomach, nausea or headaches are listed on the packaging of nicotine gum as potential side effects. In our experience, one would have to

---

[544] www.metabolicblowtorchdiet.com

[545] Jessen A, Buemann B, Toubro S, Skovgaard IM, Astrup A. The appetite-suppressant effect of nicotine is enhanced by caffeine. Diabetes Obes Metab. 2005;7(4):327-33.

[546] Sztalryd C, Hamilton J, Horwitz BA, Johnson P, Kraemer FB. Alterations of lipolysis and lipoprotein lipase in chronically nicotine-treated rats. Am J Physiol. 1996;270(2 Pt 1):E215-23.

take way too much nicotine to experience any negative side effects. As with everything, start at low dosages and gradually work your way up.

Our Recommended Dosage and Usage

Based on existing research, we know that nicotine will:

- act as a nootropic
- suppress appetite
- have its benefits enhanced by caffeine
- help mobilize fat out of cells to be used as energy

We personally use nicotine on an infrequent basis for both cognitive enhancement and fat loss, primarily during fat loss diets and fasting windows. From personal experience, nicotine is useful for increasing fat loss when stubborn fat cells stall the rate of fat loss.

Nicotine is also useful for suppressing appetite, and we use it first thing in the morning before doing fasted cardio. This helps to optimize the body's low glucose environment at that time of the day. It can also be used during the middle (or near the end) of a long fasting window to help with stubborn body fat reduction.

We usually start dosing nicotine at 1 mg per day and will work our way up to 2 mg. However, we will only use it for 4 weeks within these parameters. For example, on a 12-week fat loss diet, you would use nicotine for the last 4 weeks at 1-2 mg per piece of gum chewed on your low insulin signal (i.e. fasting) days.

Proviron

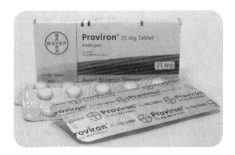

Proviron® is the trade name for the compound mesterolone manufactured by Bayer Pharma, and it is a DHT (dihydrotestosterone) derivative. This means it looks and acts in a similar way to the potent testosterone metabolite DHT. Proviron is used for men who suffer from hypogonadism and who are infertile due to low levels of androgens.

Proviron was one of the first steroid molecules on the market and was launched shortly after testosterone propionate[547]. It has never been FDA-approved for use in the United States, despite being a licensed drug throughout Europe and most other countries around the globe. It has been used to treat androgen deficiency and infertility[548]. If used alone as monotherapy, it can have a mild inhibitory effect on the hypothalamic-pituitary axis (HPTA).

Proviron has also been used to help lower the effects of aromatization (i.e. the conversion of testosterone to estrogen[549]). It acts in the same manner as DHT (dihydrotestosterone) by

---

[547] Alexandre Hohl (6 April 2017). *Testosterone: From Basic to Clinical Aspects.* Springer. pp. 204–. ISBN 978-3-319-46086-4.

[548] Gerris J, Comhaire F, Hellemans P, Peeters K, Schoonjans F. (Mar 1991). Placebo-controlled trial of high-dose Mesterolone treatment of idiopathic male infertility. Fertil Steril. 55(3):603-7.

[549] Giovanni Corona, Giulia Rastrelli, Linda Vignozzi & Mario Maggi. Emerging medication for the treatment of male hypogonadism -Expert Opinion on Emerging Drugs Vol. 17, Iss. 2, 2012.

AGENTS OF CHANGE

competing at the estrogen receptor level, and not by inhibiting the aromatase enzyme[550].

It has been favored in some fitness and bodybuilding circles due to its alleged ability to improve muscle hardness and vascularity. This may have more to do with lower levels of subcutaneous fat during the competition phase. With that said, elevated levels of androgens may help the appearance of muscle fullness when combined with lower body fat.

One study investigated Proviron as a monotherapy for hypo-gonadal men because of its androgenic properties and the lack of conversion into estradiol. Serum testosterone levels dropped slightly and free testosterone was elevated as a result of a lowered SHBG. LH and FSH levels also decreased slightly and the symptom score stayed roughly the same for the duration of the 7 year study, showing a marked improvement only upon commencement of treatment[551].

Another small study[552] demonstrated the improvement of urinary tract symptoms, which is often seen in men who are hypo-gonadal. Proviron showed improvement in prostate symptoms, independent of prostate volume. This may give credence to DHT being important for good prostate health, with the exception being those with existing prostate cancer.

---

[550] Casey RW, Wilson JD.Antiestrogenic action of dihydrotestosterone in mouse breast. Competition with estradiol for binding to the estrogen receptor. J Clin Invest. 1984 Dec;74(6):2272-8.

[551] Malcolm Carruthers, Paul Cathcart, and Mark R. Feneley. Evolution of testosterone treatment over 25 years: symptom responses, endocrine profiles and cardiovascular changes. Aging Male. 2015 Oct 2; 18(4): 217–227.

[552] Mesterolone treatment of aging male syndrome improves lower urinary tract symptoms. J Pak Med Assoc. 2014 Dec;64(12):1366-9.

How Does it Work

Proviron works by binding to the androgen receptor in much the same way DHT does. It behaves in a similar manner to an estrogen receptor antagonist, though it's much weaker than a SERM.

Side effects

Noted side effects for Proviron may include frequent erections, or erections that do not go away[553] (although this is not inherently bad if you suffer from erectile dysfunction). However, if an erection lasts too long (i.e. over 4-6 hours), then you may be at risk of priapism and would need to seek urgent medical advice as this could cause potential damage to your penis. The other potential side effect listed in the package leaflet is discomfort or pain in the abdomen. Furthermore, Proviron is not recommended by the manufacturer if you have prostate cancer or have previously had a liver tumour.

Our Recommended Dosage and Usage

It is not uncommon, and in fact recommended by the manufacturer themselves that one tablet can be taken 3 or 4 times per day. After a few months, your doctor may decide to reduce the number of tablets taken each day.

In our experience, one 25 mg tablet taken at morning and at bedtime (50 mg total throughout the day) alongside TOT helps to reduce SHBG, and may improve erection strength. Proviron is safe and effective at improving libido, and in mitigating some

---

[553] Proviron®25mg tablet Mesterolone[package leaflet]. Bayer PharmaAG, Bayer PLC marketing authorisation holder and manufacturer. Newbury, Berkshire, RG14 1JA, United Kingdom, 2014.

of the negative effects of excess estrogen when used with TOT. It's unfortunate that Proviron is not approved for usage in the United States. In Europe, it's often scripted concomitantly (along with) testosterone.

Thymosin Beta

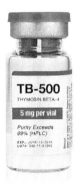

Thymosin Beta-4 (thymosin β_4) is a protein which consists of 43 amino acids and is encoded by the gene TMSB4X in the human body. It has been studied in numerous clinical trials for a wide range of healing applications. Research has shown that if the thymosin beta-4 peptide is used after a heart attack, it can reactivate cardiac progenitor cells and repair damaged heart tissue[554].

Thymosin beta-4 is a very large molecule. In fact, it is so large that it cannot fit entirely into its receptor. Due to its large size, different sections of the molecule have different activities. For example, TB-500 is the part of the thymosin beta-4 hormone which promotes many positive health effects. These include (but are not limited to) overall healing, wound repair, new blood cell and muscle cell formation. For medical applications, it is more practical to use TB-500 alone instead of the entire Thymosin Beta-4 protein.

554   Banerjee I, Zhang J, Morris TM, et al. Thymosin Beta 4 is Dispensable for Murine Cardiac Development and Function. *Circulation research.* 2012;110(3):456-464. doi:10.1161/CIRCRESAHA.111.258616.

How Does it Work?

Through the administration of thymosin β_4, TB-500 has been shown to promote the migration of cells, increase formation of blood vessels, accelerate maturation of stem cells, improve the survival of various cell types and lower the production of pro-inflammatory cytokines[555]. The main functionality of TB-500, however, hinges on its ability to upregulate cell-building proteins like actin. Upregulation of actin allows TB-500 to promote cell migration and proliferation. This not only helps build new blood vessel pathways, but it also regulates the inflammation directly involved with wound healing.

The versatility of TB-500 exists because of its molecular structure and low molecular weight, which lends to both its mobility and its ability to travel long distances through tissues. This means that when it targets injured areas (chronic or acute), TB-500 has the ability to circulate throughout the entire body, find areas of injury and take corrective action. The added benefits of improved overall flexibility and reduced inflammation in tendons have been noticed, and some users report lost hair being grown again (alongside reports of gray hairs becoming darker)[556]. In fact, some studies[557] correlate TB-

---

[555] Lee S-I, Yi J-K, Bae W-J, Lee S, Cha H-J, Kim E-C. Thymosin Beta-4 Suppresses Osteoclastic Differentiation and Inflammatory Responses in Human Periodontal Ligament Cells. Reddy SV, ed. *PLoS ONE*. 2016;11(1):e0146708. doi:10.1371/journal.pone.0146708.

[556] Gao X, Liang H, Hou F, et al. Thymosin Beta-4 Induces Mouse Hair Growth. Andl CD, ed. PLoS ONE. 2015;10(6):e0130040. doi:10.1371/journal. pone.0130040.

[557] Wei C, Kim I-K, Li L, Wu L, Gupta S. Thymosin Beta 4 Protects Mice from Monocrotaline-Induced Pulmonary Hypertension and Right Ventricular Hypertrophy. Sadoshima J, ed. *PLoS ONE*. 2014;9(11):e110598. doi:10.1371/journal.pone.0110598.

500 with healing[558] of the heart, and in select cases it repairs ventricular hypertrophy (i.e. benign enlargement of the heart).

All of these properties have provided the impetus for a worldwide series of ongoing clinical trials that investigate the potential effectiveness of thymosin β_4 in promoting the repair of wounds in the skin, cornea and heart[559]. The tissue-regenerating properties of thymosin β_4 may ultimately contribute to the repair of human heart muscles that have been damaged by heart diseases and heart attacks.

In mice, administration of thymosin β_4 has been shown to stimulate the formation of new heart muscle cells from otherwise inactive precursor cells present in the outer lining of adult hearts[560]. This is done by inducing migration of these precursor cells into heart muscle[561], while recruiting new blood vessels within the muscle[562].

[558] Xu T-J, Wang Q, Ma X-W, et al. A novel dimeric thymosin beta 4 with enhanced activities accelerates the rate of wound healing. *Drug Design, Development and Therapy.* 2013;7:1075-1088. doi:10.2147/DDDT.S50183.

[559] Philp D, Kleinman HK (April 2010). "Animal studies with thymosin beta, a multifunctional tissue repair and regeneration peptide." Annals of the New York Academy of Sciences. 1194: 81–6.

[560] Smart N, Bollini S, Dubé KN, Vieira JM, Zhou B, Davidson S, Yellon D, Riegler J, Price AN, Lythgoe MF, Pu WT, Riley PR (June 2011). "De novo cardiomyocytes from within the activated adult heart after injury." *Nature.* 474 (7353): 640–4. doi.

[561] Smart N, Riley PR (February 2009). "Derivation of epicardium-derived progenitor cells (EPDCs) from adult epicardium." Curr Protoc Stem Cell Biol. Chapter 2: Unit 2C .2.

[562] Riley PR, Smart N (December 2009). "Thymosin beta4 induces epicardium-derived neovascularization in the adult heart." *Biochem. Soc. Trans.* 37 (Pt 6): 1218–20.

Side Effects

The flu-like symptoms, lethargy or head rush associated with most peptides do not seem to be widely reported with TB-500. Everybody is different, so always follow the suggested dosing protocols and practice sterile injection techniques.

Our Recommended Dosage and Usage

TB-500, like most peptides, is a lyophilized powder that needs to reconstituted with bacteriostatic water and kept in a cool dry place. **Doses range from 2.0-2.5 mg injected subcutaneously twice a week for 4-6 consecutive weeks**. Notably, some users have reported success with doses up to 8 mg TOTAL a week.

There are others who have used **two monthly subcutaneous injections of 2.0-2.5 mg (i.e. once every two weeks) as a maintenance dose for maintaining rapid recovery and flexibility in strained areas of the body**. As already discussed, TB-500 will be distributed systemically. Therefore, injections into (or near) areas of acute injury are not necessary. Subcutaneous or intramuscular injections are both acceptable for TB-500. It is our opinion that both Thymosin Beta-4 and TB-500 show great promise in accelerating the rate of healing, especially for aging athletes with injured tendons and ligaments.

Future Agents of Change

It's important to understand that we are living in a dynamically expanding world, especially in the context of new and upcoming therapies in medicine. There are literally hundreds of new and exciting peptide hormones being studied. There are also some amazing biomedical and gene therapies that are being discovered and developed at the highest levels of biotech. The CRISPR/Cas9 gene editing technology[563] that gives us the ability to directly modify or correct the underlying disease-associated changes in our genome is truly other worldly.

Because everything is moving so quickly, we wanted to mention a few promising agents that are currently appearing on our radar. Some of these agents we may have already used, or we know of people who have experience with them. Since our familiarity with each of these agents is minimal at best, we currently don't feel confident enough to officially recommend them to readers of this book. With time, this could (and likely will) change.

As previously mentioned in the book, **Tesamorelin** (Egrifta[564]) is an amazing peptide hormone that has already been FDA

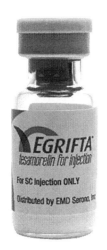

approved for the treatment of lipodistrophy (i.e. abdominal body fat reduction) and HIV. Specifically, it works by reducing visceral abdominal fat.

When used in combination with TOT and men suffering from insulin resistance/metabolic disorder, there is an enhanced fat burning effect. Tesamorelin is a growth hormone releasing hormone (GHRH) analog that has been shown to increase IGF-1 levels in men. It binds and stimulates to GHRH receptors just as well as endogenous GHRH (i.e. GHRHs that naturally exist in the body). It has a host of

---

563 http://www.crisprtx.com/our-programs/crispr-cas9-gene-editing.php

564 www.empowerpharmacy.com

other benefits, including cognitive enhancement and lowering triglyceride levels[565].

Dr. Rob Kominiarek[566] loves this peptide, and uses it with many of his patients suffering from metabolic disorder (in combination with testosterone). **The dosage used is 1 mg injected subcutaneously before bed**, and at least 90 minutes after the last meal. Neither Jim nor Jay have used this peptide hormone, but reports from the small minority of the medical community are great so far.

Ibutamoren Mesylate, also known as **MK-677** in the research peptide community, is another GHRP (like Ipamorelin) that shows great promise as it can be taken orally (avoiding the need for additional injections beyond testosterone). The most advanced, forward thinking compounding pharmacies[567] are now stocking it and various age-management doctors are prescribing it for their patients (in combination with TOT). As already discussed, GHRPs belong to a broader class of compounds, all of which share the common trait of being able to bind to the Growth Hormone Secretagogue Receptor (GHS-R) and stimulate HGH release. Ibutamoren (taken orally) increases the release of HGH and IGF-1, while also producing sustained increases in plasma levels of HGH and IGF-1.

There are a number of studies in children and the elderly that have shown the use of Ibutamoren as a treatment for reduced

---

[565] Stanley TL, Chen CY, Branch KL, Makimura H, Grinspoon SK. Effects of a Growth Hormone-Releasing Hormone Analog on Endogenous GH Pulsatility and Insulin Sensitivity in Healthy Men. *The Journal of Clinical Endocrinology and Metabolism.* 2011;96(1):150-158. doi:10.1210/jc.2010-1587.

[566] www.renuehealth.com

[567] www.empowerpharmacy.com

levels of GH and IGF-1[568]. There are also human studies showing that Ibutamoren increases both muscle mass and bone mineral density in the elderly[569]. Additionally, it also accelerates lipolysis (fat burning), which allows it to be used in the treatment of obesity[570]. Even though neither Jim nor Jay have used this oral GHRP, feedback from those who have taken it (along with the positive results from human research studies) puts it on our future radar. 25 mg taken just before bed seems to be the dosage that most people report as optimal, given that it has the ability to elevate IGF-1 levels for up to 24 hours.

NOTE Jay and his wife Monica recently attained a prescription and have started Ibutamoren at 25 mg prior to bed. Jay has experimented with a 50 mg dosage as well. After using it for 6 weeks, sleep is much deeper and pumps in the gym are noticeable. We also believe it's helping with body composition and nutrient partitioning as our diet is not the best due to the holidays.

Jim and Jay have recently been using **CBD Oil**. CBD (Cannabidiol) and TCH (Tetrahydrocannabinol) are the two most prominent cannabinoids found in the cannabis plant (this includes both

---

[568]   Adunsky, A., J. Chandler, N. Heyden, J. Lutkiewicz, B. B. Scott, Y. Berd, N. Liu, and D. A. Papanicolaou. 2011. 'MK-0677 (ibutamoren mesylate) for the treatment of patients recovering from hip fracture: a multicenter, randomized, placebo- controlled phase IIb study', Arch Gerontol Geriatr, 53: 183-9.

[569]   Bach, M. A., K. Rockwood, C. Zetterberg, G. Thamsborg, R. Hebert, J. P. Devogelaer, J. S. Christiansen, R. Rizzoli, J. L. Ochsner, N. Beisaw, O. Gluck, L. Yu, T. Schwab, J. Farrington, A. M. Taylor, J. Ng, V. Fuh, and M. K. Hip Fracture Study Group. 2004. 'The effects of MK-0677, an oral growth hormone secretagogue, in patients with hip fracture', J Am Geriatr Soc, 52: 516-23.

[570]   Svensson, J., J. O. Jansson, M. Ottosson, G. Johannsson, M. R. Taskinen, O. Wiklund, and B. A. Bengtsson. 1999. 'Treatment of obese subjects with the oral growth hormone secretagogue MK-677 affects serum concentrations of several lipoproteins, but not lipoprotein(a)', J Clin Endocrinol Metab, 84: 2028-33.

hemp and marijuana). TCH is the psychoactive part of the cannabis plant, and is responsible for the "high" that people experience when using marijuana.

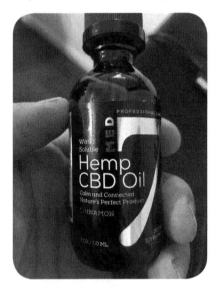

CBD, on the other hand, has no psychoactive properties. Hemp strains with high CBD to TCH ratios (i.e. there is much more CBD than TCH in the strain) are used to make CBD products, while strains with high TCH to CBD ratios are given to users that want a psychoactive product. The version that's available to most people over the counter is the CBT-only version. This makes it a safer and far less contro-versial alternative to marijuana, while still offering significant health benefits.

CBD affects the endocannabinoid system (ECS), which is present in the central and peripheral nervous system of mammals. It's a key player in regulating many cognitive processes such as mood, memory, perception of pain, appetite, and fetal development[571,572,573]. In the past decade or so, there

571 Klein C, Hill MN, Chang SCH, Hillard CJ, Gorzalka BB. Circulating Endocannabinoid Concentrations and Sexual Arousal in Women. *The journal of sexual medicine.* 2012;9(6):10.1111/j.1743-6109.2012.02708.x. doi:10.1111/j.1743-6109.2012.02708.x.

572 Wang H, Xie H, Dey SK. Endocannabinoid signaling directs periimplantation events. *The AAPS Journal.* 2006;8(2):E425-E432. doi:10.1007/BF02854916.

573 Morena M., Campolongo P. The endocannabinoid system: An emotional buffer in the modulation of memory function. Neurobiology of Learning and Memory, Volume 112, 2014.

have been over 23,000 studies published in peer-reviewed medical journals that detail the effects of cannabis, cannabis oil, and cannabinoids on the body[574].

The most common uses for CBD (and the ones we are experimenting with) are as follows: improving mood, reducing pain and inflammation, aiding with sleep issues and anxiety. **The typical starting dosage starting is 25 mg taken 1-3x per day**. But for people in extreme pain, the dosages can be much higher.

Imagine a drug that has the potential to reduce the risk of heart attack and stroke[575,576,577,578,579], improve dementia[580], reduce

574 https://www.medicalmarijuanainc.com/education/

575 Pentoxifylline for vascular health: a brief review of the literature. McCarty MF, O'Keefe JH, DiNicolantonio JJ. Open Heart. 2016 Feb 8;3(1):e000365. doi: 10.1136/openhrt-2015-000365. eCollection 2016. Review.

576 Pentoxifylline influences acute-phase response in acute myocardial infarction. Lechleitner P, Genser N, Mair J, Maier J, Herold M, Beimpold H, Föger B, Dienstl F, Puschendorf B, Tilg H. Clin Investig. 1992 Sep;70(9):755. No abstract available.

577 Windmeier C, Gressner AM. Pharmacological aspects of Pentoxifylline with emphasis on its inhibitory actions on hepatic fibrogenesis. Gen Pharmacol 1997;29:181–96. doi:10.1016/S0306-3623(96)00314-X [CrossRef] [Medline] [Web of Science] Google Scholar.

578 Herskovits E, Famulari A, Tamaroff L, et al. Preventive treatment of cerebral transient ischemia: comparative randomized trial of Pentoxifylline versus conventional antiaggregants. Eur Neurol 1985;24:73–81. doi:10.1159/000115765 [CrossRef] [Medline] [Web of Science].

579 Herskovits E, Famulari A, Tamaroff L, et al. Comparative study of Pentoxifylline vs antiaggregants in patients with transient ischaemic attacks. Acta Neurol Scand Suppl 1989;127:31–5. doi:10.1111/j.1600-0404.1989.tb 01808.x [Medline].

580 Torigoe R, Hayashi T, Anegawa S, et al. Effect of propentofylline and Pentoxifylline on cerebral blood flow using 123I-IMP SPECT in patients with cerebral arteriosclerosis. Clin Ther 1994;16:65–73.

plaque in the penis of patients with peyronie's disease[581,582,583], improve blood sugar[584], increase endogenous antioxidants[585] and mediate the toxic effects of chemotherapy[586]. The drug **Pentoxifylline** has shown promise in all of the above, but receives surprisingly little attention from the medical community. This is perhaps due to the fact that it's off patent, and so there is little money to be made from pursuing it.

Pentoxifylline, also known by the trade name TRENTAL®, is a xanthine derivative. As such, it belongs in a family of other naturally occurring compounds that also includes caffeine. It has been around for decades and its side effects are well understood. Originally, it was used for intermittent claudication (walking with a limp), which stems from blockages or narrowing of the arteries in the legs (possibly due to atherosclerosis).

---

[581]   Pentoxifylline treatment and penile calcifications in men with Peyronie's disease. Smith JF, Shindel AW, Huang YC, Clavijo RI, Flechner L, Breyer BN, Eisenberg ML, Lue TF. Asian J Androl. 2011 Mar;13(2):322-5. doi: 10.1038/aja.2010.117. Epub 2010 Nov 22. PMID: 21102473.

[582]   Pentoxifylline attenuates transforming growth factor-beta1-stimulated elastogenesis in human tunica albuginea-derived fibroblasts part 2: Interference in a TGF-beta1/Smad-dependent mechanism and downregulation of AAT1. Lin G, Shindel AW, Banie L, Ning H, Huang YC, Liu G, Lin CS, Lue TF. J Sex Med. 2010 May;7(5):1787-97.

[583]   Pentoxifylline attenuates transforming growth factor-β1-stimulated collagen deposition and elastogenesis in human tunica albuginea-derived fibroblasts part 1: impact on extracellular matrix. Shindel AW, Lin G, Ning H, Banie L, Huang YC, Liu G, Lin CS, Lue TF.

[584]   Han SJ, Kim HJ, Kim DJ, et al. Effects of Pentoxifylline on proteinuria and glucose control in patients with type 2 diabetes: a prospective randomized double-blind multicenter study. Diabetol Metab Syndr 2015;7:64.

[585]   Crouch SP, Fletcher J. Effect of ingested Pentoxifylline on neutrophil superoxide anion production. Infect Immun 1992;60:4504–9.

[586]   Toxicol Res. 2017 Jul;33(3):255-263. doi: 10.5487/TR.2017.33.3.255. Epub 2017 Jul 15. Evaluation of the Effect of Pentoxifylline on Cisplatin-Induced Testicular Toxicity in Rats. Fallahzadeh AR1, Rezaei Z2, Rahimi HR3,4, Barmak MJ1, Sadeghi H1, Mehrabi S1, Rabani SM1, Kashani IR5, Barati V2, Mahmoudi R1.

Pentoxifylline is known to inhibit TGF-Beta[9], TNF alpha[11], IL-6 and other proinflammatory cytokines that are believed to be behind atherosclerosis[587]. At the cellular level, it is considered a nonspecific CAMP phosphodiesterases inhibitor[588], essentially acting as a vasodilator (or a relatively inexpensive and non-specific PDE inhibitor). Like Cialis, it's a PDE inhibitor. However, Cialis acts directly on the PDE-5 enzyme, whereas Pentoxifylline does not. Therefore, while Pentoxifylline may not necessarily be indicated for treating erectile dysfunction, it may help.

Pentoxifylline may be useful for patients on TOT who are concerned about mild elevations in hemoglobin and hematocrit levels (which can cause one's blood to thicken). It has the ability to reduce blood viscosity, red blood cell aggregation, and reduce neutrophil activation[589,590]. This allows red blood cells to become more malleable, enabling them to move more easily through blood vessels.

On paper, Pentoxifylline appears to have several qualities that make it a suitable agent of change to TOT. Nonetheless, further studies with larger patient populations are required in order to substantiate its use.

---

[587]   Prasad K, Lee P. Suppression of hypercholesterolemic atherosclerosis by Pentoxifylline and its mechanism. Atherosclerosis 2007;192:313–22. doi:10.1016/j.atherosclerosis.2006.07.034.

[588]   Banfi C, Sironi L, De Simoni SG, et al. Pentoxifylline prevents spontaneous brain ischemia in stroke-prone rats. J Pharmacol Exp Ther 2004;310:890–5. doi:10.1124/jpet.104.067090.

[589]   Ott E, Lechner H, Fazekas F. Hemorheological effects of Pentoxifylline on disturbed flow behavior of blood in patients with cerebrovascular insufficiency. Eur Neurol 1983;22(Suppl 1):105–7.

[590]   Perego MA, Sergio G, Artale F, et al. Haemorrheological improvement by Pentoxifylline in patients with peripheral arterial occlusive disease. Curr Med Res Opin 1986;10:135–8. Soria J, Giovannangeli ML, Jolchine IE, et al. Pentoxifylline, fibrinogen and leukocytes. Blood Coagul Fibrinolysis 1990;1(4–5):485–7.

Now that you've just read an entire chapter about amazing new medications and agents to improve performance, body composition and increase cognition, you're probably wondering where it's possible to access them? Especially in a world where the Internet creates more questions and concerns about quality control than it answers!

Thankfully, there are compounding pharmacies to fill the void. Compounding is the science of creating personalized medications where drugs can be made in custom strengths, combinations, and dosage forms. Before the advent of mass manufacturing in the 1950s, the primary source of medications dispensed in the United States was through compounding pharmacies. Today, compounding pharmacies can fulfill orders for back-ordered non-commercial drugs and orphaned drugs, as well as create versions that don't contain dyes, preservatives, fillers or other excipients that patients can be sensitive to.

One of the best compounding pharmacies in North America is Empower Pharmacy in Houston, Texas. With customized healthcare playing such a powerful role, quality control becomes critical. Not only does Empower Pharmacy have a state-of-the art facility, but they also have one of the most compliant models in existence today. They are accredited, nationally licensed, and registered with the FDA, which means they manufacture their medications to similar standards that big pharmaceutical companies are required to.

With this type of pharmacy available, clinicians now have the ability to customize your prescriptions to you. If you are super sensitive to AIs and need a micro dose to attain balance, or you need access to potent erectile dysfunction medications that aren't available on the commercial market, or maybe even the latest in peptide preparations, Empower has you covered. Empower is capable of customizing your needs with precise pharmaceutical formulations based on the exact recommendations from your prescribing physician.

CHAPTER 15 KEY TAKEAWAYS

- We tell you about the supplements, medications and exotic substances that can radically alter your physique, while optimizing your performance at the same time.

- For each one, we provide a brief history on how they are typically used, along with some of the health benefits they provide.

- Every agent of change comes with a high-level description of their mechanism of action. In other words, how exactly do they work in the body and deliver their life-changing benefits?

- We also inform you of the side effects associated with each agent of change. Some side effects aren't worth worrying about, while others will be of great concern to select individuals.

- Additionally, every agent of change comes with our recommended dosages, along with instructions for usage. These are based on a mix of our decades of experience with using them, results from multiple clinical studies, and numerous reports from other patients and physicians who have used these agents of change. If you want to optimally use these agents of change and drive maximum benefits out of them, you'll want to read this! NOTE: Some of these agents of change may or may not require a doctor's prescription.

- Last but not least, there are some amazing new therapies in development that we are keeping a close eye on. We tell you all about them, but do not officially recommend them due to our lack of experience with them, and the insufficient amount of clinical research data available to draw definitive conclusions.

CHAPTER 16
TOT and Fitness

The Foundational Role of Weight Training

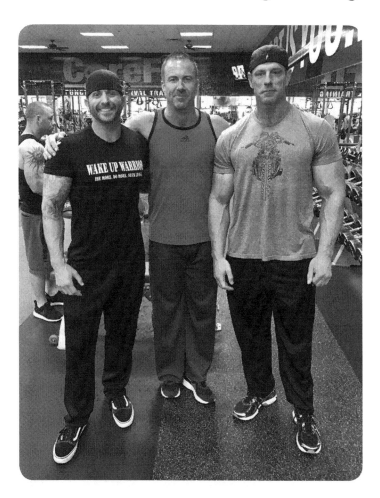

This book won't cover the science or the complex intricacies behind modern-day weight training, but it WILL provide a high-level summary of the role that resistance (i.e. strength) training should play in maximizing the success of TOT. Truthfully, talking about optimizing your testosterone levels without incorporating weight training misses the point of optimal health entirely.

Muscle is the single greatest means of prevention against the diseases of aging. Having a muscular body increases metabolic rate (BMR), improves insulin sensitivity and increases one's resistance to injury[591]. The newest research even indicates it increases the size of the human brain[592]. By now, you should understand the importance of staying lean, strong and resistant to disease as you get older.

TOT, due to its potent anabolic effects, enhances protein synthesis[593]. This ultimately leads to an increase in lean muscle tissue and a reduction of body fat[594]. WIth all of that said, please remember that testosterone is only an adjunct to a healthy lifestyle. It's not a magic bullet, nor is it 'exercise in a bottle'. As you begin TOT, you'll be blown away by how motivated you are to be in the gym, and how your body transforms itself when you regularly lift weights. Using testosterone without regular

---

[591] A Systematic Review and Meta-Analysis of Proteomics Literature on the Response of Human Skeletal Muscle to Obesity/Type 2 Diabetes Mellitus (T2DM) Versus Exercise Training.Proteomes. 2017 Nov 11;5(4). pii: E30. doi: 10.3390 /proteomes 5040030.

[592] Heather J. Ballard: Exercise makes your brain bigger: skeletal muscle VEGF and hippocampal neurogenesis. J Physiol. 2017 Sep 1; 595(17): 5721–5722. doi: 10.1113/JP274658.

[593] Anabolic applications of androgens for functional limitations associated with aging and chronic illness. Bhasin S1, Storer TW. Front Horm Res. 2009.

[594] Testosterone as potential effective therapy in treatment of obesity in men with testosterone deficiency: a review. Saad F1, Aversa A, Isidori AM, Gooren LJ. Curr Diabetes Rev. 2012 Mar;8(2):131-43.

weight training and consistent cardiovascular exercise is like driving a Ferrari and putting water in the gas tank. You don't want to be a very muscular dude who gets winded every time he walks up a flight of stairs!

Building Muscle and Strength

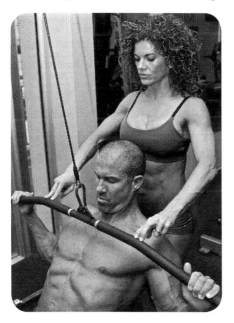

Men should learn how to train large muscle groups with foundational strength movements. **Squats, Over-head Press, Chest Press, Deadlifts, Rows, Pulldowns and Pull-Ups** are excellent weightlifting exercises for men using TOT.

Plan to exercise 3-5x per week, for 30-60 minutes per session (sessions may take longer if you're training with a partner, versus train-ing alone).

For an optimized weight lifting program, we recommend you use Jim Brown's Forged Training[595]. Forged is a system of training that allows for maximal muscle gain with minimal time spent in the gym. Later in this chapter, you'll see some sample training schedules taken directly from Forged.

---

[595]   www.advancedforgedtraining.com

One of the essential things you'll learn how to do in the gym is maximally contract your muscle fibers[596]. You do this by improving your mind-muscle connection. Here's what that means:

As you improve the communication taking place between your mind and your muscle fibers, you'll contract your muscles more effectively and build muscle faster. That's because testosterone has been proven to enhance the neurological and adaptive response of muscle fibers to weight lifting (i.e. you can better contract the right fibers, and contract them even harder)[597].

Think of the mind-muscle connection as applying the technique of *visualization* to your weight lifting. You picture yourself executing the movement in your head, while allowing your mind to truly see and feel the exercise before you perform it. Doing so requires strong mental concentration, as it will help you eliminate all external distractions, while focusing all of your energy on finishing your exercise. It also requires you to consciously control the weight, executing every single rep and set in picture-perfect form. The importance of perfect form while maximally contracting your muscle fibers can not be emphasized enough when it comes to building an amazing body.

Depending on your level of weightlifting experience, it will take time to learn how to execute perfect form. This is especially true if you are in the early stages of entering a gym. It will take

---

[596] http://fabfitover40.com/2014/05/09/do-you-know-how-to-maximally-contract-your-muscle-fibers/

[597] Ng Tang Fui M, Prendergast LA, Dupuis P, et al. Effects of testosterone treatment on body fat and lean mass in obese men on a hypocaloric diet: a randomised controlled trial. BMC Medicine. 2016;14:153. doi:10.1186/s12916-016-0700-9.

months, and sometimes years of consistent and focused training to perfect your form. If you try to remember the acronym **V-C-C** (Visualize, Concentrate and Control) and regularly make it a point of focus when performing your lifts, you'll be well on your way to attaining the physique you seek.

You can also utilize various intensity techniques like Rest Pause Training[598], supersets, varying rest intervals between each set, and four-second eccentrics[599]. Mastering these techniques is the quickest way to build muscle mass as efficiently as possible, but you should only use them once you can execute the fundamental exercises with perfect form.

It is critically important to eliminate ego and momentum[600] from your training through controlled cadence (i.e. controlling the speed at which each rep is done) and strict lifting technique. Removing ego and momentum from your training sessions will be the difference between staying average and building a world class physique.

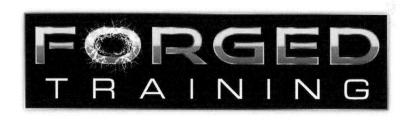

---

[598] http://fabfitover40.com/2014/09/15/ffover-40s-rest-pause-workout-explained/

[599] http://fabfitover40.com/2014/07/23/want-high-thick-ridge-clavicular-pec-muscle/

[600] http://fabfitover40.com/2014/08/01/ego-and-momentum/

Most people who go to the gym will 'work out' without any plan or strategy. As a result, they get half-assed results and look the same, even after spending DECADES in the gym. Don't be one of those people!

You've already made the decision to purchase this book, and you've already read everything up to here. Now, it's time to go ALL IN and level up your life by choosing to work with a professional. Someone who can show you how to train with weights using proper form and technique. This is exactly why Jim and Jay have created the Forged Training Video Series[601].

We've attached two separate variants of Forged ('3 Day for Maximum Fat Loss', and '4 Day for Maximum Muscle Preservation/Gain') to give you examples of how both Jim and Jay train. These weight lifting programs are designed in conjunction with our book *The Metabolic Blowtorch Diet*[602], but can also be used as basic training paradigms for your specific fitness goals (building muscle, losing body fat, maintaining, etc.).

Here is a sample day of Jay's training from a 3 Day Max Fat Loss Protocol:

---

[601]   www.advancedforgedtraining.com

[602]   www.metabolicblowtorchdiet.com

Day 1, Monday: (Chest, Back, Triceps, Abs)

EXERCISE	WARM-UP SETS	WORKING SETS TO POSITIVE FAILURE
Slight Incline Pres	1-3	2
Meadows Rows	1-3	2
Fly Machine	1-3	2
Mag Grip Inner Grip Pulldown	1-3	2
Press Machine (Decline or Flat):	1-3	2
Wide Grip Pull Ups with Band	1-3	2
Triceps Pushdowns	1-3	2
Tricep Cable Rope Extension	1-3	2
Weighted Machine Crunch	1-3	2

FOR ALL WORKING SETS: 1st working set should be in the 20 rep range (~20-30) and 2nd set should be in the 12-20 rep range. You're going to positive muscle failure (PF).

For more specific instructions (exercises, stretches, form/technique and rep ranges) on training the Forged way, sign up for the Forged training series[603]. You will also be given access to the private Facebook group where Jim and other high level fitness experts are actively involved.

---

[603]   www.advancedforgedtraining.com

For Maximum Fat Loss
(3 Days Lifting and 4 Days Fasting + Cardio)

	MON	WED	FRI
CHEST	Fly & Press		
BACK	Pulldown or Pullup Rows		
SHOULDERS			Press, Front Raises Laterals
BICEPS			Preacher Hammer Concentration
TRICEPS	Pushdown Extension Dip		
LEGS		Press or Squat Iso Quad / Hamstring	
CALVES		Knee bent or Knee Str.	
ABS	Weight Machine Crunch	Hanging Leg Raises	Roman Chair Crunches

BS

For Maximum Muscle Preservation
(4 Lifting Days and 2 or 3 Fasting + Cardio Days)
depends on level of body fat

	DAY 1 OF 7	DAY 2 OF 7	DAY 4/5 OF 7	DAY 5/6 OF 7
CHEST	Fly		Press	
BACK	Pulldown		Row	
SHOULDERS	Press		Lateral	
BICEPS		Reverse		Regular
TRICEPS		Skull Crush		Cable Ext.
LEGS		Press		Isolation Quad/ Hamstring
CALVES		Knee bent		Knee Str.
ABS	Upper	Lower		

The Cardio Equation - How Much and What Kind?

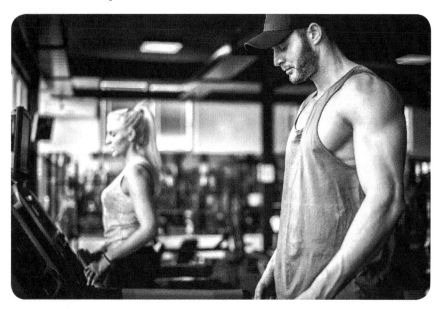

An optimal strategy for cardiovascular training is to perform *low-impact endurance exercise 3-7x per week*, depending on your body fat levels. We recommend **20-45 minutes per session at 65-80% of your maximum heart rate**. This should put you in the **125-140 bpm range**[604].

Regular endurance exercise (i.e. 'cardio') has protective effects on the vascular system[605], including nitric oxide release and reducing Low Density Lipoprotein (i.e. 'bad' cholesterol) levels, which leads to an overall reduction of inflammation. Remember:

---

[604] Please calculate your target heart rate by following the instructions found at http://www.active.com/fitness/calculators/heartrate. We are assuming you are using a low-impact cardio machine that calculates heart rate, but you can also wear things like an Apple Watch to determine your heart rate.

[605] Moderate cardiorespiratory fitness is positively associated with resting metabolic rate in young adults. Mayo Clin Proc. 2014 Jun;89(6):763-71. Epub 2014 May 5.

Inflammation leads to the chronic conditions brought on by the diseases of aging. Endurance exercise (in our opinion) reduces blood thickening (erythrocytosis) often seen in injectable TOT users.

Optimal forms include *walking outside, walking on a treadmill at an incline, riding a stationary bike,* using a *StairMaster, rowing machine* (ergometer) an *elliptical*, or *swimming.*

If you have higher body fat and want to lose it fast and efficiently, you can up the intensity of your endurance exercise by performing *interval training*, or *high-intensity interval training* (HIIT). This type of cardiovascular training increases the rate of fat loss and enhances the potential number of calories burned per unit of time. There is newer research about supramaximal interval training (SMIT) being the most effective[606] for fat loss and lean muscle tissue growth. SMIT involves interval training at 100-130% of your maximum aerobic capacity for roughly 30-60 seconds, followed by 4-5 minutes of active recovery (20-25% max capacity). To calculate your heart rate training zones, read this article[607].

Anyone choosing to perform HIIT/SMIT cardiovascular training should have a good amount of existing muscle tissue, as either form of cardio can break down muscle protein (especially in newer and less conditioned trainees). Here are some articles that demonstrate effective HIT[608] and SMIT[609] protocols. **Remember:** If you are an aging athlete, LOW IMPACT forms of cardio are best when performing HIT or SMIT to avoid potential injury to soft tissues and joints.

---

[606] https://www.ncbi.nlm.nih.gov/pmc/articles/PMC1665058/

[607] http://www.chabotcollege.edu/faculty/kgrace/FitnessCenter/TargetZones.htm

[608] https://www.topfitnessmag.com/hiit-workout-2/hiit-indoor-cycling-workout/

[609] https://www.mensfitness.com/training/pro-tips/beginners-guide-supramaximal-training

NOTE Both Jay and Jim like to do their low impact cardio and maintain a heart rate of around 135-145 BPM. Jay has a Lifecycle cardio bike right next to his bed, and a treadmill with a 15' incline on the other side, which allows him easy access to his once (or twice) a day cardio session. He normally rides his Lifecycle at an intensity of 15-16 (according to the bike's settings) for 30-45 minutes, depending on his schedule. Jim has a really nice elliptical in his home as well. Low impact cardio with variable intensity manipulation is the strategy to pursue as you age to maintain low body fat and optimal health.

We discuss all of this in in our book *The Metabolic Blowtorch Diet: How to Optimize Intermittent Fasting to Burn Fat, Preserve Muscle, Enhance Focus and Transform Your Health*[610].

☆☆☆☆☆ **I honestly can't believe this hasn't been written about before [This book shocked me]**
By Benjamin Brown on October 17, 2017
Format: Kindle Edition

As a clinical nutritionist and trainer, and having been in the industry for over 15 years, I have literally seen it all...

and I honestly can't believe this hasn't been written about before:

Jay and Jim have taken the relevant research AND anecdotal experience using their 20+ years of training and coaching in the industry to formulate an incredible resource for facilitating FAST fat loss and optimizing health long-term.

Let's be honest though, with all the B.S. quick-fix, fad diet, detox scams out there, you may be reticent and frankly skeptical about how effective this program could really be... Well, just STOP. This book is a LEGITIMATE resource in which the information is laid out in an easy to understand, yet comprehensive manner that is tried and tested to have not only measurable, but incredible body transformation results.

WARNING: if you're not willing to take the time to exercise and train 3x/week, well, then this isn't for you. There are no magic potions, powders or pills herein that will do the work for you. BUT, if you're already training, eating pretty well and READY to take a light speed approach to ramping up your fat loss in such a seemingly simple way, then quick dragging your feet and GET THIS BOOK.

---

610   https://www.amazon.com/exec/obidos/ASIN/B075YB3GQT/trtrev-71-20

I literally read it cover to cover in a couple hours and took pages upon pages of notes. Like I said, real science coupled with a lifetimes worth of invaluable experience. THESE GUYS KNOW THEIR CRAFT and have the results to back it up - AND are sharing that with you.

Do You Want to:

> Facilitate Faster Fat Loss in an easy to implement way?
> Eat the foods you want without feeling like you're constantly being restricted and starved?
> Experience more energy and BRAIN POWER and FOCUS than you've ever had?
> Learn how to eat on the road effortlessly while still honoring your weight loss goals?
> Actually turn your body into a healthier and more efficient disease fighting machine?

If you answered YES to any of these, then THE METABOLIC BLOWTORCH DIET is for you...

BUT don't take my word for it, check it out for yourself. You won't be sorry.

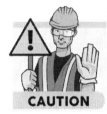

CAUTION

As an aging athlete (40+ years old), it's critically important that you minimize or avoid high-impact endurance exercises. Examples include running on hard surfaces (i.e. jogging outside) or ballistic movements (such as those found in programs like CrossFit). Those exercises can (and will) damage your soft tissues and spine, potentially leading to significant joint problems later in life. For more information on why this happens, watch Jay's video "How Running and Cardio Can Lead to Life in a Wheelchair"[611].

The Importance of Sleep

Don't try and be the type of person who doesn't get enough sleep. You CAN NOT hack sleep. Sleep is critical, period. It prevents a variety of disease processes including obesity and

---

[611]   http://youtu.be/4gDdeMLOoJs

coronary artery disease. It also prevents neurodegenerative diseases like Alzheimer's and dementia. Lack of sleep can, and does, cause inflammation[612].

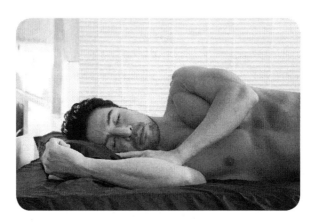

Adequate rest optimizes your recovery from the damage and stress applied to muscle fibers by intense resistance training. Most of the newest research indicates that the optimal amount of nightly sleep is between **5.5 and 7 hours**. In fact, sleeping longer than 8 hours can actually increases one's risk of death[613]. On top of getting a good night's rest, you also want to sleep with proper anatomical form to avoid stiffness and soreness in your neck and back. To learn more about correct sleeping form, read the article "Correct Sleeping Posture"[614].

---

[612] Hall MH, Smagula SF, Boudreau RM, et al. Association between Sleep Duration and Mortality Is Mediated by Markers of Inflammation and Health in Older Adults: The Health, Aging and Body Composition Study. *Sleep*. 2015;38(2):189-195. doi:10.5665/sleep.4394.

[613] Sanjay R. Patel, MD, Najib T. Ayas, MD, MPH, Mark R. Malhotra, David P. White, MD, Eva S. Schernhammer, MD, DrPH, Frank E. Speizer, MD, Meir J. Stampfer, MD, DrPH, Frank B. Hu, MD, PhD; A Prospective Study of Sleep Duration and Mortality Risk in Women, *Sleep*, Volume 27, Issue 3, 1 May 2004, Pages 440-444, https://doi.org/10.1093/sleep/27.3.440.

[614] http://www.livestrong.com/article/179141-correct-sleeping-posture/

Melatonin

You can't have a discussion about sleep without also talking about the supplement **Melatonin**. Melatonin is a derivative of the amino acid tryptophan. It is primarily synthesized in the pineal gland and released at night to make falling asleep easier (while also improving sleep quality). In addition to improving sleep, melatonin has a strong antioxidant property that's responsible for repairing cellular DNA[615]. It has also been shown to support other aspects of health, such as the immune system and brain functioning[616].

Melatonin is a hormone that is necessary for keeping our circadian rhythm in tune[617]. Many people experience difficulty falling asleep and staying asleep, and these issues occur because the secretion of melatonin declines with age, causing many of our biological functions to become impaired[618]. Furthermore, melatonin release can also be affected by jet lag, shift work, and poor vision[619]. As you already know, a good night's sleep is crucial for health and well-being.

As we've already stated, melatonin has strong antioxidant properties. It directly scavenges both hydroxyl and peroxyl free

---

[615]   Jenwitheesuk A, Nopparat C, Mukda S, Wongchitrat P, Govitrapong P. Melatonin Regulates Aging and Neurodegeneration through Energy Metabolism, Epigenetics, Autophagy and Circadian Rhythm Pathways. International Journal of Molecular Sciences. 2014;15(9):16848-16884. doi:10.3390/ijms150916848.

[616]   Shin E-J, Chung YH, Le H-LT, et al. Melatonin Attenuates Memory Impairment Induced by Klotho Gene Deficiency Via Interactive Signaling Between MT2 Receptor, ERK, and Nrf2-Related Antioxidant Potential. International Journal of Neuropsychopharmacology. 2015;18(6):pyu105. doi:10.1093/ijnp/pyu105.

[617]   Free Radic Res. 2002 Dec;36(12):1323-9.

[618]   J Pineal Res. 1994 May;16(4):178-83.

[619]   Pineal Res. 2011 Jan;50(1):1-7.

radicals, far more effectively than most other antioxidants. It also greatly potentiates the efficiency of other antioxidants (i.e. makes their antioxidant effect even stronger)[620]. Finally, melatonin has a beneficial impact on the immune system. It activates T-helper cells to trigger other immune cells, naturally boosting the immune system's responsiveness to foreign molecules[621].

The cognitive decline that occurs as we age may be directly related to the drop in melatonin[622] secretion. Melatonin supplementation can help support the brain's natural antioxidant system and potentially inhibit the factors that can lead to cognitive decline. **A typical dose taken before bed to aid sleep is anywhere from 0.3 mg to 20 mg**. If you have trouble falling asleep, you may try the regular tablet, or even opt for a sublingual. If you have even more of an issue staying asleep, then you may want to try an 'extended release' version. Some users may wake up groggy, so if that happens to you, cut back on the dosage and fine tune it to your correct dose. Some people do not respond well to the usage of melatonin. As always, self-experimentation is key.

Dealing with Injuries

It is nearly impossible to be an aging athlete and not suffer from some form of injury. Sprains, strains and tears of ligaments and tendons can (and will) happen. When it does happen to you,

---

[620]   Aging (Milano). Oct 1995;7(5):340-51.

[621]   Eur J Cancer. 1999; 35:1688-92.

[622]   Wade AG, Farmer M, Harari G, et al. Add-on prolonged-release melatonin for cognitive function and sleep in mild to moderate Alzheimer's disease: a 6-month, randomized, placebo-controlled, multicenter trial. *Clinical Interventions in Aging.* 2014;9:947-961. doi:10.2147/CIA.S65625.

the most important thing is recognition of the injury and then establishing a treatment protocol.

An aging athlete's perspective on their injury will impact how well they cope and (in some cases) how quickly they recover. Those who have a positive attitude & outlook, intrinsic motivation, and a low fear of re-injury will do best. It is also important to have a willingness to learn about your injury and be dedicated to consistently perform the rehabilitation techniques necessary to heal it.

For sprains and strains, first utilize the RICE method (Rest, Ice, Compression and Elevation). We also recommend dosing Ibuprofen up to 800 mg every 4-6 hours the first 2-3 days to reduce inflammation, depending on the level of severity of the injury. We recommend an X-Ray and/or potentially an MRI once swelling subsides. This will depend on the severity of the injury with regard to mobility and range of motion (ROM). For minor strains or sprains, the use of Penetrex[623] directly rubbed into the origin of the injury often alleviates soreness and may speed the healing process.

You then have to account for time off. Jim and Jay have a very basic rule when it comes to training and injuries:

If it hurts, don't do it

That's right. The statement NO PAIN, NO GAIN is quite possibly the DUMBEST BRO SCIENCE AXIOM ever put forth in the realm of training and fitness. The focus is always on healing and getting back to 100% as quickly as humanly possible. This will not happen if you continue to train an injured area under physical duress.

---

[623]   http://fabfitover40.com/2014/08/15/penetrex-must-topical-pain-relief-therapy/

There are many things we have used over the years to attempt to "injury proof" ourselves while maintaining our mobility and rehabbing our injuries. These are all based on either increasing or maintaining mobility in our joints, while also removing or breaking up adhesions and/or scar tissue.

For mobility, we have been following **Kelly Starrett** for years. You can find his videos all over the net and he has a site called *MobilityWOD*[624]. This is an unlimited resource for all things related to mobility, from compression bands to aspects of human anatomy you've never even heard of. Kelly provides a daily 10-15 minute mobility workout, as well as various classes and specialty videos. Each of them deal with specific limitations and issues, while also showcasing a variety of tools and how to use them to achieve better mobility.

We also recommend **yoga** for flexibility. It also has amazing spiritual benefits and helps immensely on a few different levels in terms of mobility, injury prevention and even spinal health. **Chiropractic therapies** that require adjustments (i.e. a form of spinal manipulation) to remove shifted vertebrae back into natural alignment are very effective and highly recommended, especially if you are a muscular individual.

Both Jay and Jim and been working with a certified **Active Release Technique Massage Therapist (ART)** practitioner for years and can not recommend them enough. You can find a certified practitioner in your area by visiting this active release therapy website[625].

---

[624] www.mobilitywod.com

[625] http://www.activerelease.com/

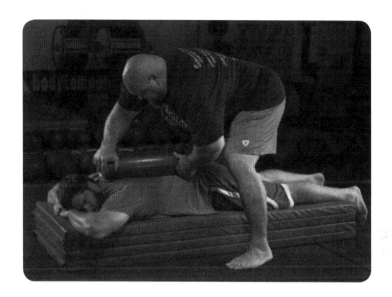

The last form of manual therapy we employ for reducing adhesions and scar tissue is body tempering. **Body tempering** is a process that uses various mechanisms to break tissue out of its adhesive state when it's placed under a crushing load. This therapy helps prevent hernias, tears, tweaks, ruptures and trauma. **Super D, Donnie Thompson**[626] created this therapy and it comes with a long line of success stories. Jim attended one of his seminars and had amazing results when applying body tempering to his own rehabilitation.

Because injuries are an inevitable part of life, it's important for us to mention new and advanced therapies to speed up and improve the healing process. New studies are being released on the therapeutic effects of **sauna heat therapy**. The regular usage of saunas can lower the risk of stroke, heart disease, and dementia.

---

[626]   https://bodytempering.com/

A Finnish study[627] that followed the sauna habits and health of 2,500 men for 20 years found that regular sauna-goers are far less likely to die of heart disease and stroke, or to develop dementia. And research from this year shows that using a sauna 4-7 times a week can reduce high blood pressure by nearly 50%, while improving chronic pain symptoms in diseases like arthritis[628]. These benefits can likely be attributed to an increased heart rate and a widening of the blood vessels, which increases circulation (similar to the effects of regular exercise).

Just as heat from sauna therapy works to speed healing, so does the super-cold temperatures produced by **cryotherapy**. Cryotherapy is a form of extreme-cold treatment that can also speed recovery, reduce injuries, increase energy and improve sleep[629]. Jay injured his back when deadlifting in the summer of 2015 and used a Cryo Chamber for 2 consecutive months to rapidly return to pre-injured form.

If you suffer from chronic pain and neurological inflammation, we highly recommend you investigate **grounding** (also known as **earthing**). There are more than 20 peer reviewed studies[630] on grounding demonstrating its profound effects on reducing inflammation. Very simply, grounding means placing one's bare

[627] Tanjaniina Laukkanen, Hassan Khan, Francesco Zaccardi, Jari A. Laukkanen. Association Between Sauna Bathing and Fatal Cardiovascular and All-Cause Mortality Events. JAMA Intern Med. 2015;175(4):542–548. doi:10.1001/jamainternmed.2014.8187.

[628] Tanjaniina Laukkanen, Hassan Khan, Francesco Zaccardi, Jari A. Laukkanen. Association Between Sauna Bathing and Fatal Cardiovascular and All-Cause Mortality Events. JAMA Intern Med. 2015;175(4):542–548. doi:10.1001/jamainternmed.2014.8187.

[629] Kadakia KC, Rozell SA, Butala AA, Loprinzi CL. Supportive Cryotherapy: A Review from Head to Toe. *Journal of pain and symptom management.* 2014;47(6):1100-1115. doi:10.1016/j.jpainsymman.2013.07.014.

[630] https://www.ncbi.nlm.nih.gov/pmc/?term=Grounding+and+Earthing

feet on natural earthen ground. For an amazing video explaining the healing power of grounding (especially in relation to reducing inflammation), watch *"Dr. Mercola says: "I'm grounded 95% of the day!" (Down to Earth - Full 15 Minutes Video)*[631]. For much more information on understanding grounding, familiarize yourself with Earthing.com's website[632].

For those of you who suffer serious joint or tendon injuries, **Protein Rich Plasma (PRP)** injections offer great hope. As a concentrated source of blood plasma and autologous conditioned plasma, PRP contains several different growth factors and other cytokines that can speed the healing of soft tissue and joints[633]. Both Jay and Jim know men who've had the PRP injections into their shoulder and knee capsules, and the effects have been miraculous. Unfortunately, there is more hype than substance with regards to studies[634] that conclusively prove the efficacy of PRP. However, because we know many people in our circles who have had the procedure done with significant long-term effectiveness, we recommend it as an effective strategy for recovering from severe soft tissue trauma or injury. With that being said, we do recommend manual therapy first before using PRP as the final solution to heal a severely damaged joint or soft tissue.

---

[631]   https://youtu.be/CSNnIg2cVjc

[632]   https://www.earthing.com/earthing-basics/

[633]   Intra-articular Autologous Conditioned Plasma Injections Provide Safe and Efficacious Treatment for Knee Osteoarthritis: An FDA-Sanctioned, Randomized, Double-blind, Placebo-controlled Clinical Trial. Patrick A. Smith, MD. The American Journal of Sports Medicine Vol 44, Issue 4, pp. 884 - 891.

[634]   Implicit hype? Representations of platelet rich plasma in the news media. Christen Rachul, John E. J. Rasko, Timothy Caulfield. Published: August 9, 2017.

Spiritual Fitness

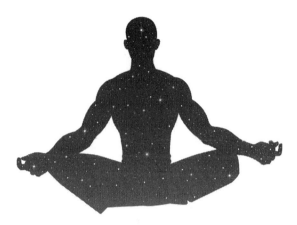

Why bother including a subsection on spirituality in a book on hormonal health? Think about it this way: What happens to a person when their hormones are optimized? Their energy increases! With increased energy, you have the capacity to fully utilize the vessel we call our body. Your body (i.e. your vessel) houses your spirit/soul (energy). Your spirit can fully express its power with a physical body that is fully energized.

Increased energy levels mean that you are more attuned to different frequencies. To understand what this means, picture a computer. If you are dealing with an old and slow computer, it is more challenging for you to search the Internet. However, if you have a state-of-the-art computer with a fast processor connected to fiber optic broadband, then you can access all of the Internet's robust videos and imagery with blazing speed!

You may choose to view this as woo-woo nonsense, and you are well within your rights to do so. But before you do, consider this: For thousands of years, spirituality was an important part of everyday life. We DO NOT define spirituality with religion. In fact, it is our understanding that the belief in the influence of a higher power starts within.

We live in a very hectic world today. Social media, in particular, is the ever-increasing cause of 'disconnection' and 'attention fragmentation'. Most of us live on the edge of stressful thoughts, anger, confusion, opinion, gossip, shame and FEAR. These thoughts and feelings control the entire existence of many people, and the world around them. There is very little wisdom and critical thinking, thus leading to little understanding and true insight. The only way to bring light to the chaos is to go within.

You need to learn to connect with your inner essence (your soul, spirit, intuition - some even like to call it 'God') through the contemplation of WHAT IS. "What is" can only be defined as pure consciousness, wisdom and love. Harnessing WHAT IS can transform your entire being by improving your confidence, wisdom, self discipline and ability to love and serve others.

Understanding this, we believe it takes a very conscious and pro-active effort to forcibly remove yourself from the negative thoughts and distractions of daily life. The best way to do this is through conscious, ritualistic and daily employment of one (if not all) of the following techniques: *Visualization, meditation, manifestation, chakra (energy centers) alignment and healing.* We have found that when you are aligned with your spiritual essence, your vehicle (known as your body) can better absorb any positive health optimization strategy you decide to implement. It's great to have the desire to be healthy and "want" to be healthier, yet if you are caught up in the busyness of life, it will be far more challenging to adopt any of these techniques and consistently use them over a long period of time.

Let's briefly discuss each of the techniques.

Visualization

This is a very powerful technique that uses the power of your mind to make any dream or goal become a reality. It is the creative force behind all of humanity's achievements. Think back to your favorite achievement: Remember how good it felt, basking in the warm glow of accomplishment and success? Jay often thinks back to the moment when the desire to write the first TRT MANual was but a tiny seed of a thought in his mind, and he chose to say "YES" to the idea (even though he had no clue what was going to happen).

What was he thinking about then? Was he worried and afraid, or excited and enthusiastic? Did he visualize the book as an amazing accomplishment? Did he say to himself, "I want this and I am going to do this," or did he say "I want this but I don't know if I could ever achieve this"? When Jay was first thinking about this goal, he was visualizing it as though it were already accomplished. This is creative visualization in action.

By repeatedly visualizing an event, situation, object or person, you tell your subconscious mind that THIS is what you will have/ be, and this is what it must seek. And it happens!

Truthfully, there's no magic to creative visualization. It's a natural process of using the power of your thoughts to imprint your desires into your mind, while projecting the right kind of energetic vibration that attracts what you desire. We have found that when you can "see" yourself accomplishing something, along with the feeling you will have once it has been accomplished, then it is easier for you to step into it. Remember, it is important to avoid getting attached to the outcome. You will always get the essence of your desire; it just may not be packaged exactly in the way you originally pictured it.

Meditation

Meditation can be defined as understanding and yielding to the power of the human spirit through an inner knowing of WHAT IS. Meditation is connecting with nature at its purest form, and it's also a place where the human form does not exist because your consciousness is free from thoughts and ignorance. Regularly meditating boosts your emotional and intellectual intelligence, allowing one to better understand the depth of life. It will provide strong self discipline to all aspects of any person's life, should they stick to it. It also provides you with the confidence and strength to serve others, acting as a beacon of inspiration and hope.

Anyone can meditate. All it takes is consistent practice every day and and an approach of inner contemplation, without the influence of ego or ambition. To start, find a place where you will not be bothered or distracted. Going into nature and planting your feet firmly in the soil (**grounding** as discussed in the previous section) will allow you to connect with the wondrous and awe-inspiring power of Mother Earth's healing energy.

We hear many people state that they can not meditate, but the truth is that everyone can meditate. Meditation is not only about sitting with your legs crossed and your hands on your lap. In fact, you can meditate while doing almost anything. You can do a walking meditation, a mindful meditation or even a prayer-based meditation. The point is this: Meditation can take many forms. Jay meditates when riding his Lifecycle.

Don't judge your meditation - simply be present to the experience of BEING. Focus on your breath, and appreciate it as it runs through your body. A great article to read about meditation and mindfulness (i.e. being fully present) is *Meditation for Beginners: 20 Practical Tips for Understanding the Mind*[635].

Manifestation

Manifestation is the intense and inward belief (i.e. knowing) in yourself to attain whatever your heart desires in life. This can be done in numerous ways. It can start with eliminating negative and limiting beliefs. When you start manifesting, approach it from the perspective of being joyous by removing your fearful and lack-based feelings. Allow yourself to believe in the power of your thoughts and truly feel your emotions. Be positive, happy and believe in the impossible. Fill every cell with love, happiness, joy, peace and let that bright energy radiate outward to attract what you want!

The more you amplify positive emotions, the higher and more powerful your body's vibration will be. Think of vibration like energy - our bodies are always emitting light, energy or frequencies that carry a specific message, information or intention! When your vibration is one of light, peace and loving kindness, you will attract others towards you and in turn this creates tremendous opportunities for joy, advancement and success.

Remember: You are whole and complete. Attachment to situations, people, or things only repels things away from you.

What you RESIST, PERSISTS!

Allow yourself to be a magnet by being a great observer in your life. Open your mind up to the numerous possibilities and ways

---

[635]   https://zenhabits.net/meditation-guide/

that things can show up in your life. It truly is amazing how our world opens up when we choose to receive what life throws at us with open arms and without judgement.

Chakra Body Alignment

Chakras are the spiritual energy centers of our body. They are the openings for our life energy to flow into and out of our soul, and they function by vitalizing our physical body and improving the development of our self-consciousness (i.e. our awareness). The chakras are associated with our physical, mental and emotional interactions with the world.

There are seven major chakras, and each is invisible to the human eye. The aura given off by all seven is often referred to as the eighth chakra. The first chakra (root) actually hangs outside of your body. It is located between your thighs, about halfway between your knees and your physical body. The seven chakra (*crown*) is located on the top of your head. The remaining chakras, (*sacral, solar plexus, heart, throat,* and *third eye*) are aligned in sequence along your spine, neck, and skull. See the accompanying picture on the next page to gain a visual understanding of the Chakra body structure.

Most people in today's world, due to mass-engineered societal living, are completely UNAWARE of their surroundings. So much so, in fact, that they are completely blocked off from receiving chakra alignment and healing. Poor physical conditioning and nutrition has lead to rampant obesity and suboptimal hormone levels. Improving your health and your physical condition will therefore allow you to maximize your spiritual energy centers.

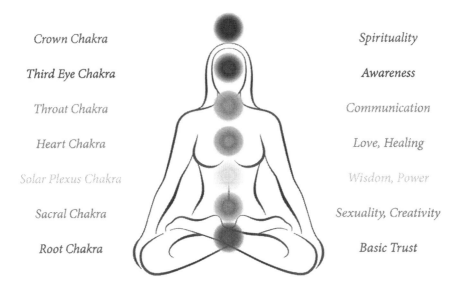

Crown Chakra — Spirituality

Third Eye Chakra — Awareness

Throat Chakra — Communication

Heart Chakra — Love, Healing

Solar Plexus Chakra — Wisdom, Power

Sacral Chakra — Sexuality, Creativity

Root Chakra — Basic Trust

Having your chakras evaluated by a trained practitioner (i.e. energy worker) is a good way to get a better understanding of how your body functions on an energetic level. A trained energy worker will be able to tell you which chakras are functioning poorly, and which chakras are working overtime. Jim and Jay use the Chakra Meditation Balancing app[636] almost daily to ensure their chakras stay in balance.

Now that you have a decent amount of familiarity with the various techniques, you can apply them to improve your spirituality. We think it's easiest if we show you how we employ some of these techniques on a daily basis. That way, you can start incorporating them into your own life.

---

[636] https://itunes.apple.com/us/app/chakra-meditation-balancing/
id886156937?mt=8

(What Jay's typical day looks like):

6:00 AM: Wake up and think of 2-5 things I'm grateful for. I also send love to 3 random people. I then turn on the Chakra Healing Guides app and connect my bluetooth headphones to my phone to listen.

For the next 3-5 minutes, as I am dressing, I think of my intentions for the day and I also take 5 deep breaths while saying the following affirmation to myself in my head:

> *"I am joy. I am love. I am gratitude. I see, hear, feel and know the purpose of my life is to optimize human health. I am powerful, persuasive, and intentional in all that I say and do, serving the Creator of All and walking the path towards spiritual enlightenment"*

If I remember to do it, I'll use the 5 Minute Journal App on my phone. I then drive to the gym for 35-50 minutes of cardio on a stationary bike (if pressed for time, I use the bike next to my bed). When I'm doing cardio, I'm always reading a new book.

6:45 AM: On days where I'm lifting weights, I will normally take a shower and say my affirmations to my shower mirror (i.e. a mirror exercise) as I shave. I'm always listening to the Chakra Healing Guides app on my bluetooth speaker while in the shower.

8:00 AM: If time allows, I will go outside and plant my feet in the grass and sun gaze for 2-3 minutes while also mentally reciting and visualizing myself as my 3 power words: **Powerful-Persuasive-Intentional.**

8:30 AM: Before training, I say a 25-second prayer and ask for an amazing training session.

10:00 AM: My calendar sends me a notification asking me: ***"What am I feeling"? "Am I feeling inspired?"*** I always stop what I'm doing and answer these questions with my eyes closed, while feeling my thoughts as much as possible (focusing on my 3 power words).

12:00 PM: Daily affirmation to my inner guidance and for greater cosmic awareness.

3:00 PM: My calendar sends me a notification asking me: ***"What Am I Creating?" "What is Successful Right Now?"*** I close my eyes and answer this, visualizing my answer as powerfully as I can.

6:00 PM: My calendar sends me a notification ***"What Am I Grateful for right now?"*** and it also asks me to focus on my 3 action words, **Powerful-Persuasive-Intentional.**

8:00 PM: My calendar sends me a notification reminding me to take 5 deep breaths right now and to focus on this statement: ***"I Choose to be Grateful and Optimistic Always."***

10:00 PM - 11:00 PM: I will get a reminder on my phone to think about my day. What were my thoughts, solutions and successes? What was great and amazing about my day? What do I desire to remember? I will then map out my intentions for the next day. I do this by clearing my mind for 3-5 minutes, and visualizing what I want to accomplish tomorrow. I may use my 5 Minute Journal app or write in my Panda Pro Planner.

Imagine if you started giving heartfelt appreciation for everything in your life. Not just the good and the happy, but also the bad, the scary, the unpleasant, the difficult, and the painful. What if you started seeing the blessings and lessons in everything, and the beauty in all people?

As we always say to one another in our inner circles:

THE GIFT IS IN THE SHIT

There is NOTHING more truthful and empowering than being able to fully acknowledge and embrace this axiom. Write it down, put it up on your wall, and engrave it in your brain.

What if you were to realize that your happiness does not depend on anything but your decision to be happy? What if you said to yourself, "I don't have to allow this to bring me down. I can deal with this situation in the spirit of optimism by enjoying this very moment?"

To finish this chapter off, we wanted to provide you with an amazing tool to use when you encounter resistance in your life. This was provided to Jay by Marci Lock[637], which she calls *The 5 Steps to Overcome Sabotage.* If you make a conscious effort to utilize this tool whenever you encounter resistance and struggle in your life, your mind will be blown at the ease and skill with which you'll handle tough times with grace.

---

[637] https://www.facebook.com/marci.lock

5 Steps to Overcome Sabotage - Quick Reference Guide

1. **What Am I Feeling Right Now? Where is It in my Body?**

   I Notice I feel....

2. **Why Am I Feeling this way? What's the thought, perception, belief or trigger?**

3. **What do I Really Want Right Now? What Questions can I use to break this down? Is it really, absolutely True? What is the feedback?**

4. **What is the NEW Belief or Perception you are now choosing to get what you want? Change it to FAITH energy! See it out of Excitement, wonderment and curiosity.**

5. **What is the ACTION you get to take NOW to give you what you want?**

   In this circumstance, what would I get to do to get what I want? What is the next step? Ask your internal self what you want and for help creating the Solution.

Change your vibe and change your state to feel good. But above all else, **choose to create the life you truly deserve.**

If you've not skipped ahead, this subsection is likely resonating deep inside your core being. It's quite possible you're ready for much more on the spiritual enlightenment path. If so, we strongly encourage you to get to know another side of Jay Campbell by joining his private Facebook group *Decoders of Truth (DOT)*[638]. We also recommend subscribing to both the TRT Revolution[639] and Decoders of Truth podcasts. Jay interviews thought leaders and authors on the esoteric, the unseen quantum world and the search for mankind's true ancestry.

[638] www.facebook.com/decodersoftruth
[639] www.youtube.com/TRTRevolution

KEY TAKEAWAYS

- We tell you about the foundational role of weight training in optimizing your testosterone levels (and your overall health), and the benefits of being lean and muscular.

- You learn about the importance of following a well-designed weight lifting program that uses foundational strength movements. As well, we teach you how to develop the mind-muscle connection and tell you why executing every rep and set of every exercise with perfect form is crucial to your success in building a world-class physique.

- We reveal an optimal strategy for cardiovascular training - exactly how many times to do it per week, how long to do it each session, the intensity to aim for at each session, the best forms of cardiovascular exercise, and the ones to avoid if you are an aging athlete (40+ years old).

- We discuss the importance of sleep in preventing common diseases and recovering from intense weight lifting workouts. On top of briefly mentioning proper sleeping form, we share our experience with using melatonin for people who have trouble falling asleep at night.

- We discuss dealing with injuries when they inevitably occur as we age. We reveal the type of therapies we apply when we are faced with an unexpected injury.

- Lastly, we demonstrate the power of spiritual fitness in improving every single aspect of your life. As well, we provide 5 proven and time-tested techniques for connecting with your inner spirit.

The State of the Science in Male Hormonal Optimization: An Exclusive Interview with Dr. Rob Kominiarek

In this chapter, Jay interviews one of the most respected thought leaders in all of Age Management: Dr. Rob Kominiarek of Renue Health in Springboro, Ohio. Dr. Kominiarek has been prescribing testosterone to patients successfully for more than 22 years. He has also been using it himself for the same length of time. What follows are his answers to the questions we believe are the most advanced and currently relevant to the clinical practice and field of age management.

Thank you so much, Dr. Kominiarek, for taking the time to answer these questions. Your contribution and serving as part of the TRT Revolution Science Team dramatically strengthens our global mission to optimize male health.

Jay: In your clinical practice, how do you manage your patient's estrogen levels from initiation of Testosterone Optimization Therapy (TOT) through maintenance?

Dr. Rob: The simplest way to manage estrogen is to leave it alone. Estrogen is a pleiotropic hormone that provides numerous health benefits, which include bone and mineral metabolism, cardiac and vascular function, cognition, memory, mood, and neuroprotection. There is rarely a need to decrease estrogen with an aromatase inhibitor (AI) in an individual on TOT. Excess estrogen symptoms can easily be managed by reduction of the testosterone dosage and/or frequency, or short-term low-dose AI usage.

There is no study in existence that demonstrates any benefit to AI usage, only harm. The use of aromatase inhibitors is ubiquitous in the body-building community, as testosterone abuse and the supraphysiologic testosterone levels that follow require intervention with aromatase inhibitors by these individuals. They will all pay the price eventually, most developing osteopenia and osteoporosis. Both disease processes remains unseen until they see a doctor versed in hormone management who understands the potential perils of long-term AI use.

Jay: Let's talk about the prevalence of subclinical thyroid disease (i.e. hypothyroidism)? How do you identify and treat it in your patients?

Dr. Rob: Subclinical hypothyroidism is quite prevalent and underdiagnosed. The devil is in the details when it comes to the diagnosis of subclinical hypothyroidism. Listening carefully to the patient's symptoms, in combination with specific questionnaires designed to discover this often-subtle diagnosis, often makes this diagnosis possible. Careful interpretation of TSH, free T4, free T3, reverse T3, TPO, TSH index, and T3/rT3 ratio will provide additional guidance that will lead to the diagnosis. An individual suffering with thinning hair, sensitivity to cold, dry skin, muscle fatigue and weakness, fatigue, feeling depressed and/or moody, apathy, difficulty losing weight, and periods of constipation has symptoms of low thyroid function. A trial of combination therapy may be used to relieve these symptoms.

Recent studies have confirmed that even mild thyroid disease can affect metabolism. Despite normal laboratory results, patients with subclinical hypothyroidism warrant treatment of their symptoms. Evidence of an association between subclinical hypothyroidism and cardiovascular disease is mounting. The impact of thyroid hormone on lipid levels is primarily mediated through triiodothyronine (T3). The resulting decrease of T3 levels seen in hypothyroidism may result in increased serum cholesterol levels. Current data suggest that normalizing even modest TSH elevations may result in improvement of the lipid profile.

As essential elements of DNA-binding proteins that regulate transcription, thyroid hormones influence the utilization of essentially all substrates, vitamins, and hormones. Replacement doses of T3 sufficient to return levels to normal enhance left ventricular function of the heart and normal expression of T3 responsive genes, thus supporting the therapeutic utility of combination therapy. The Journal of Endocrinology and Metabolism found that even suppressive doses of levothyroxine therapy that lowers TSH to hyperthyroid levels has no significant effect on bone metabolism or bone mass.

Additionally, genetic variants of deiodinase activity are associated with decreasing activity at various end organs as a result of one of two common single nucleotide polymorphisms (Thr92Ala). These changes in deiodinase activity play an important role in an individual's response to replacement therapy. A significant reason as to why some individuals fail to respond to L-T4 therapy alone and feel significantly better on combination L-T4/L-T3 replacement therapy. This is why many of the Dessicated Porcine thyroid medications discussed in Chapter 15 are the optimal therapeutic solutions due to their having a combination of all 4 forms of active thyroid hormone.

In patients with subclinical hypothyroidism, the presence of thyroperoxidase (TPO) antibodies is associated with an increased risk of developing overt hypothyroidism. Many physicians use the TPO antibody test as a diagnostic tool in deciding whether to treat a patient with subclinical hypothyroidism, and the Mayo Clinic (along with numerous studies) endorse this practice. Thyroid disease may be present for years before the clinical manifestation of hypothyroidism becomes evident. The highest TPO levels are observed in patients suffering from Hashimoto's thyroiditis.

Jay: In your own clinical practice, is your TOT for males under the age of 30 different from an older patient? If so, how?

Yes and No. Every man is evaluated as an individual, and based on their medical need, a treatment plan is devised. What therapy we choose to start with depends on numerous individual factors. A young male may take a "ladder approach" to therapy, starting with enclomiphene or HCG, and evaluating the response to therapy before proceeding to testosterone. A 55-year-old male with metabolic syndrome is a "metabolic emergency" and an interventional endocrinology treatment plan with testosterone (along with other hormones, medications, and supplements) will be needed.

Jay: Discuss your thoughts on the importance of monitoring the levels of pregnenolone at initiation and during maintenance of TOT?

Dr. Rob: Whether at the beginning of treatment or sometime after the initiation of therapy, pregnenolone replacement may/will become necessary to offset the eventual disruption of pregnenolone production, due to the loss of the gonadotropin called luteinizing hormone. Luteinizing hormone (LH) stimulates steroidogenesis by up-regulating the rate limiting transport of cholesterol into the inner mitochondrial membrane. LH increases the expression of the P450 cholesterol side-chain cleavage enzyme, which then catalyzes the conversion of cholesterol into pregnenolone.

When on testosterone replacement therapy, you will suppress the production of LH, which is critical for the conversion of cholesterol into pregnenolone and its metabolites. Pregnenolone, progesterone, alloprogesterone, allopregnenolone, and allopregnanolone are hormones that are responsible not only for short-term memory but also for cognition, mood, inflammation, mitochondrial function, and keeping us calm. When you take testosterone, you are altering brain chemistry. Many individuals, after the initiation of therapy, develop anxiety due to the loss of these hormones.

Jay: Knowing that human endocrine systems are under siege via endocrine-disrupting chemicals and a polluted modern day environment, is there any real option right now (i.e. today, in large populated areas) to optimize your health without also undergoing some form of hormonal optimization?

Dr. Rob: Yes. Eat organic, drink plenty of water, exercise daily, limit sugar, avoid alcohol and drugs, use saunas, and perform a monthly detox. Avoid heating foods in microwaves in any plastic containers, use glass containers instead.

Jay: What's the percentage of people you see who respond to lifestyle changes (better nutrition, reduction of cortisol, inflammation, alcohol, improving exercise) in bringing up hormones into optimal ranges, versus those who you place on a TOT protocol?

Dr. Rob: It's extremely low, as there are probably 2 out of 100 men over the age of 50 (and fewer than 20 out of 100 between the ages of 30-50) that can reach upper quartile hormone levels. It takes a truly disciplined type-A individual to implement this type of recovery plan, but it can be done. Type-A men don't ever let it get that far from a metabolic standpoint, unless there has been some serious injury or disease process that was out of their control. However, these lifestyle changes are important for ALL men to adopt. You may not be able to reach upper quartile numbers, but your body will still benefit enormously from these positive health initiatives.

Jay: Is the usage of Exemestane (Aromasin) any better than Arimidex (Anastrozole), from a bone mineral density standpoint, in men when used for estrogen management? Is there ever a time to use an aromatase inhibitor in men when undergoing TOT?

Dr. Rob: The data regarding the use of aromatase inhibitors is not good. All studies only demonstrate harm, and no benefit in the long term. **An appropriately managed testosterone replacement therapy program should rarely require the use of an aromatase inhibitor. If they become necessary to control unwanted side effects, then they should only be used at the minimum effective dose (MED) for a short period of time.** I strongly advocate having a bone densitometry scan (DEXA) performed prior to the initiation of therapy, and at 1 year thereafter. Not a week goes by that we do not see men with severe osteopenia and osteoporosis (i.e. bone deformation and breakdown) from the non-judicious use of aromatase inhibitors. They may "look" good, but they have the bone health of a 90-year-old woman.

Jay: What are your thoughts on the power of TOT to alleviate depression in lieu of SSRI treatment? Can TOT replace the need of an SSRI in most instances?

Dr. Rob: Amazing! If you look at the data over the past decade alone, there have been over 450,000 studies conducted on the use of hormones to treat mood disorders. Studies looking at thyroid, testosterone, estrogen, progesterone, DHEA, pregnenolone, and growth hormone for the treatment of mood disorders. It makes one wonder what in the hell is standard medicine thinking and doing! While psychotropic medications are a valuable tool for treatment in some individuals, they have generally been grossly over-prescribed to treat the symptoms of "life." Neurosteroids and neuroactive steroids have a profound effect on the treatment of mood disorders when replacing the use of psychotropic medications, and there is literally hundreds of thousands of studies that provide evidence to that fact.

Jay: What are your thoughts on the usage of Human Growth Hormone (HGH) in combination with TOT for Age Management? What do you think of GHRP's? Which ones do you use in your clinical practice?

Dr. Rob: Next to thyroid, HGH is probably the most misunder-stood and irrationally feared hormone. HGH can have profound mental and physical effects in those individuals identified through testing to be deficient.

In adults, when using HGH in a clinical dosage, the goals are to restore normal body composition, improve muscle and cardiac function, normalize serum lipid concentrations, and improve quality of life. HGH, in randomized placebo-controlled studies, has shown to enhance energy, self-esteem, social function, general well being, improve memory and cognition, normalize lipid profiles, improve body composition, increase physical capacity, improve heart function with increased myocardial mass and reduced left ventricular size with improvements in hemodynamics, energy and metabolism, reduced CIMT, and improve bone mineral density. An increased incidence in cancers or re-growth of tumors has never been found in any study to date when HGH is used in clinical dosage fashion.

Peptide therapy is the future of medicine: Incredibly safe and effective therapies to intervene in a disease process, or slow the unwanted effects of aging. Peptide therapy aimed at normalization of the serum IGF-1 is associated with significant improvements in serum triglycerides, LDL-C, total cholesterol, total cholesterol/HDL-C ratio, decrease in Carotid intima media thickness and visceral adipose tissue, and atherogenic lipid profile, increase in cardiac output, increase in ejection fraction, decrease in cardiovascular disease, increased lean body mass, decreased inflammatory visceral fat, improvement in energy levels and emotional reaction, improved psychological well-being, improved skeletal mass and osteopenia/osteoporosis scores, decreased fatigability and greater vitality.

My preferred peptide hormone for the reduction of visceral adipose tissue, high sensitivity-c reactive protein (hs-CRP), triglycerides and carotid intima media thickness and the improvement of cognitive function is **Tesamorelin**. The only GHRP to exhibit interaction with the growth hormone releasing hormone (GHRH) receptor and ghrelin receptor and does not induce insulin resistance. It also benefits important age-related processes affecting cardiovascular morbidity and mental functioning, and in my opinion, is superior to any other peptide currently on the market for these reasons.

Jay: How do you identify a patient with metabolic syndrome, and what is your preferred treatment protocol?

Dr. Rob: Well, living in the Midwest that's easy! 8 out of 10 men over the age of 40 have metabolic syndrome, that's a personal observation. So, pretty much almost every man that walks through the door. Which is quite sad, really. Metabolic syndrome is considered to be present if 3 or more of the following 5 criteria are met: waist circumference over 40 inches (men) or 35 inches (women), blood pressure over 130/85 mmHg, fasting triglyceride level over 150 mg/dl, fasting high-density lipoprotein (HDL) less than 40 mg/dL in men or less than 50 mg/dL in women, and elevated fasting blood sugar of 100 mg/dL or higher.

My preferred and immediate treatment plan includes substantial lifestyle changes and interventional endocrinology with all the necessary hormones, medications, and supplements. Metabolic syndrome is a "metabolic emergency" that requires immediate and aggressive intervention.

CHAPTER 17 KEY TAKEAWAYS

- We provided you with an exclusive interview between Jay and Dr. Rob Kominiarek, a respected thought leader in Age Management who has had over 22 years of personally using therapeutic testosterone for himself and his patients.

- Dr. Kominiarek tells us how he manages a patient's estrogen levels throughout lifelong TOT administration, while also revealing how he identifies and treats subclinical thyroid disease in his patients.

- Jay and Dr. Kominiarek discuss how TOT is used for males under the age of 30 versus his older patients, and dives deep into the importance of monitoring pregnenolone levels at all stages of TOT.

- Dr. Kominiarek provides some quick tips for optimizing health in the absence of hormonal optimization, and reveals the shocking truth about the miniscule number of patients who can bring up their hormones into optimal ranges using nothing more than natural lifestyle changes.

- Dr. Kominiarek lays the smackdown on the dangers of using aromatase inhibitors, and why he isn't a fan of using SSRIs in alleviating depression.

- Jay quizzes Dr. Kominiarek about the use of Human Growth Hormone in combination with TOT, and gets him to discuss his methods for identifying and treating patients with metabolic syndrome.

BONUS CHAPTER 18

Hormonal Optimization Therapy (HOT) for Women: Doing it the Right Way

by Jim Meehan MD and Monica Campbell

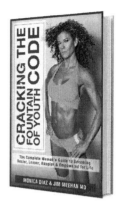

This is a preview chapter from the upcoming women's HOT book titled *Cracking the Fountain of Youth Code: The Complete Women's Guide to Becoming Sexier, Leaner, Happier and Empowered for Life* by Dr. Jim Meehan and Monica Campbell. In this exclusive sneak-peek, you will be getting two unique point of views: One from the scientific side (Jim), and the other from the practical side (Monica). They both serve separate yet equal purposes for women to get the full story on optimizing their hormone levels for superior levels of health.

Monica Campbell:

Ladies...

- Do you want to look great well into your 40's, 50's, 60's and beyond?

- Do you want to get to know your own body so well, you help your doctor determine what is best for you?

- Do you want to have energy and vitality well into your 70's and 80s?

- Do you want to be told the truth about the medical industry and if it is really working for or against you?

- Do you want to be mentally sharp?

- Do you want to truly embrace the years as they come without resisting the effects of aging?

Now don't get me wrong, I am by no means stating you won't age. Time will inevitably pass and one day we will all experience death. So the question to ask is not about how you can avoid death, but rather "How can I live longer enjoying this life experience, while rocking my sexy, kick-ass body, according to my personal definition of success and fulfillment?"

At the time of this writing, I am a 46 year old mother of 5 children (3 biological and 2 bonus girls).

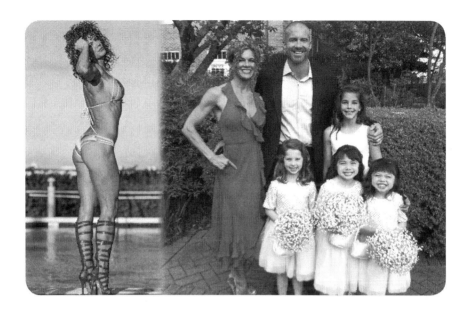

Although I was thin for most of my life, I was never an athlete. I was very awkward and clumsy growing up. I constantly dealt with disappointment, never being good enough to make it on any of the sports teams I tried out for. The one time I had an opportunity to join gymnastics, my mom, a single woman raising 4 kids on her own while working full-time, decided it would be too much stress for her. As a result, I got my exercise by playing on the neighborhood streets.

As a young girl, I grew up with the belief that aging is a death sentence. Once you get older, everything gets worse. Women get fatter, less attractive, and crazier. Men get bellies and lose their hair. On top of going downhill physically as you age, people seemed to get moodier and unhappy. Add a complete lack of energy to the mix, and you might as well start planning the funeral!

Now, in my late 40's, I realize that aging is NOT a death sentence. We now live in a time where we can truly age "gracefully," but it's not as easy as it sounds. The modern medical industry teaches people how to treat sickness and diseases instead of helping others stay healthy. If you go to the doctor as a healthy person and tell them you want to maintain optimal levels of health, they'll have no idea how to help you!

We are writing this book to give a voice to all the women who want to understand their bodies inside and out. In the process of writing it, we've learned how to become our own best practitioners while working with our doctors. Furthermore, we wanted to see if we could crack the "Fountain of Youth" code and be the best possible version of ourselves at any age.

I am NOT a scientist, nor will I provide any scientific data (that's Dr. Jim Meehan's job). However, I will give you real-world knowledge on the tools I have found to be the most helpful in aging with energy, vitality, sexiness, and beauty (both inside and out).

Additionally, I can help you understand what all the complicated medical jargon means. After all, we're getting lost in a system where doctors treat us like a number with a diagnosis attached to it. It's hard to even find a doctor who can invest more than 15 minutes of their time to discuss your health. Heck, most of us don't have millions of dollars to hire the best doctors in the world who would give us their undivided attention. What's a woman to do?

Our intention is to help women all over the world understand their bodies, get in touch with their soul, and crack the Fountain of Youth code so that they can live their lives to the absolute fullest.

This book is about far more than the latest cutting-edge science in female hormone optimization: It's also about living life to our personal best, loving our bodies, our souls and our spirit. It's about how we can age beautifully, full of vitality and energy.

However, we should never forget that our bodies house our spirit. When our bodies aren't healthy, it becomes challenging to have the zest for life needed to expand our spirit. Add in all the emotions we get to experience as we age, and it's no wonder that some women are thought to get crazier as they get older!

Dr. Jim Meehan

My name is Dr. Jim Meehan. Hormone therapy became my passion when my own struggles with health nearly cost me my career, my marriage, and my life. By the age of 40, I had gone from an elite athlete to someone I did not recognize when I looked in the mirror: I was fat, sick, depressed, and suffering non-stop. And I had no idea why. All I knew was that I felt lost in a never-ending fog.

At the time, I was at the height of a successful surgical career. By all accounts, I should have been happy and content, and yet I could feel my life slowly slipping away from me. My health was deteriorating, my weight was increasing, I felt depressed, and my relationship with my wife and kids was severely damaged.

Knowing I could not stand to live like this a moment longer, I sought the care of the best doctors in the midwest region of the United States. They all missed the underlying cause and treated me for a long list of symptoms with a cocktail of multiple drugs. Ultimately, a blood test that I ordered for myself showed my total testosterone levels to be 138 ng/dL - WAY below the bottom end of the reference range for normal testosterone levels. After a number of imperfect, marginally effective treatments (much like those still being delivered by most doctors in America today), I was getting better. However, I knew that the testosterone pellets, gels, and 1-2x/month injections of large dosages of testosterone were not optimal approaches. Therefore, I dedicated myself to learning everything I could about my disease, known as testosterone deficiency.

I sought out thought leaders and subject matter experts in hormone therapy. I read the work of physicians like **Abraham Morgentaler, MD, John Crisler, DO, John Lee, MD,** and **T.S. Wiley.** I trained with every expert (sometimes begging them to mentor me) and consumed every program that I could attend or buy with my own money. I trained in every program, from The American Academy of Anti-Aging Medicine to Cenegenics, and even the Age Management Medicine Group. To say I'm fully versed in the fields of Age Management would be a massive understatement.

As a former medical journal editor with extensive clinical experience in female hormonal health, I'm concerned about the future of a society whose mothers, daughters, and sisters are being diminished by misguided treatments using synthetic hormones. These treatments are dosed in amounts and patterns that obliterate any semblance of the natural rhythms and beautiful balances of the natural female hormonal cycle. These synthetic hormones are also metabolized in the liver and form harmful by-products, resulting in the creation of unhealthy hormonal imbalances.

In the chapter that follows, Monica and I will discuss how the female menstrual cycle is being diminished, disrupted and destroyed by failed approaches to female hormone optimization therapy (HOT) that do not honor the cycle's perfect design and purpose. We will also discuss the key principles, essential elements, and advanced strategies that are necessary for optimizing a woman's hormone levels.

The stark reality is that the overwhelming majority of the most commonly prescribed hormonal treatments for women are guilty of violating key principles of natural hormonal health. These principles are not mysterious, elusive, or yet to be discovered. They have always been right in front of us because they are based on the natural physiology of healthy, vital, and resilient young women.

I come to this process, not only as a medical practitioner of hormone optimization, but as a patient myself. Testosterone Optimization Therapy restored my health and zeal for life. Monica and I both write this book as practitioners of hormone optimization therapy, in the service of women everywhere. The medical industry must do better for the women in our lives. We must recognize and stop the decline of women's health in America (and the world) before it's too late.

Female Health is Neglected

Women's health, especially their hormonal health, has been terribly neglected by modern medicine. If women and their symptoms are not ignored, they are often misdiagnosed and ultimately mistreated. The evidence of mistreatment ranges from peer-reviewed analyses published by the Women's Health Initiative[640], to public records of medical liability lawsuits. Tens of thousands of women have been paid hundreds of millions of dollars in damages for injuries caused by synthetic hormones

---

[640] Manson JE, Chlebowski RT, Stefanick ML, et al. The Women's Health Initiative Hormone Therapy Trials: Update and Overview of Health Outcomes During the Intervention and Post-Stopping Phases. JAMA: the journal of the American Medical Association. 2013;310(13):1353-1368. doi:10.1001/ jama.2013.278040.

dosed to destroy the normal female hormone cycle (and with it, a woman's health).

For the last two decades, our mothers, wives, sisters and daughters have been stripped and forced to don blue paper gowns. They are then herded into cold medical exam rooms to have their complaints minimized and their symptoms of hormone deficiency neglected. Their attempts to convince doctors that they need something other than another prescription for depression, anxiety, or sleep have been simply ignored.

Monica Campbell:

At the same time, women can also have a tendency to neglect their own health. Many of them do not fully appreciate the joys and wonders of being a woman! I get it, because I grew up as a tomboy. I hated wearing a dress and wondered how much easier it would to be a boy. However, being a woman is SO MUCH MORE than wearing a dress.

Being a woman is a privilege and with it comes a huge responsibllity. I mean, just look at our bodies - we can carry other humans within our bodies, all while still functioning in society! We are expected to carry an enormous amount of responsibility on our shoulders. With the high expectations that women have to live up to, it's easy to see why they may end up neglecting their own health.

Remember: You are THE only one who lives in your beautiful skin and can feel as only you can feel. Depending solely on an outside doctor to make you "whole" is delusional, so you should take the time to get to know who you are and how you tick.

Learn how to trust your own instincts and decide whether something is right for you or not. As we age, our bodies prepare themselves to stop being the carrier of another human being, and the female body diminishes much of its restorative and reproductive powers as it ages. To make matters worse, our medical industry is now heavily influenced by the pharmaceutical industry. We easily second-guess ourselves because a doctor recommends a synthetic hormone to help us, but we have no idea if they are more loyal to us, their patient, or to the pharmaceutical representative.

Hormone Deficiencies are a Disease at Any Age

Dr. Jim Meehan:

Proper recognition and treatment of hormone deficiency is essential to good health, vitality, and longevity. Hormone imbalances and deficiencies occur at all ages and represent a serious threat to a woman's health.

The treatment of a woman's hormone deficiencies or imbalances should NEVER involve the ingestion of synthetic, hormone-like analogues administered in dosages and patterns that looks nothing like the healthy, normal rhythms of the female hormone cycle. If you learn nothing else from this chapter, please appreciate the truth in that statement.

Hormone disruption in youth increases a woman's risk of experiencing serious and difficult-to-treat health consequences later in life. After all, a young woman's hormones are increasingly imbalanced and deficient. Mood swings, painful and irregular menstrual cycles, trouble sleeping, brain fog, low energy, anxiety, depression, and weight gain are common signs of insufficient or imbalanced hormones. The earlier these abnormal hormonal patterns present themselves, and the longer the imbalances and deficiencies are allowed to persist, the more difficult they are to treat. This can lead to serious, health-destroying consequences. That's why early diagnosis and proper treatment are essential for young women everywhere.

Monica Campbell:

KNOW THYSELF. You don't have to be old to be hormone deficient. In fact, since we are all uniquely created, some may start having hormonal imbalances at an early age.

Just after high school, I had a friend ("Jill") who had very irregular periods. Her hormones were completely out of whack. Her mother continually used scare tactics on Jill to get her to act the way her mother wanted her to act. Jill's mother would also make her feel ashamed for how she was dealing with the stresses in her own life. The added stress and pressure from her mother did not help her, and she struggled throughout her adult life dealing with health issues. Unfortunately, she never invested the time to know THYSELF. She continually went to the doctor, allowing them to diagnose her and treat her with numerous antidepressants and birth control pills.

On top of receiving the wrong medical treatments, we also live in a world filled with toxins. Toxins in our food, air, water and clothes - everywhere!

Not only are we exposed to external toxins, but we create our own mental toxins as well. All of these toxins are poisoning our bodies. It's no wonder we start having hormonal imbalances at younger ages.

If you are in your 20s or 30s, and are suffering from mood swings, painful/irregular menstrual cycles, trouble sleeping, brain fog, low energy, anxiety, depression and weight gain (as Dr. Meehan mentioned above), get your hormone panels checked as soon as possible. If you aren't hormone deficient, then a lifestyle change involving diet and exercise will surely help.

Hormone Deficiencies are a Health Priority

Balanced hormones are essential to healthy aging, preventing chronic disease, and decreasing the likelihood of cancer. Unfortunately, this realization is just dawning on the medical industry right now. It is well known by experiential based practitioners (i.e. doctors) of age management medicine that hormonal imbalances and deficiencies not only accelerate aging, but are also at the root of many chronic health problems.

For example, an estrogen and/or testosterone deficiency leads to many symptoms that not only affect a woman's quality of life negatively, but also expose her to an increased risk of degenerative diseases including heart disease, osteoporosis, Alzheimer's disease, diabetes and colon cancer[641].

Sadly, everyday women in America are having their ovaries and uterus surgically removed at alarming rates. Painful fibroid tumors and endometriosis (a condition resulting from the appearance of tissue outside the uterus that can cause pelvic pain) can result from this common form of female castration[642]. Women are also being placed on forms of birth control that render their natural endocrine systems dysfunctional. However,

---

[641] Fishman JR, Flatt MA, Settersten RA. Bioidentical Hormones, Menopausal Women, and the Lure of the "Natural" in U.S. Anti-Aging Medicine. *Social science & medicine* (1982). 2015;132:79-87. doi:10.1016/j.socscimed.2015.02.027.

[642] Commandeur AE, Styer AK, Teixeira JM. Epidemiological and genetic clues for molecular mechanisms involved in uterine leiomyoma development and growth. *Human Reproduction Update.* 2015;21(5):593-615. doi:10.1093/humupd/dmv030.

even more alarming than the frequency of total hysterectomies (removal of a woman's uterus) is the rate at which these women are left with dangerous hormonal imbalances.

It is medically unwise to remove a woman's ovaries without having a treatment plan for lifelong hormone replacement. Removing the primary organs of hormone production leaves a woman vulnerable to the slow erosion of health she invariably faces after the surgical removal, which is a pointless tragedy in and of itself. Dr. Philip Sarrel, emeritus professor in the Departments of Obstetrics, Gynecology & Reproductive Sciences, and Psychiatry at Yale University, estimates that the widespread rejection of estrogen therapy after the 2002 Women's Health Initiative (WHI) study has most likely led to almost 50,000 unnecessary deaths over the last 10 years among women aged 50 to 69 who have had a hysterectomy[643].

Monica Campbell:

Have you had a hormone panel done recently? If so, how often do you have it done?

Do you understand how to read it, or have someone you trust who can help you read it?

Did you know that women need certain levels of estrogen and testosterone to be healthy?

If your body is not functioning optimally, then what is going on with you?

How you deal with stress in your life can either break your body down or make it stronger. A major part of cracking the

---

[643] American Journal of Public Health. https://news.yale.edu/2013/07/18/women-hysterectomies-estrogen-may-be-lifesaver-after-all

Fountain of Youth code involves understanding your hormones and what optimization protocol works best to allow you to look and feel better. If you follow the advice in this book, you will be empowered to take charge of your own health, to listen to your body, and restore your health, vitality, and sense of beauty.

Birth Control is NOT Hormone Restoration: Hormonal Contraception Methodologies are a Potentially Dangerous Adulteration of Female Hormonal Physiology

One of the most damaging medical mistakes made with young women's overall health and hormone levels today is the use of hormonal contraceptives as a form of hormone therapy. There is not a single hormonal contraceptive on the market that should be prescribed for female hormone restoration or optimization. It doesn't matter what mechanism of delivery you use, whether it's a birth control pill (BCP), implant, patches, rings, or intrauterine devices (IUDs).

It is a terrible mistake and a tremendous disservice to women when birth control pills or contraceptive devices are prescribed, as they often are, to address <u>symptoms</u> of hormonal imbalance. Symptoms such as cramping, spotting, irregular periods and acne are signals that the body is out of balance, under stress, or otherwise deficient in some essential element.

It is a testament to the failure of too many doctors today that, instead of identifying and treating the underlying cause of a young woman's hormone imbalance, they opt for the quick fix. They ignore the cause, treat the symptoms and lazily expose a young woman to the serious risks that every contraceptive product on the market today holds. We encounter this scenario time and again at all levels of society. In chapter 20 of this book, we will see how U.S. Veterans suffer a similar fate at the hands of the healthcare system.

I have heard the testimonies of too many young women that end up telling the same story. Their doctor rushed them through a five minute office visit, hard-sold them on the doctor's preferred birth control method (usually the brand that gets their office the most free lunches), and fail to mention the method of delivery used and/or the brand's serious risks to their health or life.

The symptoms are most often the result of a combined assault from multiple sources: stress, processed foods, bisphenol-A (BPA) laden food packaging, endocrine disrupting chemicals in our personal care products, and an environment full of chemicals, toxins, glyphosate and pollutants that disrupt the hormonal physiology of all women.

At some point in every woman's life, usually in the early to mid 50s, these uncomfortable and unhealthy indicators of unstable hormone levels will be labeled "menopause." Unfortunately, because menopause is considered an inevitable event in every woman's life, it's often not even considered a medical problem, let alone treated as one.

Monica Campbell:

Welcome to the 21st century's instant gratification society! We are now conditioned to believe that a quick visit to the doctor can yield us fantastic results without even having to understand our own bodies.

When I was 18 years old, I decided to go on BCPs to avoid getting pregnant. I went to a clinic that dealt with low-income women. At that time, the doctor at the clinic never discussed what hormones were, or the impact they had on my overall health. I was only told there may be side effects associated with taking the pill. However, I easily dismissed them without a second thought because my main concern was not getting pregnant at a young age.

I stayed on birth control for 5 years. During those 5 years, I had some cysts removed but they were not found to be cancerous. Once I became married, I wanted to give my body a break because my gut instinct told me that the chemicals coming from the pill would not help my body in the long run. Honestly, it seems like we are being fed so much disinformation to the point where it's hard to tell the lies apart from the truths.

If a woman goes to the gynecologist today, chemical birth control methods are quickly pushed as a primary option. Believe me, I know how much easier it was to be on the pill and not have to worry about getting pregnant. But how many women truly understand the real side effects of chemical birth control methods?

When I was approaching 40 years old, my periods were increasingly heavy. The young male doctor I saw kept pushing me to go for an IUD, or ablation surgery. He really liked the ablation surgery, and tried to hard-sell me on the benefits. He kept emphasizing how it wasn't normal to bleed as much as I did during my menstrual cycle and how great my life could if I didn't have any more periods. I opted for the IUD as I knew I didn't want a permanent solution to a temporary problem.

I kept the IUD in for about a year and upon removing it, I bled like a dying animal each time I had my period for the next 6 months. Fortunately, my periods are now very regular and I am not bleeding as heavily as I once was. Interestingly enough, not once did my doctor mention anything about a hormone panel. I didn't even understand what it meant to have female-oriented hormone optimization therapy until I met my husband.

Looking back, I am beyond grateful that I did not go for ablation surgery. Although the thought of having no periods sounds amazing, I trusted my instincts and feel great about my decision. Ablation surgery, for those of you who don't know, involves burning the inside of a woman's uterus lining. This is done for women who want to stop their menstrual cycle. If you burn the inside of your uterus, it ultimately becomes scar tissue inside of your body. How can that be healthy or productive as you age? Think about it: You now have a permanent, irreversible solution to a temporary issue. To make matters worse, there is no way to know what type of side effects may occur until after the procedure.

Doctors do not live in your body and they offer solutions primarily based on your complaints. Additionally, they are trained to deal with specific issues while offering specific solutions for those issues. A patient presents their issue and then the doctor presents one solution, if not multiple solutions. In that scenario, you should always ask questions about the solutions presented to you. If you still don't understand the doctor's answers, then get a second opinion and always do your own research. It's PERFECTLY OK to doubt the solution a doctor is giving you if you don't "get it." Just don't expect ignorance to be tolerated if you aren't willing to investigate things for yourself.

Pre- and Perimenopause

The signs of hormone imbalance and deficiency are occurring in women who are too young for menopause. The evidence for this increasing disruption of women's hormone levels lies in factors such as stress, poor nutrition, lack of exercise and the hundreds of environmental toxins that find their way into a woman's body on a daily basis.

Early signs of hormonal deficiencies, such as weight gain and depression, are commonly ignored, misdiagnosed, and utterly mistreated in women today. For example, prescribing antidepressants to treat the symptoms of an estrogen, progesterone, or testosterone deficiency won't do anything, other than mask the symptoms. It's more likely to make matters far worse as the underlying problem(s) remains untreated.

Women are born with a finite number of oocytes (eggs) stored in their ovaries. This "ovarian reserve" is typically depleted between the ages of 40 and 50. Once a woman's ovaries have released their final egg, her production of health-supporting hormones is lowered and chronic diseases (including diabetes) begin to rise. This is why low estrogen levels are commonly experienced by menopausal women.

In fact, there are many detrimental effects of low estrogen levels. For example, low estrogen levels can increase insulin resistance, increase carbohydrate cravings, and lead to weight gain[644]. With that being said, women suffering menopausal hormone decline need to know that ALL hormone therapies (whether for estrogen or some other hormone) carry some risks. However, the risks are fewer with bioidentical hormones delivered topically (i.e. through your skin) than they are with synthetic hormones delivered orally.

Women need to be aware of the fact that their risk of contracting chronic diseases increases when hormones like estradiol, progesterone, and testosterone decrease. You can even make a strong case for the risks of declining health being far greater than the risks associated with hormone replacement therapy.

---

[644]   Suba Z. Interplay between insulin resistance and estrogen deficiency as co-activators in carcinogenesis. Pathol Oncol Res. 2012 Apr;18(2):123-33. doi: 10.1007/s12253-011-9466-8. Epub 2011 Oct 9.

Monica Campbell:

As the years pass by and we get older, it becomes crucial to understand our bodies and our behavior. Depression is a real problem that is difficult to treat, especially if women are not taking care of themselves, both mentally and physically.

Whenever someone thinks of a woman, the hormone that easily comes to mind is estrogen. Little do they know that testosterone is also important for women who want to age optimally - imbalanced testosterone levels (just like in men) can also be a root cause of depression[645].

It's my belief that a woman should get their hormone panels done as early in their lives as they can, because it gives her and her doctor a better understanding on what is optimal for her. Remember: It's vitally important for a woman to know how they FEEL at any given point in time.

Hormones are NOT precise, and can affect each woman differently depending on her unique biochemistry. Therefore, a woman should not be treated based solely on her age. Rather, she needs to be treated as an individual human being with her own unique needs and problems.

Medications can help with some symptoms and they certainly have their place in an overall treatment strategy, but they won't destroy the source of the problem. Once again, this is why knowing what is most optimal for a woman can help her and her doctor discover what is best for her. In an ideal world, a woman would get her hormone panels done in her 20's so she can get a baseline. This will help her as she ages to determine

---

[645] Cappelletti M, Wallen K. Increasing women's sexual desire: The comparative effectiveness of estrogens and androgens. *Hormones and behavior.* 2016;78:178-193. doi:10.1016/j.yhbeh.2015.11.003.

what kind of hormone optimization therapy would be best for her long-term health and vitality.

If a woman is in her 40's (or older) and dealing with depression, she MUST get a comprehensive hormone panel done to rule out hormone deficiency. DO NOT take anti-depressant medications without first understanding the root cause of your problem. Often times, doctors are trained to use standard medications before dealing with the actual root cause of the issue. If you are concerned about quality of life as you get older, don't rob yourself of a potentially wonderful life by taking antidepressants before checking your hormone levels.

In addition to monitoring and tracking your hormone levels as you age, it's also important to take a good account of what's going on in your life. If a woman eats a horrible diet and finds herself gaining weight, then it's easy to blame age: "I am getting older and my metabolism has slowed down." "It is harder and harder to keep the weight off because I am heading into menopause."

What are you trying to convince yourself of? Are you trying to defend your right to get older while being overweight, depressed and/or emotional? Fundamentally, we are all a result of the accumulated choices we have made on a day-to-day basis. The only time the past really matters (and should matter) is when you look in the mirror and see how you are showing up, both physically and mentally. After all, you can't expect to be in great health if you are eating fast food every night while watching the news!

Key Principles in Female Hormone Optimization Therapy (HOT)

The key principles to remember for any female hormonal optimization protocol are as follows:

- **Bioidentical -** Restoring optimal hormone levels requires the use of hormones that are identical to those produced in the (human) female body.

- **Biorhythmic -** Optimizing a female's hormone levels should replicate (i.e. mimic) the rhythmic waves of a young woman's natural hormone cycle.

- **Balanced -** Optimizing a female's hormone levels should lead to a hormonal balance that allows the female to feel youthful again.

- **Bioavailable/Transdermal -** Female hormone optimization should be administered in transdermal form (i.e. on the skin), or in a similar form that avoids the negative consequences of first-pass metabolism in the liver (consequences such as potential damage to the liver from metabolizing the active ingredients found in the oral medication).

Let's explore each of these key principles in greater detail.

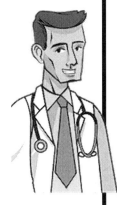

Principle #1 - Bioidentical

Optimizing a female's hormone levels requires the use of hormones that are identical to those produced in the (human) female body. For example, estradiol and progesterone are natural human female hormones. Conjugated horse estrogen (also known as Premarin), however, is not human estrogen. Neither are ethinyl estradiol, levonorgestrel, etonogestrel or norelgestromin. Progestins, the term given to the large variety of synthetic progesterone-like analogues found in pharmaceutical prescription drugs, are not equivalent to human progesterone.

The pharmaceutical industry has repeatedly and miserably failed to improve on nature's design of human hormones, despite all of the clever marketing they use to make you think otherwise. Making very slight modifications to a natural human hormone might make it patentable, prevent market competition, and command a higher retail price, but these same modifications may increase inflammation, increase the potential for blood clots, and can also increase the risk of developing cancer[646].

That's exactly what we learned in the late 90's, when the National Institutes for Health (NIH) decided to test the most commonly prescribed

---

[646] LaCroix AZ, Chlebowski RT, Manson JE, et al. Health Risks and Benefits after Stopping the Women's Health Initiative Trial of Conjugated Equine Estrogens in Postmenopausal Women with Prior Hysterectomy. *JAMA: the journal of the American Medical Association*. 2011;305(13):1305-1314. doi:10.1001/jama.2011.382.

hormonal therapies used for menopause (Premarin, PremPro, and PremPhase) in the largest study of women's health ever conducted. It was called the Women's Health Initiative[647].

The pharmaceutical and medical industries do not want the public to discover an inconvenient yet undeniable truth: Whenever these new drugs are released, we have next to no awareness of the negative side effects they might have. These consequences often avoid detection (and sometimes any real form of scrutiny) until the public has used these drugs long enough to piece together the complete picture regarding the potential damage they cause to one's health. By the time the truth is known, tens of thousands of women have already suffered or died in an experiment that they never knew they were a part of.

To shed some light on the truth about the hormones you SHOULD be using (i.e. *Bioidentical hormones*), here are some quick facts you need to be aware of[648]: (All the following bullet points are cited from the study in citation 645)

- Bioidentical hormones are identical in composition and chemical structure to human hormones.

- Bioidentical hormones are made from botanical sources such as Mexican yams or soy.

- Bioidentical estradiol, progesterone, and testosterone are FDA-approved. In fact, FDA approval is required for all medications marketed to the public.

647　Manson JE, Chlebowski RT, Stefanick ML, et al. The Women's Health Initiative Hormone Therapy Trials: Update and Overview of Health Outcomes During the Intervention and Post-Stopping Phases. *JAMA: the journal of the American Medical Association.* 2013;310(13):1353-1368. doi:10.1001/jama.2013.278040.

648　Fishman JR, Flatt MA, Settersten RA. Bioidentical Hormones, Menopausal Women, and the Lure of the "Natural" in U.S. Anti-Aging Medicine. *Social science & medicine* (1982). 2015;132:79-87. doi:10.1016/j.socscimed.2015.02.027.

- Bioidentical hormones have been used in Europe (and the U.S.) for over 60 years.

- Bioidentical hormones are not patentable, thus the pharmaceutical industry is not interested in them (i.e. they can't make a profit off of them).

- With very few exceptions, the hormones manufactured by the pharmaceutical industry and supplied for contraception (i.e. birth control), or the treatment of menopause, are synthetic hormone analogues.

- Bioidentical hormones have been extensively re-searched and are repeatedly shown in scientific studies to be safer than synthetic analogues. Additionally, bioidentical hormones have been shown to have fewer health risks than conventional, industrial, or synthetic hormone replacement therapies.

Now that you know more about bioidentical hormones, here are some useful facts to know about *synthetic hormones*:

- Synthetic progestins (ex. Provera) increase the risk of breast cancer, heart disease, and clot formation, potentially leading to a blood clot, pulmonary embolism, heart attack, or stroke[649].

- Progesterone does not increase the risk of breast cancer[650].

---

[649] J Obstet Gynaecol Can. 2002 Sep;24(9):711-5. The relevance of the Women's Health Initiative results on combined hormone replacement therapy in clinical practice. Lemay A.

[650] Eur J Cancer Prev. 1997 Oct;6(5):473-8. E3N, a French cohort study on cancer risk factors. E3N Group. Etude Epidémiologique auprès de femmes de l'Education Nationale. Clavel-Chapelon F, van Liere MJ, Giubout C, Niravong MY, Goulard H, Le Corre C, Hoang LA, Amoyel J, Auquier A, Duquesnel E.

- Synthetic progestins increase fluid retention, edema, and weight gain[651].
- Synthetic progestins negatively affect mood, mental status, and well being[652].
- Synthetic progestins also increase the risk of[653]:
  - Dementia
  - Headaches
  - Birth defects
  - Hair loss
  - Acne, skin discoloration
- Synthetic testosterone (Methyl-test, estratest, etc.) increases the risk of breast cancer[654].

Monica Campbell:

So now that you've just read all the medical jargon from Dr. Meehan, everything you've been told about female hormone optimization therapy (HOT) might seem confusing. Allow me to translate that jargon into plain English for you. :)

Mother Nature made you perfect, whole and complete. That means you are perfectly made, so don't screw it up by putting

---

651   Chlebowski, Rowan T., 2009. Breast cancer after use of estrogen plus progestin in postmenopausal women, New England Journal of Medicine, February 5, Volume 360:573-587.

652   Kahn, Linda S., Halbreich, Uriel, 2005. Oral Contraceptives and Mood. The Journal of Expert Opinion on Pharmacotherapy; Vol 2, 2001; pp 1367-1382.

653   Ibid.

654   Tamimi RM, Hankinson SE, Chen WY, Rosner B, Colditz GA. Combined estrogen and testosterone use and risk of breast cancer in postmenopausal women. Arch Intern Med. 2006 Jul 24;166(14):1483-9.

crappy stuff in your body! The best way to avoid doing that is by using bioidentical hormones, which are most similar to the hormones naturally produced in your body. Make sure you're using bioidentical hormones when starting female HOT, and remember: "Synthetic Sucks!"

The pharmaceutical drug companies are trained and taught to sell - you guessed it - DRUGS to the general public! As long as they get sold, it doesn't really matter which ones are bringing in the bucks.

If you are going to use a study or controlled test to help you decide what hormone(s) you should take, make sure you know who the study/test was funded by. By all means, ASK...ASK... ASK if you are not clear on anything. Make sure you know if your doctor is recommending a bioidentical hormone or a synthetic hormone.

Once you have all the necessary information, make an informed choice for yourself. If you decide to go with a synthetic hormone, only do so because it is YOUR choice alone and you fully understand (and accept) the potential health consequences that come with using synthetic hormones.

Principle #2 - Biorhythmic

Optimizing a female's hormone levels should replicate (i.e. mimic) the rhythmic waves of a young woman's natural hormone cycle. I'm always shocked at how the medical-pharmaceutical industry manages to continually ignore this basic, fundamental principle. When in the history of the world has man's creations EVER surpassed those of nature and the Creator?

I'm sure there are many justifications for using arbitrary and never-changing dosing regimens that greatly affect a woman's natural hormone cycles, but I cannot imagine a HEALTH reason. It is impossible to argue against the principle of treating a hormonal disorder by restoring one's natural hormone cycles. Optimal (and natural) hormonal cycles are typically experienced by women when they are young and vital. Therefore, any hormone restoration program should attempt to replicate the hormonal patterns seen in a young woman's natural hormonal cycle.

Examine the diagram of the female hormone cycle shown below. Notice the rhythms, waves, peaks (i.e. high points), and valleys (i.e. low points). There are most certainly variations from one woman to another, but that variation is not as great as many believe. In fact, there should not be much variability when it comes to optimal hormonal health.

The rhythmic waves and patterns seen in each of the hormones involved in the female hormonal cycle are there for a REASON. This cannot be ignored! It must be honored and replicated when using HOT. Otherwise, hormonal dysfunction and bodily diseases will eventually come about.

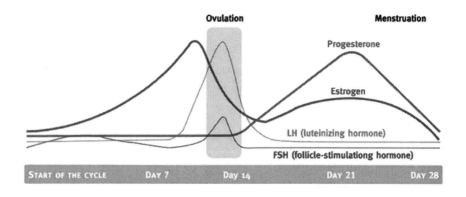

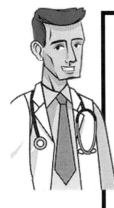

For example, over the course of a normal 28-day menstrual cycle, there should be a predictable rise in blood estrogen levels (to a peak height) that typically occurs around day 12 in a woman's cycle. This rapid ascension is believed to be a key event for estrogen-activated DNA transcription that results in, among many other things, receptor formation for both testosterone and progesterone. Without this important rise in estrogen levels (and overall rhythm of the cycle), the body may be unprepared to receive the important health benefits (more vitality, energy, muscle tone, etc.) of testosterone and progesterone.

If we fail to recognize this biorhythmic principle, along with the important peaks and valleys of the hormone cycle, we miss the valuable opportunity to improve our health. And if your doctor prescribes and maintains low doses of estrogen every single day (as commonly seen in the symptom-based treatment of menopause), then the important health-boosting effects of testosterone and progesterone won't be fully received by the body.

Similarly, if a woman is prescribed hormonal therapy that continuously releases high levels of estrogen into the blood (as seen in many birth control pills and devices), the brain and body may be deceived into believing that it is pregnant. The body would not be deceived in the same way if it had the optimal rhythms of health, youth, and life.

Monica Campbell:

There is a beautiful order within the woman's body. All of your hormones have a natural flow to them, and therefore they can fluctuate depending on where you are within your monthly cycle. When you are getting closer to ovulation, your estrogen could be higher. Remember: A woman's body functions around whether or not she is pregnant.

However, synthetic hormones don't factor in your natural hormone levels during the monthly cycle. They also don't account for WHERE you are within your cycle. They just keep releasing high levels of estrogen without accounting for the other hormones that play an important role in your menstrual cycle. It's no wonder why a woman's emotions might be all over the place, depending on where they are within their cycle!

Principle #3 - Balanced

Dr. Jim Meehan:

Optimizing a female's hormone levels should lead to a harmonious hormonal balance that allows her to feel youthful again.

Put simply, every biological system in the body seeks stability and balance; your metabolism and your hormone levels are prime examples. In fact, the body's drive to maintain normal cycles, rhythms and an overall balance is called homeostasis. Homeostasis is such a powerful physiological response that it can even fight the medications being given to the body! For example, trying to alter your serotonin levels with an SSRI to treat depression might slightly alleviate your symptoms. However, in doing so, there is a very high risk of drug dependency and eventual chronic disease[655].

Many people have used the analogy of a symphony orchestra to illustrate the principle of balance and harmony in the female hormone cycle. One section being out of tune, or even a single instrument, is enough to ruin the musical performance and sound of the entire orchestra. Similarly, maintaining the natural balance and harmony within the female hormone cycle is imperative for excellent mental and physical health. Chronic imbalances in estradiol, progesterone, and testosterone result in poor health at best, and chronic disease or cancer in the worst-case scenarios.

In the previous principle, we discussed the negative effects that occur when females are given dosages of estrogen that are too high or too low. Not only do these commonly-prescribed estrogen treatments disrupt the normal biorhythms, they also disrupt hormonal balances, resulting in hormonal excesses or deficiencies.

It is my belief (based on more than a decade of clinical experience) that balanced hormones are critical to improving health and preventing disease, while offering protection against bodily dysfunction and cancer. Hormone imbalances, however, increase one's risk of cancer[656]. For example, high levels of

---

[655]   Wang S, Yang L, Wang L, Gao L, Xu B, Xiong Y. Selective Serotonin Reuptake Inhibitors (SSRIs) and the Risk of Congenital Heart Defects: A Meta-Analysis of Prospective Cohort Studies. *Journal of the American Heart Association: Cardiovascular and Cerebrovascular Disease.* 2015;4(5):e001681. doi:10.1161/JAHA.114.001681.

[656]   Diep CH, Daniel AR, Mauro LJ, Knutson TP, Lange CA. Progesterone action in breast, uterine, and ovarian cancers. *Journal of molecular endocrinology.* 2015;54(2):R31-R53. doi:10.1530/JME-14-0252.

estrogen increase one's risk of breast cancer[657]. The good news is that balanced progesterone levels balance and oppose the potentially cancerous effects of estrogen, thereby lowering the risk of cancer[658].

Monica Campbell:

If you keep screwing up your natural system, you're going to cause more health issues for yourself. This means that when you add drugs to your body, your hormonal functions go out-of-whack. If you're unlucky enough, you'll also have an unhealthy addiction to these drugs as they'll temporarily make you feel better when you take them.

I LOVE Dr. Meehan's music analogy. Our bodies must flow with all of the beautiful instruments (hormones) that cause our music (health) to sound beautiful (be healthy), just like an inspirational song (a productive life). If one of those instruments (hormones) is out of tune, the frequency of the music (a productive life) won't sound as beautiful.

You have a choice when it comes to your body:

1. You can choose to IGNORE your hormone levels and deal with the inevitable health decline and bodily dysfunctions as you age.

---

[657] Costa M, Saldanha P. Risk Reduction Strategies in Breast Cancer Prevention. *European Journal of Breast Health.* 2017;13(3):103-112. doi:10.5152/ejbh.2017.3583.

[658] Cekic M, Sayeed I, Stein DG. Combination Treatment with Progesterone and Vitamin D Hormone May Be More Effective than Monotherapy for Nervous System Injury and Disease. *Frontiers in neuroendocrinology.* 2009;30(2):158-172. doi:10.1016/j.yfrne.2009.04.002.

2. You can choose to UNDERSTAND how your body functions best, and know how to manipulate your hormone cycle to make it function productively.

No matter what you pick, there will be consequences. Number 1 will most likely yield negative consequences because you are not taking an active role in your health and longevity. Number 2 will most likely give you a productive and fulfilling life with better health and longevity. Number 1 seems easier until you get a life-threatening illness and you try doing anything you can to stay alive. Unfortunately, the long-term effects of Number 1 can be so severe that you won't make it out alive. Even if you do, you will be be permanently and negatively affected by your choice.

Principle #4 - Bioavailable/Transdermal

Dr. Jim Meehan

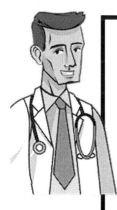

Female HOT should be administered trans-dermally (i.e. in a cream or gel applied to the skin) in order to avoid the negative conse-quences of first-pass metabolism in the liver (some oral medications, due to the way they break down in the liver, may cause specific liver enzyme issues). That's because trans-dermal hormone formulations are the safest way to deliver female hormones. In partic-ular, transdermal estrogen has repeatedly been shown to be safer than oral forms of estrogen[659]. By blending bioidentical hormones into special-ly-formulated carrier creams, we can reliably deliver these hormones across the skin, into the subcutaneous tissue, and ultimately into systemic circulation (i.e. your bloodstream). Once in the bloodstream, the bioidentical hormones will bind to receptors throughout the body and 'deliver' their positive health effects.

It should be common knowledge that administering hormones orally is a bad idea. When hormones like estrogen are administered orally, they are absorbed into the intestinal circulatory system and delivered directly to the liver. This is called "first-pass metabolism" or the "first-pass effect." The first-pass effect ensures that the liver is the first line of defense in protecting us from drugs, hormones, or any toxic substances we might swallow. The liver "transforms" the substances it encounters to make them more water-soluble, and easier to remove from the body.

This "first-pass effect" dramatically reduces the amount of hormone that leaves the liver to enter the bloodstream. To counter this effect, the amount of hormone that is delivered to the liver needs to be so high that it overwhelms the liver's metabolic capacity to process the hormone, and a sufficient amount of the hormone makes it past the liver to reach the target tissues and exert its intended effect.

Due to this "first-pass effect," orally delivering hormones is inefficient, but the extremely high levels of hormones in the liver can have serious negative consequences. Put simply, overwhelming the liver to overcome the "first pass effect" is risky business. Forcing the liver to tie up much of its metabolic capabilities to deal with an orally-delivered hormone means

---

[659] North American Menopause Society (NAMS) 22nd Annual Meeting: Abstract S-4. Presented September 23, 2011.

that it is less capable of dealing with other toxins that enter the body.

Oral hormone therapies also increase the production of sex hormone binding globulin (SHBG)[660]. SHBG tightly binds to the sex hormones, including testosterone and progesterone, and thus diminishes the positive health-protective effects of these hormones.

Additionally, hitting the liver with the super-high levels of hormone necessary to make it through to the bloodstream means that the liver is unable to devote adequate resources to the production of proteins that decrease inflammation, support immune function, or break down blood clots. Oral hormones markedly increase the number of blood clots that form in the deep veins, dislodge, and float downstream with the potential to obstruct blood vessels in the lungs[661].

In short, transdermal estrogen hormone therapy is far safer than oral estrogen therapy[662]. By avoiding first-pass metabolism, transdermal hormone therapy may have less pronounced effects on the production of important proteins, such as inflammatory markers, markers of coagulation and fibrinolysis, and steroid binding proteins.

---

[660] Edlefsen KL, Jackson RD, Prentice RL, et al. The effects of postmenopausal hormone therapy on serum estrogen, progesterone and sex hormone binding globulin levels in healthy post-menopausal women. *Menopause (New York, NY)*. 2010;17(3):622-629. doi:10.1097/gme.0b013e3181cb49e9.

[661] J Womens Health (Larchmt). 2012 Feb;21(2):161-9. doi: 10.1089/jwh.2011.2839. Epub 2011 Oct 19. Are all estrogens created equal? A review of oral vs. transdermal therapy. Goodman MP.

[662] Shufelt CL, Merz CNB, Prentice RL, et al. Hormone Therapy Dose, Formulation, Route of Delivery, and Risk of Cardiovascular Events in Women: Findings from the WHI Observational Study. *Menopause (New York, NY)*. 2014;21(3):260-266. doi:10.1097/GME.0b013e31829a64f9.

Monica Campbell:

In general, you should avoid taking a pill when it comes to HOT. The application (i.e. how the hormone is delivered) depends on your doctor and what they have been accustomed to prescribing. For example, I know women who are prescribed testosterone injections at extremely low doses and have excellent results. Again, all of this depends entirely on the individual and what works best for them.

I highly suggest trying different options, while working with an experiential-based physician, to see what works best for you. I personally don't like transdermal delivery as it causes me to have acne breakouts.

Applying the Key Principles

Dr. Jim Meehan

Understanding the key principles necessary for a safe and effective HOT program will protect women from the common mistreatments perpetrated by well-meaning providers.

As a result of understanding and applying the key principles discussed in this chapter, we can arrive at the following state-of-the art, compounded female HOT solution:

- **Bioidentical estradiol (i.e. estrogen), progesterone, and testosterone** equivalent to the hormones produced naturally in a woman's body.

- **Compounded formulations** of each of these bioidentical hormones blended in optimal hormonal base creams.

– As an alternative to individual dispensers for each hormone (i.e. one separate cream per hormone), I will sometimes prescribe one dispenser that contains both estradiol and testosterone.

– Because the testosterone peak typically occurs on days 14-16 of a woman's menstrual cycle, the timing of the testosterone and estradiol peaks (relative to one another) allows for a reasonable compromise. This leads to a dosing regime that is affordable, more convenient and less complicated. By combining testosterone with estradiol, there will be two applicators (estradiol and testosterone in one, progesterone in the other) rather than three separate ones.

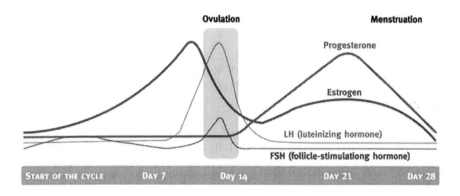

– NOTE: Please consult with a compounding pharmacist[663] regarding the preferred 'base' for each formulation.

• A **transdermal dispenser/applicator system** capable of reliably dispensing controlled dosages of compounded hormonal cream (preferably in dosing increments of 0.05 to 0.1 mL).

---

[663] www.empowerpharmacy.com

- — I like the "Ticker" transdermal applicator manufactured by BiosRx[664]. It holds a month's worth of cream in an easy-to-use dispenser. The dispenser is calibrated to deliver 0.05 mL of hormone cream per "tick" of its base.

- — The "Topi-click" dispenser is a great alternative[665]. It has the advantage of being on the market longer, and therefore it is more familiar to many compounding pharmacies. However, it does not provide as much control over the amount of cream per click. The Topi-click dispenses 0.25 mL per "click."

- — My third choice is a standard syringe in a 3, 5, or 10 mL size. In this case, you will need multiple syringes to hold a month's worth of hormonal cream. Furthermore, the syringes need to be capped with an end cap made of a material that does not 'leach' into the cream.

- A **biorhythmic and balanced dosing schedule** that replicates the natural rhythmic peaks and valleys of hormones in the youthful prime of a woman's life.

  - — **Calendar/schedule** - varying doses of each hormonal cream (estradiol, progesterone, and testosterone) that correspond to the appropriate day in a woman's menstrual cycle.

    - ▪ Women who know the first day of their last menstrual period may use that knowledge to establish a "day one" of their new HOT cycle.

---

[664] https://www.biosrx.com/collections/featured-tees

[665] http://doselogix.com/product/topi-click-35

- Women with no menstrual cycle (due to surgical or natural menopause) can consider using the lunar cycle to guide their cycle schedule.
- **Estradiol** (or estradiol plus testosterone)
    - Days 1-12: Estradiol dosages are increased over the course of the first 12 days of the cycle to create the first and most important peak on day 12.
    - Days 12-16: Estradiol dosages decrease to a trough (valley) on day 16.
    - Days 17-21: Estradiol dosages progressively increase to a secondary, smaller peak on day 21.
    - Days 21-28: Estradiol dosages decrease in order to return to baseline levels on day 28. Menstruation should occur.
- As previously mentioned, I often prescribe a combination formula that contains both estradiol and testosterone in a single dispenser. I do this as an alternative to using individual dispensers for both estradiol and testosterone.
- **Progesterone**
    - Progesterone is not applied during the first half of the cycle (days 1-12).
    - Progesterone is only applied in the second half of the cycle, beginning around day 13.
    - Days 13-20: Progesterone dosages progressively increase to a peak on day 21.
    - Days 22-28: Progesterone dosages progressively decrease to baseline levels by the last day of the cycle (on or around day 28).

Cycle Day	Estradiol /Testosterone # of Clicks				Progesterone # of Clicks				Symptom Tracker
1	2	AM	2	PM	No Progesterone				
2	2	AM	2	PM	No Progesterone				
3	2	AM	2	PM	No Progesterone				
4	2	AM	2	PM	No Progesterone				
5	2	AM	2	PM	No Progesterone				
6	2	AM	2	PM	No Progesterone				
7	2	AM	2	PM	No Progesterone				
8	2	AM	2	PM	No Progesterone				
9	3	AM	3	PM	No Progesterone				
10	3	AM	3	PM	No Progesterone				
11	3	AM	3	PM	No Progesterone				
12	3	AM	3	PM	No Progesterone				
13	1	AM	1	PM	3	AM	3	PM	
14	1	AM	1	PM	3	AM	3	PM	
15	1	AM	1	PM	3	AM	3	PM	
16	1	AM	1	PM	3	AM	3	PM	
17	1	AM	1	PM	5	AM	5	PM	
18	1	AM	1	PM	5	AM	5	PM	
19	1	AM	1	PM	5	AM	5	PM	
20	1	AM	1	PM	5	AM	5	PM	
21	2	AM	2	PM	3	AM	3	PM	
22	2	AM	2	PM	3	AM	3	PM	
23	2	AM	2	PM	3	AM	3	PM	
24	2	AM	2	PM	3	AM	3	PM	
25	2	AM	2	PM	2	AM	2	PM	
26	2	AM	2	PM	2	AM	2	PM	
27	2	AM	2	PM	2	AM	2	PM	
28	2	AM	2	PM	2	AM	2	PM	

Figure 3. Hormone Optimization Therapy (HOT) Dosage Calendar. This calendar is based on the use of the Topi-Click dispenser.

- **Laboratory testing** should be used to periodically monitor hormone levels. Women undergoing treatment should measure specific hormones on specific days of their cycle:

- Estradiol on day 12
- Testosterone on day 14
- Progesterone on day 21
- Make sure you order tests which use high sensitivity (LC/MS) lab methodologies whenever possible, especially for measuring testosterone levels.
- It is VERY important to always note the day within the menstrual cycle at which any hormonal lab test is obtained. Without the cycle day reference point, the lab results are near meaningless.

- **Monitoring symptoms**

  - Be sure to note unusual symptoms such as migraines/headaches, cramping, spotting, breakthrough bleeding, etc.
  - These symptoms, and where they fall in the timeline of your therapeutic cycle, will suggest the underlying hormonal cause and the possible treatment.

Monica Campbell:

The truth is that none of you will be able to correctly and consistently apply any of Dr. Meehan's principles unless you're working with an experienced HOT physician. Working with a doctor who is inexperienced in HOT is a recipe for disaster! It's important to remember that you won't fit with every doctor, so practice on them like they do on you. However, if you keep having issues with doctors, then you should start looking inward and examine why you aren't syncing with them. There are enough HOT-trained doctors in the world to go around, so you should be able to find one who is willing to listen and work with you.

Let's skip forward in time and say that you've located an experienced and successful HOT doctor who has prescribed you HOT. You can have the BEST doctor in the world who implements the 4 key principles of Dr. Meehan, but if you continue to have bad habits such as excessive drinking and experiencing high stress levels, it will be MUCH harder to get optimal results.

Take full responsibility for your health, monitor how you feel and how your body is reacting. If you don't notice any improvements from the therapy, then why not? Are you following the instructions properly? Did you become lazy and forget to administer the therapy exactly as instructed? You could keep a journal and write down how you are doing on a daily basis. In any case, have realistic expectations and give yourself an adequate amount of time to determine how the therapy is working. You are not going to transform into the 25-year-old version of yourself overnight. Make sure you identify with the kind of results you are expecting, and communicate with your doctor on a regular basis to make sure they understand what is working for you (or not working).

We all want easy solutions in life because we want to understand what everything means. At the same time, don't get stuck in the confusion. Realize that YOU are the one living in your body, and only YOU can understand how it functions best. However, you can only achieve this understanding when you pay attention.

In every single aspect of life, you get what you focus on, and your health is no exception to this rule. If you CHOOSE to focus on the younger and healthier version of yourself, HOT will become much easier to understand. But when you choose to focus on feelings of resentment, rage or revenge, you are biochemically poisoning your body. These feelings create cortisol spikes in your body, which greatly affects your hormonal balance in a negative way.

Being healthy, and being your own best advocate for your body, soul and mind takes time and effort. Therefore, I will ask that you be patient with your progress. Don't buy into the magic pill that will cause you to lose weight in 2 weeks and get you the bikini body you've been dreaming of. Doing the minimum amount of work and expecting the maximum amount of results is unrealistic.

Above all else, enjoy the ride and remember that time is on your side! Understanding and implementing female HOT will definitely get you on the right track to cracking the 'Fountain of Youth' code. If you stick with the key principles of HOT and apply them, you'll find yourself rocking the sexier, leaner and more beautiful version of YOU before you know it.

To conclude my bit in this chapter, I'd like to share 10 tips that I've found to be extremely helpful when used alongside female HOT. These will be explored in far greater detail in our book coming out in 2018.

1. **Love yourself.** Look at yourself in the mirror and truly love who you are. You will make better choices for yourself when you love 'you' for who you are. It will also be easier to follow the HOT protocol your doctor prescribes for you when you love yourself.

2. **Invest time for yourself.** For me, I love taking time in the early morning to simply appreciate being in my skin.

3. **Delegate.** Don't put it all on you. It's great to be a Wonder Woman, but it's also great to be a normal woman!

4. **Exercise.** We will go into more detail on the types of exercise to perform in our book.

5. **Appreciate.** Look at your life with eyes of appreciation. A grateful heart is a healthy heart.

6. **Nutrition.** Eat good foods. Again, much more on this in our upcoming book.

7. **Have fun.** Laughter is the best medicine. Do the things you truly enjoy!

8. **Get comfortable and cozy with change.** Your body and skin will change over time. Be OK with its changes.

9. **Get comfortable with the truth.** The truth is not always comfortable, but it will set you free.

10. **Pray/Meditate.** Getting in touch with your inner spirit and soul is a great way to lower your stress levels and improve your overall mood.

Dr. Jim Meehan:

There are many more topics we've talked about that deserve a much deeper discussion before even scratching the surface of female HOT. The topic is extremely broad, and it's exactly why Monica and I are writing a book that offers a comprehensive look at advanced strategies for HOT in women. We will be publishing it in 2018.

Through the use of progressive compounding pharmacies, bioidentical hormones delivered in a biorhythmic fashion can not only provide women with much-needed relief from uncomfortable symptoms, but also safely and effectively protect them from the devastating diseases that result from hormone deficiencies. And through medically-supervised treatment, a female hormone optimization program can provide women with the most natural approach to a better life filled with health, wellness, and vitality.

Many thanks to my cherished friend, T.S. Wiley. Were it not for her brilliant mind, indomitable spirit, tireless research, outstanding contributions to the science of female hormone therapy and chronobiology, as well as her courageous defense of compounding pharmacies, women in America would have few or no options beyond the mostly unnatural and unhealthy products contrived by the pharmaceutical industry.

CHAPTER 18 KEY TAKEAWAYS

- Monica and Dr. Meehan share their personal journeys into discovering the world of hormonal optimization, and how they discovered that aging DOES NOT have to be a death sentence!

- They discuss how female health is dangerously neglected by the medical community, especially when symptoms are ignored. Instead, harmful prescriptions are given to them, which don't do anything to solve their hormone-related problems. Thus, WOMEN need to step up and own responsibility for their own health!

- Hormone deficiencies are a disease at any age, and both Monica and Dr. Meehan discuss the long-term health consequences that people face if they do not fix their hormone imbalances immediately. Balancing your hormones should be your #1 health priority!

- Birth control (i.e. hormonal contraceptives) can be potentially dangerous to your overall health, and may actually do more harm in restoring an optimal balance of hormones within your body.

- The hormonal imbalances seen within pre-menopause and peri-menopause are discussed, along with the early signs to detect said imbalances and why you should get comprehensive hormone panels done as early in your life as possible. It's important for both you and your doctor to work together and see what is most optimal for YOU!

- Monica and Dr. Meehan reveal the 4 key principles for female hormonal optimization therapy (Bioidentical, Biorhythmic, Balanced, Bioavailable) and discuss each one in greater detail.

- You are provided with a state-of-the-art, compounded female HOT solution for applying all of the key principles discussed in the chapter.

- Finally, Monica concludes the chapter with 10 quick empowerment tips that she's found to be extremely helpful when used alongside female HOT.

The Stone Cold Truth about Anabolic and Androgenic Steroids (AAS)

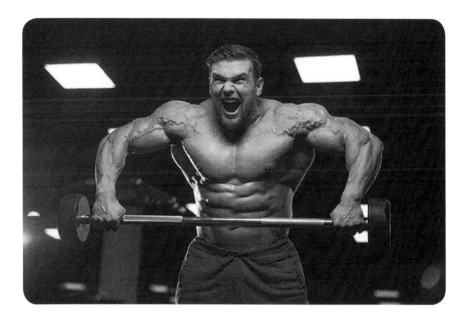

This chapter is a very high-level summary and analysis of Anabolic and Androgenic Steroid (AAS) use in the bodybuilding and performance enhancement communities.

I highly recommend that you read BOTH of the articles I'm about to mention before reading this chapter. The Birth of a Demon[666] is an in-depth article by John Romano that discusses how and

---

[666]   https://www.t-nation.com/training/steroids-the-birth-of-a-demon

why steroids became such a taboo subject of discussion to the general public. The S-Word[667] is an excellent article about an elite-level, super-heavyweight powerlifter named Chad Eichs. He recounts the story of how he arrived at using steroids, the effects he got from them, and reflects on his personal experience with using them.

I am asking you to read these because I think steroids should be legal. I also want to dispel any misconceptions you might have about steroids being used by evil muscleheads who apparently hate women and turn into raging hate-filled demons. Most of these stereotypes created by mainstream media outlets are largely bullshit. I'm going to run through this bonus chapter in a Q&A format to make things simple. It will keep my points clear and allow you to develop a holistic understanding of the subject.

Don't Ask About Steroids Until You Understand Steroids

What are steroids? The term 'steroid' refers to an entire class of organic compounds which have many different effects. For example, cholesterol is a steroid. You already know that testosterone is a steroid. Estrogen is a steroid. Various anti-inflammatory drugs like prednisone are corticosteroids.

Steroids are BIOLOGICAL compounds created by your body. They perform two main functions:

1. They form part of the structure that makes up cell membranes (your cells are basically made up of fats and proteins).

---

[667] https://www.elitefts.com/education/the-s-word-what-ive-learned/

2. They are "signaling" molecules for THOUSANDS of pathways and processes.

Many times, people (including medical professionals) confuse 'catabolic' (growth-destroying) steroids, labeled as corticosteroids, with 'anabolic' (growth-promoting) steroids. It happens so often that 95% of society doesn't even know the difference between the two, but the difference is extremely large in size.

So understanding this, what are people specifically referring to when they ask about steroids?

Answer: Steroids, the way most people use the term, refers to testosterone and its derivative anabolic hormones (otherwise known as synthetics, or AAS)

NOTE: I am going to use the terms 'steroids', 'drugs', 'anabolics', 'juiced', and 'geared' interchangeably from this point on. Again, these terms refer to the use of AAS.

A Brief Mention of AAS Drugs (The Most Popular Synthetics)

We will keep referring to different drugs, so you might wonder what I'm really talking about. First, understand that there are many different forms of AAS. Testosterone was the first to be synthesized, but there are many 'synthetic' versions of it. There are also variations that act very fast in the body, versions that act slower, and versions that are "long lasting."

Aside from testosterone, there are other steroids that are alternate, man-made versions of testosterone and have difference effects. The most common are: Trenbolone, Masteron, Winstrol, Dianabol, Deca-durabolin, Equipose, Anavar (Oxandrolone),

Oxymethelone, Primobolan and Turanibol. This book is not the place for analyzing the effectiveness of each of these compounds. William Llewellyn has written prolifically on the subject, so if you are interested in informing yourself about AAS use to the highest level, buy his book *Anabolics*.[668]

Do Anabolic Steroids Work?

Absolutely! This question is nonsensical, as it's an awful lot like asking if oxygen is important. Your body PRODUCES its own "steroids," as they are a basic part of the biochemistry found in every living creature on earth. If they didn't "work," they wouldn't exist.

What I think this question is asking, is whether AAS make a true difference when they are used.

Once again: When the majority of people talk about steroids, they are referring to testosterone and its derivatives. These steroids are classified as AAS. And as I said before, anabolic means 'growth-promoting'. 'Growth-promoting' in this context means promoting muscle growth, neurological growth, and cellular regeneration. The "Androgenic" in AAS refers to the promotion of MALE secondary sexual characteristics.

The effects that people typically associate with steroids are as follows: bigger muscles, greater strength, and increased physical power. These are the result of the anabolic and androgenic effects of this particular class of steroids (i.e. AAS).

---

[668] https://roidtest.com/products/anabolics-11th-edition?variant=32558126083

The Biological Differences Between Testosterone in Men and Women

The biological reality is that men and women are different on a cellular level, cognitive level, skeletal level, and so on. Any postmodernist protesting to this can kindly stop reading. Brushing the politics aside, testosterone is the hormone largely responsible for the differences between men and women. The anabolic and androgenic effects of testosterone are what produce the following:

- bigger muscles
- stronger connective tissue
- stronger nervous systems
- stronger motor coordination
- improved spatial awareness
- testicle growth
- deeper voice
- masculinized features

Women DO have testosterone in their body, but at much lower levels compared to men. If you give women more than minor amounts of testosterone, they will masculinize (i.e. experience some of the effects described above) because testosterone has very strong androgenic effects in women.

Testosterone is both anabolic and androgenic, and it is the "base" for practically every other steroid in existence.

Does TOT Count As Steroids?

If you use TOT (more commonly called TRT), are you using steroids? YES! TOT involves the use of testosterone to raise your testosterone levels to optimal levels (i.e. the high-normal range). Testosterone levels are usually measured in 'total testosterone', which ranges anywhere from 200-1000 ng/dL (depending on what lab measurement company is being used).

Our opinion is that anything under 400 ng/dL should be considered 'low' and confirmed clinically by a knowledgeable physician in the presence of the relevant symptoms. As Jay and Jim already discussed in Chapter 6, the medical establishment has LOWERED the normal range as testosterone levels have dropped in the last 40 years, all due to a variety of reasons (all previously discussed in this book).

As such (and I KNOW many intelligent and informed doctors who would agree with me), the current range for normal levels is skewed. The majority of men would be vastly healthier in the normal to high range of 600-1400 ng/dL.

Difference Between TOT and AAS

The difference is in the DOSAGE and the compounds used. In other words, there's a huge difference between therapeutic dosages for optimization, and supraphysiological (i.e. much higher) dosages.

As you already know, a dosage of testosterone under TOT is typically 100-200 mg delivered weekly via various optional delivery systems. A supraphysiologic dose of testosterone is more than double, triple, quadruple, or even quintuple that. Put another way, a 'steroidal' dose of testosterone involves injecting yourself with anywhere from 500-1000 mg (or more) of testosterone on a weekly basis. It is administered in a variety of ways with a mixed bag of testosterone esters, not to mention that there are often other anabolic agents involved in the mix. There's a MASSIVE difference between the two dosages.

When men use TOT, they report improved mood, libido, and energy levels. If they are also engaging in frequent and consistent resistance training, strength and muscle mass will improve. Testosterone affects EVERY system in the body, plain and simple. A dose of testosterone under TOT will NOT add 40 pounds of muscle to your frame or yield insane strength gains. Instead, you'll feel like you are young again, while noticing significant improvements in the gym.

A steroidal dose, though? Depending on the individual and the hormones used, a typical response involves greatly enhanced strength and faster post-workout recovery (compared to those not using steroidal doses). Your body weight increases, your sex drive goes up and your muscles will respond with growth if you are eating and training in a semi-intelligent manner.

Testosterone normally follows a linear dose-response curve (i.e. the more you take, the greater the results). Based on anecdotal evidence, the benefits seem to max out around 700-750 mg dosed weekly. However, dosages up to 1000 mg and higher aren't uncommon. Both professional and aspiring pro bodybuilders have been known to take 2-3 GRAMS (2000-3000 mg) of testosterone per week. And let me be very clear: Past a certain point, you do NOT feel great at all.

Given all of the positive benefits of using high doses of testosterone, why not just jump right in?

Put simply, there ARE potentially negative side effects. They are not guaranteed to happen but there is a definite possibility of them happening. However, the extent of side effects varies among individuals. There is no real way of knowing how the side effects will affect you until you take high doses of testosterone. As Jay and Jim have stated throughout this book, we're all biochemically unique.

Potential Negative Side Effects

Here is a quick rundown of the type of side effects produced by a supraphysiologic dose of testosterone[669].

Acne and oily skin - Testosterone affects everything, including speeding up the rate of skin growth and oil production. Many guys experience acne, especially on their backs and shoulders (commonly referred to as 'bacne').

Hair loss - If you are genetically prone to baldness, AAS will speed this up. Again, some guys get ZERO hair loss while others will quickly go bald. All of this comes down to genetics. I personally have a good friend who has used AAS since he was a teenager, and he went bald by the age of 20. There is no real way to counteract this, and the higher the dose you use, the faster this process happens.

Increased blood pressure - the higher the dose, the worse your blood pressure tends to get. This can be readily fixed by doing cardio, and even then some guys will still have chronically

---

[669] Wu BW, Berger M, Sum JC, Hatch GF, Todd Schroeder E. Randomized control trial to evaluate the effects of acute testosterone administration in men on muscle mass, strength, and physical function following ACL reconstructive surgery: rationale, design, methods. BMC Surgery. 2014;14:102. doi:10.1186/1471-2482-14-102.

elevated blood pressure. If you gain a lot of weight, which is almost inevitable with a high dose of testosterone, your blood pressure will go up due to the increase in hematocrit and hemoglobin levels (high doses of testosterone also stimulate red blood cell production).

Increased estrogen levels - Allow me to explain: Testosterone and estrogen are structurally similar, and some of that injected testosterone gets converted into estrogen. If you have high body fat levels and a lot of aromatase (remember that aromatase is the enzyme responsible for converting testosterone to estrogen) in your body, a greater amount of testosterone will convert into estrogen. This can result in gynecomastia (a.k.a. bitch tits), erratic and unbalanced moods, water retention and bloating. There are anti-estrogen compounds that most heavy steroid users take to counteract this, but again, the exact extent of the estrogenic side effects is hard to pin down. Some steroids convert to estrogen more than others, so you MUST KNOW what you are taking.

Insomnia, or trouble sleeping - For some people, their sleep will be negatively affected. This happens because your central nervous system (CNS) is dramatically elevated, which is caused by the full frontal assault of testosterone on most biological systems. The end result is your CNS working overtime from every measurable capacity.

The Effects of AAS on Mood

Is 'roid rage' a real thing? Do steroids turn men into assholes? Trying to answer these questions requires context, like all other things. With respect to roid rage, there is no doubt that high doses of testosterone and other AAS will cause changes in mood. That said, the vast majority of changes are POSITIVE. The negative changes are rare events that happen to a select few. I believe it is irresponsible to place the blame solely on the drugs without also considering the user who is taking them.

If you are an asshole before you're geared up, you'll be more of an asshole after you're geared up. In plain English, steroids amplify your preexisting personality. The only "angry" steroid users I've encountered were narcissistic, selfish men who were already assholes to begin with. The steroids did not make them that way, because they were ALREADY that way.

Speaking from personal experience, the only difference between "juiced" and "natural" men is assertiveness and energy. That's it. Not anger, not getting upset, or any other negative characteristic. Bluntly, it's hard to feel passive when your hormones are supercharged.

As such, I would not call roid rage a "myth." Rather, it's a rare phenomena that naturally arises when you sample a large population.

What About the Increased Strength and Size?

This is what most men care about. Unfortunately, there is no guarantee as to how much muscle you will gain because everyone responds differently. In more technical terms, each of us has a unique genetic androgen receptor (AR) specificity in our muscle cells. The better your muscle cells' receptors are at binding to the active metabolites in the AAS you are using, the better of a response you'll have to the drugs. This leads to bigger muscles and greater strength. While you can take higher doses, your RESPONSE to the dose is highly individual. If you have average genetics and/or a lack of AR sites, your response to AAS will be minimal at best (regardless of the dose).

With steroids, the FIRST cycle you ever run is always the most powerful because your ARs are not used to such a strong level of binding. This means that your first cycle has the highest possibility for the greatest muscular gains, as the steroid molecules will bind to your ARs for the first time. If your nutrition and training are dialed in (i.e. done properly), your body will theoretically increase the net amount of skeletal muscle proteins in your body, leading to more muscle. For this reason, a common recommendation is to "blast" high doses of testosterone when you first start using it.

How Much Muscle Can I Expect To Gain?

This depends on the dose used, your AR specificity, your nutrition and your training. I've never heard of anyone gaining less than 10 lbs of muscle tissue on their first cycle when using a moderate dose of 400-600 mg of testosterone per week, and a 20 lb weight gain is common.

On the higher end, I've also known guys who gain 40+ lbs on their first cycle while taking more than 1000 mg of testosterone a week. That's a BIG shift in weight! Imagine going from 180 lbs of body weight to 220 lbs in just 2-3 months - it's insane to even think about. But as I've previously said, you cannot guarantee how much muscle you'll gain. It's also important to realize that some of this weight gain can be attributed to increased water retention and glycogen storage. Contractile proteins (i.e. skeletal muscle tissue) do not magically appear without substantial and productive resistance training.

Generally, you have three categories of people who respond to AAS (these explanations are also given in context of first exposure to using AAS):

Low Responders - These are guys with poor to average levels of AR expression. Their muscle gain will be minimal at best. They are definitely bigger and stronger after dosing, but their results are nothing to shout home about. However, they often end up ABUSING steroids because they have to take high dosages in order to keep their size and strength. Additionally, low responders tend to have A LOT of side effects (not always, but it happens). These are the guys that get acne, lose their hair, and get gynecomastia (bitch tits). In some cases, they don't even look like they are on AAS despite taking copious amounts of gear!

Some men just don't respond at all to fairly substantial doses (ex. 750 mg of testosterone a week, plus an anabolic) and they STILL don't look like they take steroids. This can be very disappointing for men, as they have to juice up just to look like they "lift weights."

Moderate Responders - You might call this the middle ground. You can potentially gain 20+ pounds on a moderate to high dose (your first cycle only), you are definitely bigger and stronger after dosing, and you get more results if you take even higher doses. Side effects are minimal to moderate, or you might not even get any at all. For these men, AAS are awesome as they see great results while being on gear and maintaining these moderate-to-high dosages.

High Responders - These are the guys who have an extremely high affinity for AAS. This means that the drugs they use will maximally bind to the ARs in their muscles, allowing for their muscle cells to rapidly increase in size. They become massively bigger and/or stronger on AAS, ultimately turning into ungodly machines of muscle. These are the extreme, mesomorphic mutant types that you find competing for the Mr. Olympia title. They'll potentially put on 40 lbs of mass (first cycle), while their strength skyrockets through the roof. And all of this comes from nothing more than MODERATE dosages.

If you've never known pro bodybuilders types, this is hard to truly understand. It has to be seen to be believed, and there's no way around it. I've seen guys go from 200 lbs to 240 lbs or even 250 lbs of body weight, from bench pressing 275 lbs as a 1-rep max to bench pressing 375 lbs for reps. It's insane to witness! These men are genetically blessed in their biochemical response to AAS, and they generally don't experience bad side effects either. Often times there are NONE at all!

The Downside to Taking Steroids

Remember that this is a BONUS chapter, and as such it is strictly for informational purposes only. Our aim is to prevent men from reading and believing information from locker rooms and internet forums (where the majority of 'knowledgeable posters' are often the drug dealers who own or sponsor the forum itself) that turns out to be erroneous (and even potentially damaging to your health).

<u>NOTE:</u> Jim and Jay recommend you DO NOT USE AAS for ANY reason, unless your goal is to become a professional bodybuilder. And even if that is your goal, we HIGHLY RECOMMEND you consult with a doctor who is understanding of this goal and willing to help you in your pursuit of staying healthy (and ultimately NOT DYING)!

Aside from the short-term side effects, which there are many, there is an unavoidable long-term side effect: You LOSE the muscle and strength you gain once you stop taking supraphysiologic dosages of AAS. While there is some evidence that steroids can raise your "natural" strength and size levels even after you stop, the reality is that there is NO WAY to maintain your substantial size and strength gains without being "juiced" all year long.

Speaking with experienced and knowledgeable steroid users, and intimately knowing human biological systems myself, a pragmatic truth emerges for many bodybuilders using AAS at supraphysiologic doses:

Once you are ON, you do NOT come OFF. Once you are using, you don't stop using. You can lower your dosage to a TOT dose (i.e. a therapeutic dose) with time, and many guys do this for health reasons, but you can never come off completely (if you want to retain the muscle mass and size gained from using supraphysiologic dosages of AAS).

The idea of "cycling" is a myth. Taking steroids for a "cycle" and then never taking them again would be idiotic and pointless, as the positive effects go away completely. What cycling actually means is that you go through periods of higher doses and lower doses (also known as 'blasting and cruising'), while taking different compounds at different times. Every steroid user I've known who went completely "cold turkey" has returned to their natural levels of size and strength. **Every single time.**

This is why most men never come off: They cannot accept the idea of becoming big and strong, and suddenly going back to being normal again. So before considering the use of AAS, ask yourself this question (think LONG AND HARD about your answer):

Where is this road ultimately taking me?

Do all bodybuilders take massive amounts of steroids? What if someone takes only low doses?

Over the decades, bodybuilders have gradually used higher dosages. If you study bodybuilding history, you can spot TRENDS in historical data that provide some insight into the effects of different dosages. Numbers will begin to emerge:

1900-1940s - The biggest bodybuilders during this time were about 200 lbs, and lean. Excluding some outliers who were taller and bigger-boned, it was very uncommon for any 'ripped' man to be over 200 lbs. 200 lbs is about the maximum amount of lean body mass that a "normal" sized man can carry on his skeleton. Normally, in this context, this is not defined as 'genetically elite'.

1950s - This is when the first few bodybuilders over 200 lbs started to emerge. Steve Reeves, a notable Mr. America, was approximately 210 lbs. While it is possible that men were using testosterone (or certain testosterone analogs), they were still not widely available. If you look at body weights from this era, you begin to see more genetically gifted men that started getting into bodybuilding. Keep in mind that bodybuilding was 20 years away from becoming mainstream, and that bodyweights of 200-210 lbs WERE still "naturally" conceivable.

1960s - During this decade, you begin to see bodybuilders well over 220 pounds. Sergio Oliva, known as "The Myth," was the first "freak" in bodybuilding at 230 lbs. At this point, most competitive bodybuilders are using AAS. Their doses, however, are MUCH lower than what guys take today, and the range of drugs available was very limited. Testosterone, and the oral drug Dianabol, were the primary drugs they took.

1970s - This is the 'Arnold Schwarzenegger' Era. At this point, drug use was pretty much accepted but the dosing was still moderate. Drug cycles from this era basically consisted of moderate testosterone dosages, an oral medication to be used for a few weeks during a bulking phase, and TOT-level dosing any time one stopped cycling. During the 1970s, almost everyone is over 210 lbs, and you have the first guys emerging that weigh 240 lbs or more (Lou Ferrigno being the most notable).

1980s - This was when BLASTING (higher doses of drugs) really began to take off, along with STACKING (running multiple compounds at once). Steroids were entirely legal during this time, and so guys could take whatever they wanted. This is also the decade when growth hormone started being used, and when it was discovered that exogenous INSULIN (i.e. insulin that is injected into your body) could promote muscle growth. Lee Haney, the most popular Mr. Olympia of the 1980s, weighed 250 lbs on stage (he was the biggest Mr. Olympia to date).

1990s - This decade gave rise to the "Mass Monsters." Everyone began blasting drugs, and you begin to see steroid cycles that involved taking 3-5 different drugs at once (plus insulin and growth hormone). Dorian Yates, who held the title of Mr. Olympia for most of the 1990s, weighed 260 lbs on stage at 4% bodyfat. Everyone else was trying to compete with him! At this point in time, if you did not weigh at least 240 lbs, you were not competitive.

2000s - Ronnie Coleman becomes Mr. Olympia. He possesses perhaps the greatest muscular genetic profile of any human being to have ever lived. He weighs 290 lbs at 4% bodyfat. His closest competitor, Jay Cutler, weighed 270 lbs. The drug usage at this time is entirely out of control, and bodybuilders are freakishly unhealthy. The massive drug use, combined with the stacking of multiple compounds, continues to this day.

Putting Pro Bodybuilding History Into Perspective

Taking into account the timelines discussed in the previous section, we think you can make some general estimations about drug use in each time period:

1950s to early 1970s - Low dosages of compounds, much less than 1000 mg per week total between all AAS used. This equates to 10-25 lbs of muscle beyond genetic limitations.

1970s to early 1980s - Moderate dosages of all AAS compounds, approaching 1000 mg per week. This equates to 15-40 lbs lbs of muscle beyond genetic limitations.

Late 1980s to Modern times - High dosages of MULTIPLE AAS compounds (plus growth hormone and insulin) in the range of 1500 - 4000 mg (or more) per week. This equates to 40-60 lbs of muscle beyond genetic limitations (in those who are genetically capable).

Today, you have 5'9" bodybuilders that weigh 280 lbs and are under 10% body fat. Put that into perspective!

Does the use of supraphysiologic doses of AAS lead to premature death?

You may occasionally read about bodybuilders, professional wrestlers or NFL players dying young. It should be noted that the vast majority of them use steroids. Did steroids kill these men? In my opinion, no. What killed them was either:

A) How they used steroids, the kinds of steroids they used and the dosages (i.e. amount + frequency) of each.

B) An unhealthy lifestyle, likely consisting of abusing alcohol and other recreational drugs that accompanied their abuse of AAS.

C) In the case of wrestlers and NFL players, a hell of a lot of brain damage from the high-impact collisions their bodies suffered from years of participation.

D) The most common cause of death, however, is cardiovascular -related complications. This results from being unaware of your genetic predisposition, or ignoring it. Using high amounts of testosterone and growth hormone are both known to increase the size of the heart. We know that common side effects include high blood pressure, a negative impact on blood lipid levels, and (for older users) a rise in hematocrit levels that becomes uncontrollable. All of these are common contributing factors to cardiovascular problems.

As such, we don't think it is reasonable to say that steroids kill people. ABUSE of them, combined with living an unhealthy lifestyle, does.

For a man using TOT, however, you might expect him to live LONGER than a man with suboptimal testosterone levels. And we are quite confident that the majority of recent empirical studies[670] regarding TOT in aging men[671] will verify my assertion.

[670] Almehmadi Y, Yassin AA, Nettleship JE, Saad F. Testosterone replacement therapy improves the health-related quality of life of men diagnosed with late-onset hypogonadism. *Arab Journal of Urology.* 2016;14(1):31-36. doi:10.1016/j.aju.2015.10.002.

[671] Bassil N, Alkaade S, Morley JE. The benefits and risks of testosterone replacement therapy: a review. *Therapeutics and Clinical Risk Management.* 2009;5:427-448.

CHAPTER 19 KEY TAKEAWAYS

- We provide a high-level overview of what steroids are, how they work in the body, and a brief investigation into Anabolic and Androgenic Steroids (AAS). The next time someone talks about 'steroid' use, you'll know what they are specifically referring to.

- We tell you the stone cold truth about whether anabolic steroids work or not, and explain the subtle yet important differences between TOT and AAS.

- We give you a quick rundown of the side effects produced by supraphysiologic (i.e. much higher than therapeutic) doses of testosterone, while discussing how 'roid rage' comes about in steroid users.

- Does AAS use actually lead to increased strength and size? There's no guaranteed one-size-fits-all answer to this question, as it depends on a large variety of factors. For those of you wondering how genetics plays a role in getting the most out of steroid use, you're going to want to read this!

- There's one major downside to taking steroids and maintaining the gains they provide that most people don't want to talk about, or admit to. (Hint: Once you go ON, you never go OFF).

- An extensive look into the history of drug use by bodybuilders from the 1900s to the present decade reveals patterns and trends in the number of drugs taken, the amounts of said drugs that were taken, and the emergence of physiques that contain an ever-increasing amount of muscle mass (beyond genetic limitations) at ridiculously low body fat percentages.

- Do steroids kill people? Not exactly - we told you about the other factors present in the premature deaths of steroid users that significantly contributed to their eventual demise.

TOT and US Military Veterans: The Problem and Solution

After reading this book, you will hopefully have drawn two main conclusions. First, that the healthcare system in the United States and the Western world is broken. And secondly, that you are the captain of your own ship and are therefore responsible for your own health. Today, more and more people are waking up to the fact that the healthcare system is only there to treat you when you're sick. We call this the "Sick Care Patient Model." To get a feel for this, try scheduling an appointment with your local physician. Tell them you feel amazing, and then tell them you'd like to stay that way for the rest of your life. Their reaction will be a good indicator of whether they're into healing people, or into the very profitable BUSINESS of treating symptoms.

Sadly, most physicians these days are busy treating symptoms. But why is this happening? We could sit here and debate the point all day. Doctors are under intense scrutiny and pressure, and with limited time and resources, it's often easier to give out pills instead of investigating root causes. Some doctors have become jaded and cynical after dealing with countless patients who cry wolf too many times. And a small minority have become 'drug dealers in lab coats', either incentivized by Big Pharma to prescribe pills[672] or too preoccupied with reimbursements from insurance companies. Regardless of the cause, it's clear that our healthcare system is broken.

---

[672] https://www.nytimes.com/2017/10/18/opinion/opioid-pharmaceutical-addiction-pain.html - 'Drug Dealers in Lab Coats'

However, this scenario is not just confined to the civilian population. It's also happening on a grand scale to our Veterans, and if anything, it's worse. Despite the fact that we have institutions like Veterans Affairs (VA) that are specifically set up to help them, veterans aren't getting the treatment and attention they need and deserve. What's more, we have tens of thousands of Veterans returning to civilian life on the back of multiple tours in Iraq and Afghanistan. Many of them have suffered unspeakable tragedies, both mental and physical. Despite all of these things, the Sick Care Patient Model doesn't know what to do with them.

In this chapter, we look at how the "Sick Care Patient Model" has failed our Veterans and how testosterone has the power to heal the deepest wounds. We also interviewed two of the foremost and respected experts on healthcare for Veterans; ex Special Forces Green Beret Andrew Marr of the Warrior Angels Foundation[673], and Russ Scala, the Founder of Precision Health[674] and author of *American Biohacker*[675].

Tales From the Blast Factory: A Veteran's Story

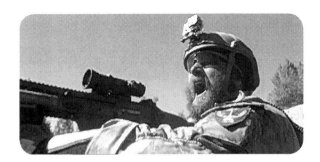

[673]   http://waftbi.org/

[674]   http://scalaprecisionhealth.com/about-us/

[675]   https://www.amazon.com/American-Biohacker-Russ-Scala/dp/1981250220

Andrew Marr is a medically retired Special Forces Green Beret who served multiple tours of duty in Afghanistan. In his fantastic book **TALES FROM THE BLAST FACTORY: A Brain Injured Special Forces Green Beret's Journey Back From The Brink**[676], he describes his journey that involves going from a high-performing Special Forces operator, to taking 13 different medications every day and drinking from the time he woke up until he passed out in the evening. The effects of having his brain jarred repeatedly through the course of his career finally caught up with him. He was told he couldn't afford to take one more blow to the head, and was given a service connected disability rating of 100% with well over twenty documented and rated disabilities.

One of Andrew's specialties in the military was explosives. Indeed, he was in and around countless low-level blasts and explosions on a routine basis for roughly a decade. He was knocked unconscious only once in combat, and it was during a tour in Afghanistan when he came in close proximity to a detonation. Everything went black, and he was unconscious only for a brief moment until he came to. Suddenly, bullets cracked and zipped over his head, and rocket-propelled grenades thundered by. But he quickly regained his senses, his muscle memory kicked in and he did what he was trained to do: **Take the fight to the enemy and win.** During deployment, Andrew didn't notice anything wrong with his health because his high level of foundational training enabled him to carry on. Unfortunately, all of this masked a greater problem taking place. To make matters worse, this is a familiar story among Veterans.

It wasn't until six months after returning home from deployment that he realized something was drastically wrong. In 2014, his

---

[676]   http://www.amazon.com/exec/obidos/ASIN/B073ZQCHCD/trtrev-71-20

health took a nosedive and nobody could figure out what was wrong. His memory was fading, he suffered psychological issues and he felt multiple migraines that resulted in double vision. Maintaining balance and walking straight was a major struggle for him. His life was spiralling out of control; he had reached rock bottom, and turned to heavy drinking in an attempt to cope with the pain.

Testosterone and the Road to Recovery

Eventually, Andrew came to terms with the fact he had a problem, and in the Special Forces they have a tried-and-true saying: 'You can either bitch about something or you can find a way to fix it'. And as Andrew knew, better than anybody else, the Special Forces have no time for bitches. With that saying in mind, he went out in search of a solution. He visited physicians who prescribed him a cocktail of mind-bending antidepressants and anti-anxiety medications. Yet in spite of this, he was still battling terrible anxiety and depression. With the side effects from all the medications, in combination with the everyday drinking, he was worse off than before.

One day, he went to see an army endocrinologist who ran some tests, which included checking his testosterone levels. The reading for testosterone came back so low that the endocrinologist accused him of taking anabolic steroids and thought was trying to replenish his supply! Sick of being treated like a criminal, Andrew asked the endocrinologist if he thought that being in close proximity to thousands of low-level blasts could disrupt the hypothalamic-pituitary axis (i.e. the main control system for our hormones). The endocrinologist replied: "Not in my experience." Unbelievable! Here he was, a senior Special Forces operator, and yet he couldn't find anyone in the military to take him seriously. The "Sick Care Patient Model" couldn't (and wouldn't) treat him.

The journey back to optimal health came from finding physicians who took the time to truly understand his situation and the events that lead to his condition. Eventually, Andrew ran into Dr. Mark L. Gordon of the Millennium Health Center[677]. Dr. Gordon has a unique protocol that employs various medical tests to identify and treat the underlying condition, unlike the Sick Care Patient Model that only treats symptoms. The tests on Andrew indicated that he had a Traumatic Brain Injury (TBI). His brain was riddled with chronic neuro-inflammation, and severe damage to the hypothalamus and pituitary gland. The tests also revealed that Andrew was deficient in a number of hormones, particularly testosterone.

For those of you who don't already know, a TBI is a two-phase injury. Phase 1 is the actual physical trauma to the brain and/ or body. This can come about in any number of ways, such as a slip-and-fall, a blunt force trauma (for example, getting hit hard by an object, or an explosive blast wave). But it's the second phase, the "silent wound," that can be the real killer. It is the post-traumatic neuroinflammation that's caused by the initial injury. This inflammation can lower the levels of key hormones that are produced in the body. The slow process of inflammation, coupled with the down-regulation of hormones, can set Veterans up to be ticking time bombs of collapsing health.

The "silent wound" (neuro-inflammation and loss of hormones) produces disastrous side effects like fat gain, loss of focus, depression and many more. The central nervous system that controls your cognition, emotion, and physiology starts to

---

[677]   http://www.millenniumhealthcenters.com/

short-circuit and malfunction. However, given that the "silent wound" can remain hidden from detection for years, it is very difficult to diagnose the condition accurately. It is very rare for one to do so before the problems get much worse.

Andrew eventually underwent Dr. Gordon's protocol to reduce systemic inflammation, which involved the administration of testosterone. According to Dr. Gordon, testosterone is connected with one's inflammatory chemistry and repair of the body, and so it was important to administer it. After the first testosterone injection, Andrew reported that he "felt like Cinderella for sixty hours." It was an incredible turnaround: The depression-induced darkness and anxiety he had lived with for so long were gone. He was FINALLY on the road to recovery.

Eventually, all of Andrew's symptoms were completely reversed and today he is off all forms of medication. He already knew what it was like to defeat the enemy and win, so this was just another battle he needed to fight. As a result of his experiences, he set up the Warrior Angels Foundation, a non-profit specifically created and designed to help treat other Veterans.

"When there is a deficit of testosterone, we pay a steep price: our minds, our families, and our lives."
- Andrew Marr

Looking After Our Veterans

For every Veteran like Andrew Marr who gets successful treatment, there are countless others who end up being victims of medical negligence. In many cases, there are also Veterans who don't get any treatment at all! In 2014, an average of 20 Veterans per day committed suicide, and suicide is 20%

higher among Veterans than the civilian population. If that wasn't shocking enough, male Veterans who used the Veterans Health Administration (VHA) services were 22% more likely to die by suicide than those who didn't use it all[678]. Just think about it: This is the VERY administration designed to help these poor veterans!

We have failed our Veterans, and our pathetic attempts to help them aren't working. They did their duty to protect the freedoms we all hold dear, now we need to do our duty and look after them. **The systematically poor treatment of Veterans needs to end right here, right now.**

Hardwired

Being in the military means you may end up in the line of fire, or even make the ultimate sacrifice. In order to take the fight to the enemy, military personnel undergo rigorous training and develop courage, discipline and an iron will to succeed at all costs. In a war zone, fighting could erupt at any moment, which means that soldiers need to be ready at all times. This state of hypervigilance works well in combat situations, but when Veterans try to integrate back into civilian life in this mental state, things start to go wrong.

In addition, Veterans often have to deal with multiple personal issues. They fall into depression and develop addictions to alcohol and opiates, just so they can forget some of the things they've seen. Anything to shut their brains off will do, because they haven't been given the tools needed to integrate back into

---

[678] https://www.mentalhealth.va.gov/docs/2016suicidedatareport.pdf - Suicide Among Veterans and Other Americans 2001-2014.

society. As a consequence, Veterans are highly stressed and their cortisol levels are off the charts.

According to **Russ Scala, Founder of Scala Precision Health,** when you elevate cortisol, whether through physical, mental or emotional stress, you suppress the Hypothalamic Pituitary Testes Axis (HPTA). This leads to suppressed thyroid and adrenal function, diminished growth hormone and **low testosterone levels.** Elevated cortisol also damages neurological architecture, meaning that Veterans begin to lose their short-term memory.

To make matters worse, many Veterans join the military at a young age. At the tender age of 18, the prefrontal cortex is still not developed; it doesn't fully develop until your late 20s. Subsequently, high-stress combat scenarios rewire brain chemistry, meaning that the feel-good neurotransmitters (adrenaline, dopamine and serotonin) are out of balance. This results in fluctuating mood swings, and a strong craving for carbohydrates. Therefore, many Veterans resort to alcohol in a subconscious effort to raise serotonin and dopamine levels. They may also end up using opiates or marijuana, just to feel good (or even 'normal') because their brain chemistry is so imbalanced.

Getting Treated

Veterans are used to taking orders and respecting authority, and they take this modus operandi into civilian life. So when they visit their physician for treatment, they respect them as authority figures and rarely question their judgement. It's easy to feel intimidated! Indeed, the default option is to show someone their due respect when they've studied long and hard to become an expert in their field. However, this becomes a problem when the doctor has no understanding of the underlying condition and doesn't make an attempt to treat it. Instead, they prefer to throw pills at the problem in the hopes that it will go away. Even worse, they may dismiss the problem altogether!

Therefore, as a Veteran you must be very discerning because few doctors will truly understand your plight. The VA might be there to help you, but that doesn't mean they know how to treat you. So, if you're not getting the answers you want, be willing to look outside of the military. Often times, it's not that doctors want to obstruct you. They are merely hesitant to practice outside of 'standard care' out of the fear of being sued. So do your homework, and be willing to show your doctor the latest research. Show them the work of leading doctors like Russ Scala and Mark Gordon, who demonstrate how optimized hormone levels can reduce neuro-inflammation and save lives.

However, if they still refuse to play ball, don't tolerate doctors who just want to treat you as nothing more than a lab number. Symptoms come FIRST, and the lab results are a guide. Going down this road may result in expensive treatment costs, but there are incredible organizations like the Warrior Angels Foundation or Mission 22 that can help you.

Out with the Old and In with the New

The current paradigm of treatment is to treat PTSD-stricken Veterans with Xanax or Prozac, and then 'talk it out' with a counsellor. However, this just masks the deeper issue. If you've gotten this far in the book and still doubt the power of testosterone, remember that testosterone is a hormone produced by the human body, and that it also acts as a natural anti-depressant. We have testosterone receptors ALL OVER the body, and yet there **is not a single** Prozac receptor in the body. Let that sink in for a moment.

The "Sick Care Patient Model" compartmentalizes healthcare and treats the body in isolation. The cardiologist only looks at the heart, and the neurologist only looks at the brain. As a result, physicians fail to see the entire picture when treating veterans. The human body works synergistically (i.e. all of the parts work in harmony with one another), and so a holistic approach is required in order for treatment to be successful.

Russ Scala states that one of the keys to the healing process for Veterans is the development of new brain tissue and brain cells, particularly in the hippocampus (via neurogenesis). And central to neurogenesis is Brain-Derived Neutrophic Factor (BDNF), a protein that triggers the process. BDNF promotes improved mood via antidepressant activity and lowers cortisol levels, two crucial outcomes that Veterans desperately need.

Another key point to consider in your treatment is your diet. What's your doctor's view on nutrition? Having a predominantly fat-based diet, for starters, will help you develop new brain tissue because the brain will respond to fat more efficiently than glucose. In a bodily environment where there is already a lot of neural-inflammation, the goal is to minimize carbohydrate intake in order to prevent the release of free radicals that cause further damage.

This leads us to the importance of a healthy gut microbiome, and entire books have been written on the subject. The intestinal tract, a major part of the gut, regulates serotonin, dopamine and oxytocin levels[679]. Therefore, if your intestinal tract is out of balance, this will greatly affect your brain chemistry. Can you now see the importance of treating the body as a unit, and how everything is linked to one another?

Furthermore, if your intestinal tract is out of balance, you won't absorb any nutrients from your food (and nutrients play a vital role in the healing process). Therefore, it's critical to avoid consuming things that might affect your gut flora, such as the pharmaceuticals from the "Sick Care Patient Model" that destroy them. We would do well to remember what Hippocrates said over 2000 years ago: 'Let food be thy medicine'.

On a final note, Veterans train in teams where they develop iron-tight bonds between one another, and a strong sense of brotherhood. After extensive experience with treating Veterans, Russ Scala believes it's crucial for Veterans to also heal as a team. Being left to cope alone can have serious repercussions, as your surroundings can have a profound effect on whether your recovery goes well or not (also known as 'social-neurobiology'[680]). Therefore, it's fundamental to ensure that you're spending time with the right crowd. As the saying goes, 'Show me your friends and I'll show you your future'.

Additionally, the chronic head injuries of footballers and the traumatic brain injuries of veterans are both devastating conditions. Yet only one group of people (NFL football players) gets extensive media coverage, whereas the other group barely

[679] Thomas S, Izard J, Walsh E, et al. The Host Microbiome Regulates and Maintains Human Health: A Primer and Perspective for Non-Microbiologists. Cancer research. 2017;77(8):1783-1812. doi:10.1158/0008-5472.CAN-16-2929.

[680] Knudsen, Eric I. et al. "Economic, Neurobiological, and Behavioral Perspectives on Building America's Future Workforce." Proceedings of the National Academy of Sciences of the United States of America 103.27 (2006): 10155–10162. PMC. Web. 6 Nov 2017.

gets a mention. Some kneel to the flag, while others give their lives for it.

If you're a U.S. military veteran reading this book, you have the information that you need to take personal charge of your own recovery and your long-term health. Don't wait a moment longer!

CHAPTER 20 KEY TAKEAWAYS

- We talk about the "Sick Care Patient Model" and why it has failed our US Veterans in helping them get the recovery and treatment they need. Additionally, you'll see why institutions like the Veterans Affairs (VA), set up specifically to help Veterans, are not providing them with the treatment and attention they both need and deserve.

- Andrew Marr, a medically retired Special Forces Green Beret, tells the tragic story of how his health rapidly deteriorated and his life spiralled out of control after returning home from deployment.

- Fortunately, after years of receiving poor treatment from various physicians, he finally found a doctor who understood his situation and the events leading to his poor health. Dr. Mark L. Gordon provided Andrew with the tests and treatments needed to restore optimal levels of health and completely reverse his symptoms.

- We discuss why thousands of Veterans have become victims of medical negligence, and how these Veterans end up dealing with multiple health issues after leaving the military.

- We tell you how to to find the right physicians who will treat Veterans and their underlying conditions, instead of merely dispensing pills. It involves a combination of doing your homework, showing your doctor the latest research, optimizing your nutrition and spending time with a community of Veterans who will help you with the healing and coping process.

CHAPTER 21
Conclusion

Since the beginning of time, the ability to resist the effects of aging and prolong life has been a universal human desire. For thousands of years, alchemists sought in vain for an elixir of life, and their wishes were eventually manifested into reality when scientists synthesized the testosterone molecule in the 20th century.

Millions of men in modern society are needlessly suffering from low sex drive, loss of energy, an inability to focus, soul-crushing indecisiveness and a diminishing enthusiasm for life. All of this is happening because of chronically low levels of testosterone. There are many prominent voices in society, and far too many physicians who know next to nothing about TOT and continue to be mystified by numerous misconceptions[681]. They don't truly understand testosterone's profound effects on human biology and behavior, or the vital role that TOT can play in optimizing an adult male's life.

If you've learned anything from this book, you've seen how we've conclusively, yet scientifically, proven the mainstream-accepted and negative propaganda on therapeutic testosterone to be patently false. In the same vein, we offer you this consensus position statement from the Mayo Clinic International Expert Panel[682] regarding testosterone deficiency and treatment:

---

[681]   http://m.embor.embopress.org/content/18/1/11.long

[682]   Mayo Clin Proc. n July 2016;91(7):881-896 n http://dx.doi.org/10.1016/j. mayocp.2016.04.007. www.mayoclinicproceedings.org

(1) *Testosterone Deficiency (TD) is a well-established, clinically significant medical condition that negatively affects male sexuality, reproduction, general health, and quality of life;*

(2) *Symptoms and signs of TD occur as a result of low levels of testosterone (T) and may benefit from treatment regardless of whether there is an identified underlying etiology;*

(3) *TD is a global public health concern.*

(4) *T therapy for men with TD is effective, rational, and evidence based.*

(5) *There is no T concentration threshold that reliably distinguishes those who will respond to treatment from those who will not.*

(6) *There is no scientific basis for any age- specific recommendations against the use of T therapy in men.*

(7) *The evidence does not support increased risks of cardiovascular events with T therapy.*

(8) *The evidence does not support increased risk of prostate cancer with T therapy.*

(9) *The evidence supports a major research initiative to explore possible benefits of T therapy for cardiometabolic disease, including diabetes*

Testosterone optimization therapy is a verifiable and scientifically-proven way to dramatically enhance your life. It should also be quite apparent by now that "normal levels" of testosterone can be readily optimized using the simple TOT protocols of progressive and well-informed physicians. Doing so will radically improve your health, vitality, and zest for life.

It is important to thank the small number of dedicated physicians, scientists and active researchers who have devoted their lives to understanding testosterone's numerous effects on male life spans, and on building an evidence-based myth-destroying approach to TOT. This book is the result of close to 20 years of trial-and-error research, testing, refining, and a ton of blood (literally and figuratively) to deliver what we KNOW is THE authoritative research bible on not only using testosterone in a therapeutic manner, but also optimizing your lifelong health.

The TOT protocols in this book represent efficient strategies that are known to bring blood testosterone values to the highest end of the range, while minimizing side effects and maintaining optimal health and safety at the same time. Even though this book represents years of work from a team of people, we're just getting started. We will be at the forefront of the latest therapeutic protocols that contribute to the betterment of men (and women) worldwide for as long as we can breathe.

You should now be informed enough to speak intelligently with your TOT doctor. Together, you should be able to formulate a plan for using TOT that will positively transform your life.

The ball is in your court to take action and become the man you've always wanted to be.

Remember: **He who hesitates is lost (and likely the victim of low testosterone).**

The Golden Rules of TOT

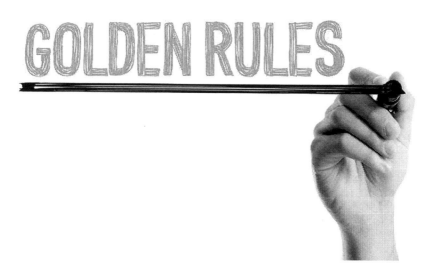

1) Testosterone Optimization Therapy SHOULD ONLY HAP-
    PEN when there is a real clinical need - diagnosed as a
    Partial Androgen Deficiency (PAD) - that is proven by
    symptoms <u>first</u> and blood work second.

2) Before initiating TOT, you must take an accurate account
    of your habits, your lifestyle and your fitness goals:

    • Are you fat?

    • Do you lift weights?

    • How important is augmenting your lifestyle in the
      game of life to you?

    • Are you willing to commit to fixing everything else
      (naturally) before beginning TOT?

    • Are you willing to pursue TOT as a lifelong course of
      action?

TOT is not an "I'll try it out and see if it works for me" approach. You are disrupting your body's natural production of testosterone, and SERIOUS SIDE EFFECTS can occur by carelessly cycling on and off (or discontinuing therapy altogether).

3) **YOU MUST work with a progressive physician who has an experience-based practice (ideally more than 5 years), and has successfully worked with men and women to help tweak and optimize their testosterone therapy.**

DO NOT WORK with a physician who has a GOD COMPLEX (i.e. a know-it-all), or even worse, no experience whatsoever with prescribing TOT. It is important to vet your TOT-prescribing physician thoroughly with the questions found in Chapter 8.

4) **If you live in an area of the world where you can't find a qualified TOT-prescribing physician, are you willing to commit to learning the concepts espoused in this book and apply them to yourself (where legal to do so)?**

Are you willing to pay for expert advice from physicians outside of your country who can guide you and tweak your therapy when necessary? Will you do your research in advance to ensure you are in a position to make informed decisions on your own health?

5) **Testosterone Optimization Therapy, done correctly, uses testosterone ONLY to establish a baseline for your blood work and correctly evaluate your vital biomarkers.**

This rule also applies to men of reproductive age and capacity. hCG should not be started with TOT until 6 weeks AFTER you establish baseline lab work. This allows your physician to properly understand what is happening to your endocrine system when exogenous testosterone is used by itself.

6) **Aromatase Inhibitor (AI) medications are ONLY used when there is a CLINICAL NEED to do so, based on blood work and pronounced side effects. AIs can cause serious negative effects to bone mineral density over time.**

When they are dosed, the MED (Minimum Effective Dose) principle should be applied, with the end goal of gradually eliminating AI use as soon as a therapeutic range of both testosterone and estrogen is established. This therapeutic range is said to be reached when there are *no side effects and the patient feels happy and balanced.*

Starting a patient on hCG, testosterone and an AI at the same time is not only INEFFECTIVE, but also unnecessary FOR BIOMARKER EVALUATION. When therapy is initiated with all three of these medications, there is a total lack of understanding when it comes to identifying what each medication is doing in combination with the others.

If anything, the patient is playing a "guess the problem" game with his endocrine system for months (usually years) because they can't properly evaluate biomarkers. There is nothing good than can come from it, plain and simple.

7) **The usage of medications to increase luteinizing hormone (LH) levels (hCG, hMG, clomiphene) and consequently raise testosterone levels without disrupting your body's homeostatic mechanisms (HPTA/HPGA axes) should NORMALLY be the front line treatment with men who are of prime reproductive age (18-35 years old).**

If a patient over 35 agrees to it, the usage of a LH stim- ulating medication alongside TOT is acceptable. The patient must be aware of the risks posed to fertility when using testosterone, which are minimal. For men who wish to have children in the future, the ULTIMATE strategy involves having the patient attain a measured sperm count and freeze their sperm before they start TOT. This strategy allows men to have easy access to viable and motile sperm when they are ready to have children.

8) There is no such thing as a one-size-fits-all TOT delivery system.

In our opinion, based on decades of experience and consultation with the top progressive physicians all around the world, injectable testosterone is the best way to optimize blood levels of testosterone in the fastest and most efficient way possible.

Some men will be needle-phobic (i.e. scared of needles), and in those instances, transdermal delivery is the best alternative strategy for maintaining lifelong patient adherence. Beyond those two delivery systems, EVERYTHING else is suboptimal with respect to the likelihood of potential issues and the added inconveniences to your daily lifestyle.

9) You must regularly perform blood work and become familiar with YOUR specific biomarkers to assess your overall health when undergoing TOT.

You should understand the specific tests to run, the ranges you should be within for each biomarker, how often to run each test, and any exceptional circumstances to watch out for. Since TOT is a lifelong treatment, that means you'll be regularly running these tests and tracking the results for the rest of your life.

Phlebotomy (donating blood) should only happen when there is an elevation of platelet count (as clearly explained in this book), along with high levels of both hemoglobin (+20 g/dL) and hematocrit (+54%).

10) **Your physician should know how to quickly alleviate common TOT side effects. These effects include high or low estrogen readings, itchy nipples (gynecomastia), water retention, lack of erectile strength, and mood imbalances.**

The potential side effects of TOT are minimal in scope, simple to detect and easy to safely correct when managed by a qualified TOT physician. Front-line treatment options should first involve changing the dose of testosterone (usually lowering) and the frequency of said doses before introducing medications that are specifically used for alleviating side effects. This rule is especially important when it comes to introducing AI medications into one's TOT regime, which can cause bone mineral density issues over time.

11) **Therapeutic dosages of testosterone can completely change your physique by decreasing body fat and increasing muscle mass, but ONLY when living a dialed-in lifestyle.**

This lifestyle MUST CONSIST of a clean insulin-controlled diet, in combination with productive resistance and cardiovascular training. If you think you can hack life with TOT while eating Cheetos and laying down on the couch all day, you are DEAD WRONG!

TOT is NOT a magic bullet. Also, if you think you can get away with skipping cardio and doing nothing else but training with weights, think again. You'll end up getting average to below average results at best. You must do cardio on a regular basis to keep your blood supply oxygenated, and decrease the thickening of blood (via increased red blood cell counts) often caused when using injectable testosterone.

12) If Your body fat is over 30% (i.e. you are obese) and you start TOT without a FIRM COMMITMENT to reducing body fat, you will fail miserably.

There are too many biological systems that are not functioning properly when you are obese. As a result, using testosterone in isolation can create additional problems. As discussed in the book, obesity and high aromatase levels go hand in hand with low testosterone levels. Dr. Rob Kominiarek says that when you are a 'metabolic emergency' due to things like insulin resistance and metabolic disorder, nothing will work 'as expected' until all systems are operating normally. Therefore, GET RID OF YOUR BODY FAT or accept inevitable failure as the likely result.

13) Almost every single "testosterone boosting" supplement sold today is a complete scam.

The cold hard truth is that there's little to NO SCIENTIFIC EVIDENCE which supports the claims made by supplement companies about their testosterone boosters actually raising testosterone levels. The only proven way to raise and optimize testosterone levels is through pharmaceutical means (i.e. utilizing TOT).

This is because powerful factors in our modern-day environment are constantly placing our endocrine systems under siege. This environmental assault overshadows most men's natural ability to produce testosterone, and their efforts to fix low testosterone levels. It is the opinion of the most advanced and progressive physicians, that only Type A personality types can fix their issues naturally, due to their commitment and their militant attention to detail.

14) **There is nothing morally wrong, unethical or illegal about optimizing your body's testosterone levels. It's the exact same thing as having Lasix, or an artificial hip replacement surgery.**

Using TOT productively is a lifelong strategy, and so you need to be financially stable in order to start therapy. Being able to pay for your treatment and any additional medications (when necessary) MUST BE factored into your daily expenses.

15) **When using injectable testosterone as a delivery system, the optimal protocols to choose from are as follows:**

- **Option 1A: 10-30 mg of testosterone injected daily.** This provides the most stable testosterone levels (i.e. mimicking endogenous production of testosterone as closely as possible), and it will also help to minimize aromatization (thereby minimizing side effects) and erythrocytosis (blood thickening). Normally, this type of protocol works well for individuals with a Type A personality.

- **Option 1B: 50-70 mg of testosterone injected every other day (EOD).** This is a nice compromise between injecting yourself daily and injecting yourself twice a week. This protocol is best for individuals who cannot bring themselves to administer daily injections.

- **Option 2: 50-100 mg of testosterone injected twice a week (preferably every 3rd day).** This option is the MOST POPULAR CHOICE, and is preferred by most patients because they don't have to inject themselves too often. Additionally, this protocol is still more advantageous than once per week therapy.

16) **Injecting yourself is a learned art form that takes time, patience and consistent practice.**

Smaller gauge needles (i.e. thinner needles) are a NECESSITY when you're poking your body full of holes over the course of your life. You MUST EXPERIMENT with both intramuscular and subcutaneous injections to learn what works best for you and your body.

17) **Baldness and acne can, and often, manifest themselves when using clinical dosages of testosterone.**

Baldness (a.k.a. Androgenic alopecia) is a genetic condition, and TOT can accelerate the rate of hair loss (via conversion of testosterone into DHT).

Causes of both mild and severe acne are multifactorial (i.e. multiple factors are at play). Sometimes acne can arise due to issues related to nutrition, and other times it can arise due to high levels of stress. There are some people who believe that acne can be caused by an imbalance between testosterone and estrogen. Whatever the cause, please be aware that it can happen, and we highly recommend having strategies in place to cope with it. Speak to your physician about this.

18) **Mainstream media will scare you into believing that there are many harmful side effects which arise from using TOT (heart disease, increased vascular incidents, prostate**

issues, cancer, reduction in penis size, loss of emotional control, etc.)

However, these side effects are either entirely false, or outright fabricated when TOT is used properly in normal population groups. Our book clearly presents substantial evidence that proves our statement.

19) **You MUST understand the three specific types of physical fitness goals (fat loss, maintenance, muscle gain) and the amount of calories you need to eat in order to achieve each of them.**

You must also understand your body type, and its unique insulin sensitivity. Finally, you must be aware of the 3 primary macronutrients (protein, carbohydrates, fats) and the importance of each one in relation to your overall health and your success with TOT. This includes knowing the exact amounts of each macronutrient to eat, depending on your fitness goals and your body type.

20) **To fully optimize your TOT, you should also include additional supplements and medications in your overall health regimen.**

As discussed in "Chapter 16 - Agents of Change," they go hand in hand with reducing your insulin signal (ultimately decreasing your body fat and levels of inflammation), improving your focus, increasing your energy levels and resistance to age related disease. They also can enhance your performance in the gym, build muscle mass and accelerate your rate of recovery.

Frequently Asked Questions

Q: What is the optimal form of TOT for a newbie starting out for the very first time?

A: Listen to your physician and the diagnosis they make based on your lab results, presenting symptoms, and your unique lifestyle needs and wants. Optimally, using injectable testosterone for a total dose of 80-200 mg per week (preferably divided up in at least two injections per week) should be more than enough for any adult male to optimize their testosterone levels. However, every man is different. There is no one-size-fits-all approach to hormonal optimization. It requires the observation of an experienced physician who can intervene if (and when) necessary.

Q: I recently started Testosterone Optimization Therapy (2 weekly injections of 60 mg testosterone cypionate) and I'm suffering from extreme and severe panic attacks. My doctor is unable to help. Do you have any idea what might be happening to me? We already tried lowering the dose but it didn't help. I would truly appreciate your thoughts in helping me find out what's going on.

A: Dr. Rob Kominiarek[683] has seen this issue with some of his patients. It's very unfortunate and problematic, but select individuals with **Monoamine oxidase A Single Nucleotide Polymorphism**[684] have a genetic predisposition to a slow

---

[683] www.renuehealth.com

[684] Study on the correlation between single nucleotide polymorphism of monoamine oxidase A gene and anger regulation. Zhongguo Zhong Xi Yi Jie He Za Zhi. 2012 Oct;32(10):1354-7.

degradation of neurotransmitter pathways. As soon as these patients take a shot of testosterone, they have full-blown panic attacks. Some attacks are so severe that they are unable to leave their homes, or even function properly. He offers a couple of reasons as to why this may happen, including depletion of pregnenolone or magnesium. If restoring both pregnenolone and magnesium to healthy levels doesn't help, there's a good chance that the patient doesn't tolerate estrogens or androgens very well (if at all). As a result, any dose of testosterone will likely lead to panic attacks, some of which may be profound. If you are one of these men, make sure you work with a physician who truly understands this condition. At the very least, have your doctor reach out to Dr. Kominiarek at RenueHealth.com.

Q: My doctor recommends Nebido, and argues it is far superior to all other testosterone esters. He is an author of a standard endocrinology textbook, and the head of the WHO Center for andrology. What do you think about Nebido or Aveed?

A: We are very familiar with Professor Eberhard Nieschlag and his comprehensive 2012 textbook **Testosterone: Action, Deficiency, Substitution**[685]. There are actually citations from his research in this book.

Nebido and Aveed are actually brand names for testosterone undecanoate. It's an old-school version of testosterone re-engineered as an injectable form of delivery. It used to be available under the trade name 'Andriol', and was available in capsule form. Although it's a very weak (and expensive) form of testosterone, there are no observed side effects from its use on the HPTA (Hypothalamus-Pituitary-Testes-Axis), also

---

[685]   http://www.amazon.com/exec/obidos/ASIN/1107012902/trtrevbook-20

known as the HPGA (Hypothalamic–Pituitary–Gonadal-Axis). Apparently, it doesn't disturb follicle-stimulating hormone (FSH) or luteinizing hormone (LH) levels either.

Nebido has been used in parts of Europe for more than a decade, and Aveed in the USA for close to 4 years. As we already wrote in Chapter 6, practice-based knowledge tells us that this medication looks great in theory but fails in what is most important: The end-user experience. Besides the issues previously discussed that most patients complain about, another massive issue we have is with the injection volume used for the initial dosing (750 - 1,000 mg). That is a *lot* of injection volume. With that much fluid making its way into your body, there is a great risk of pain at the injection site, or accidentally injecting into a blood vessel (leading to a potential pulmonary embolism). We don't want that!

Q: On a long enough time horizon (i.e. months), is there really any difference between testosterone cypionate and testosterone propionate if you inject both at least 3x/ week, given that you use the same dosage of testosterone equivalently?

A: As far as efficacy, milligram for milligram it probably won't matter as much. Injectable testosterone is injectable testosterone, plain and simple. We'd bet that if you did blood work for 7 days in a row, you'd have elevated testosterone levels for each day that you injected propionate (due to the shorter half life of the propionate ester, as previously discussed). Likewise, you'd have days without elevated levels when injecting cypionate (due its longer half life). Therefore, there may or may not be a marginal benefit to using propionate, since you'd be at higher levels every day. The days of having higher levels should avoid any low points (troughs) potentially experienced by patients using the longer-acting testosterone esters (i.e. Cypionate or Enanthate). This is another reason why injecting daily is a recommended option, especially for patients who have lifestyles where it makes sense to do so, as there will never be any troughs throughout a 7 day week.

Q: I'd really like for you to answer this question for me (as the bro and doctor insights are all over the place). How long will it take for testosterone to show effects? FYI, I use a compounded cream at 200 mg without AI or hCG.

A: There was an excellent study[686] done in 2011 that investigated this very same question. Here is what the study found, verbatim:

- **Effects on sexual interest appear** after **3 weeks plateauing at 6 weeks,** no further increments beyond.
- **Changes in erections/ejaculations may require up to 6 months.**
- **Effects on quality of life manifest within 3-4 weeks,** but maximum benefits take longer.
- **Effects on depressive mood appear after 3-6 weeks with a maximum after 18-30 weeks.**
- First effects on **erythropoiesis (increased red blood cell count) after 3 months, peaking at 9-12 months.**
- **Prostate specific antigen and volume rise, marginally, plateauing at 12 months;** further increase related to aging rather than therapy.

---

[686] Onset of effects of testosterone treatment and time span until maximum effects are achieved eur J Endocrinol EJE-11-0221, doi: 10.1530/EJE-11-0221 First published online 13 July 2011.

- **Effects on lipids appear after 4 weeks, maximal after 6-12 months. Insulin sensitivity may improve within few days, but effects on glycemic control become evident only after 3-12 months.**

- **Changes in fat mass, lean body mass and muscle strength occur within 12-16 weeks, stabilize at 6-12 months, but marginally continue to improve over years. Effects on inflammation occur within 3 to 12 weeks.**

- **Effects on bone mineral density detectable after 6 months but continue for at least 3 years.**

Q: I've listened to your podcasts and I want to understand your final stance on hCG.

A: Experimenting, and measuring the results of said experimentation, is the only guaranteed way to find out what works for your body because we are all biochemically unique. **hCG** monotherapy (discussed in more detail in Chapter 10) is used by physicians to elevate testosterone levels (by increasing luteinizing hormone). There is research indicating that it works especially well with younger men who don't want to disturb their endogenous (natural) testosterone production while maintaining their fertility at the same time. Dr. Crisler (interviewed in Chapter 12) recommends using **hCG** at 250-500 IU (international units) per shot as part of his injection protocol (a.k.a. *The Crisler Method*[687]). **hCG** can also be used daily at 100 IU with great success, due to its ability to produce randomness in the serum androgen profile at varying points in the day. As we noted earlier in the book, this dosing strategy mimics your body's natural testosterone production. If retaining your

---

[687] Testosterone Replacement Therapy-A Recipe for Success-Dr. Crisler pg.71 Milestones Publishing (March 13, 2015).

fertility is important to you, it is one of the top medications to use in combination with testosterone. Using **hCG** also prevents testicular atrophy for men who prefer having full testicles. If you do not use **hCG**, you will still retain gonadal function. Your testicles will be less full, but you will still be able to ejaculate and reach orgasm as normal.

Jay and Jim DO NOT use **hCG** as they have experienced increased E2 conversion, acne flares and an imbalance between testosterone and estrogen levels. They are also in their mid-40's and have no interest in fathering any more children. However, it's important to note that experiences on **hCG** can be very subjective. Some users feel great without **hCG** and others feel great on it. If you are using it when first starting TOT, it may be difficult to determine what its effects are, especially in comparison to testosterone administered by itself (i.e. without any other drugs or medications). The only thing you can do is experiment on yourself, noting any physiological changes or side effects, while also drawing labs to document variations over time. There are clearly luteinizing hormone (LH) receptors all over the body, and theoretically, using hCG can work well to restore improved mood and well being (for those who respond well to it). Although LH and **hCG** bind to a common receptor, emerging evidence suggests that LH and **hCG** have different biochemical downstream effects[688]. Understanding that we are all biochemically unique, this study substantiates why not all men will respond in a uniform (i.e. positive) fashion when using **hCG**.

---

[688]   Janet Choi, Johan Smitz, Luteinizing hormone and human chorionic gonadotropin: Origins of difference, In Molecular and Cellular Endocrinology, Volume 383, Issues 1–2, 2014, Pages 203-213, ISSN 0303-7207, https://doi.org/10.1016/j.mce.2013.12.009.

Q: When on injectable TOT and preparing for a blood test, how long should I wait after doing the injection before going to the lab for the test?

You want to get your labs done based on what your physician is specifically looking for. Most of them want to see your levels when peak plasma values are attained. Peak values are generally attained 1.5 to 3.5 days after the injection, depending on the ester being used. Propionate would be 36-48 hours post-injection, and the longer-acting esters (cypionate or enanthate) would be 48-72 hours post-injection. For example, if you're using testosterone cypionate and your doctor wants to see your peak plasma levels, take your dose on Monday morning and get blood work done on Thursday morning.

Q: I hear the term HRT (hormone replacement therapy) a lot. Is that for women? How is TOT different from (or the same as) HRT?

Here is the definition of HRT, as defined by Wikipedia:

> "...any form of hormone therapy wherein the patient, in the course of medical treatment, receives hormones, either to supplement a lack of naturally occurring hormones, or to substitute other hormones for naturally occurring hormones."

The term is definitely more visible in women's circles, referring to hormone replacement for pre- and post-menopausal women. In this instance, it involves the use of one or more medications designed to artificially boost hormone levels. The main types of hormones involved are estrogen, progesterone/progestins, and usually testosterone. Just as we changed the acronym TRT to TOT in men, Dr. Jim Meehan and Monica Campbell are doing the same for women by changing HRT to HOT (Hormone Optimization Therapy).

Hormone Optimization Therapy (HOT) can be just as effective for women as TOT is for men, from a treatment standpoint. As we stated in the preface of the book, there is plenty of scientific evidence showing that HOT for women[689] is highly effective and safe[690]. There are WAY too many popular myths surrounding women and HOT that can be easily debunked, and we believe this topic warrants an entire book unto itself. And that's exactly why Monica Campbell and Dr. Jim Meehan are releasing their companion series book titled *Cracking the Fountain of Youth Code: The Complete Woman's Guide to Becoming Sexier, Leaner, Happier and Empowered for Life* in 2018.

Q: I was diagnosed with varicoceles in my left testicle, and I'm going to have the microsurgery. Will I need TOT post-surgery to maintain optimized hormone levels for the rest of my life?

A: As many as 15% of men have varicoceles, which are masses of enlarged and dilated veins in the testicles. There is new evidence showing that varicoceles, long known to be a cause of male infertility, interfere with the production of testosterone[691]. In your situation, it depends on how well your testes are producing LH, both before and after the surgery. You need to work with an experienced and progressive doctor who will monitor important biomarkers, before and after your surgery,

---

[689]   Tuiten A, Von Honk J, Koppeschaar H, et al. Time course of effects of testosterone administration on sexual arousal in women. Arch Gen Psychiatry. 2000;57(2):149-153.

[690]   Davis SR. Cardiovascular and cancer safety of testosterone in women. Curr Opin Endocrinol Diabetes Obes. 2011;18(3):198-203.

[691]   Dabaja AA, Goldstein M. When is a varicocele repair indicated: the dilemma of hypogonadism and erectile dysfunction? *Asian Journal of Andrology.* 2016;18(2):213-216. doi:10.4103/1008-682X.169560.

to effectively determine if you will need TOT for the remainder of your life. There are multiple cases in the scientific literature showing men who have recovered without having to use TOT.

Q: How much of a hassle is it to go from self-medicating your testosterone therapy (grey market) to being under a doctor's care?

A: This is an excellent question. It really depends on where you're being self-medicated. Are you in the USA? How much does it cost you to get your hands on testosterone, acquire ancillary medications and get your blood work done regularly? It is crucially important to find a doctor who is not only willing to prescribe testosterone, but who will also monitor you and your blood work properly.

We highly recommend working with doctors via telemedicine providers[692] who can treat you remotely. Having an outside perspective on your blood work, and receiving treatment from someone who is qualified and objective, will only benefit your health.

If you have medical benefits, many of the anti-aging medications (Metformin, Dessicated Thyroid, etc.) and TOT ancillaries (Arimidex, hCG, Nolvadex or Clomid, etc.) discussed in the book can be billed through insurance. Some of the medications will be more expensive than others, and sometimes you will be denied access on the basis of certain factors. Said factors can include (but are not limited to) your individual diagnosis, your age and the level of coverage you currently have.

Having a physician who can counsel you through your attempts to find a balance between testosterone and estrogen is critical.

---

[692]   www.bodhd.com

No dosage, or any reaction to said dosage, is universal to all humans. Any hormone therapy is, as Dr. Crisler states, 'dropping a pebble into an ocean'. In other words, optimizing your body can be a complicated process. The more you know about using TOT and how it may or may not affect your individual biochemistry, the higher your chances of long-term success.

ONCE MORE: If you live in a country or state where it is illegal to administer testosterone without a doctor's prescription, then choosing the route of self-administration without a legitimate prescription is breaking the law.

Q: Will it be an issue going through airports and countries while traveling with testosterone and syringes? Do I need to have a prescription with me?

A: You should have a copy of your prescription, or at the very least have your medications indicated with the prescription labeling on the packaging and storage bag. It is unlikely to ever be an issue. For convenience purposes, however, pack your TOT equipment in your checked baggage using something like this diabetic organizer bag[693].

Q: After researching TOT, it seems that lots of bodybuilders have died of renal failure - will testosterone damage my kidneys?

A: Absolutely not. Do not confuse the supraphysiologic (i.e. excessively high dosages of many drugs, including testosterone) that professional bodybuilders use with the therapeutic dosages of testosterone found in TOT. There is not a single study found in medical literature which proves that

---

[693]   http://www.amazon.com/exec/obidos/ASIN/B00KXNK7CA/trtrevbook-20

testosterone causes issues with the kidneys. The bodybuilders that come to mind with kidney issues were either genetically prone to these issues from the start, or using other kidney-affecting drugs (such as diuretics and NSAIDs) while ignoring the increasing warning signs.

Q: What if I develop a rash around my injection site?

It is possible to experience an allergic reaction from the chemical that keeps the testosterone ester stable in injectable solution form (usually ethyl oleate or propylene glycol). Very rarely, an allergic reaction to an injection will lead to a localized skin infection. Often known as cellulitis, it appears as a burning sensation at the point of injection. Sometimes, the skin turns red or fills up with white blood cells. If you are experiencing any of these symptoms, it may be a good idea to see your doctor right away. In the worst case scenario (and this is rarely seen or experienced), your doctor might have you do a round of antibiotics for several days to treat the cellulitis.

Q: About a day after injection, I'm getting some soreness/ bruising at the place where I injected. Is that normal? I just recently started TOT.

A: Yes. As a newbie to TOT, when first receiving intramuscular injections, you may experience minor soreness at the point of injection several hours later. It feels just like the soreness you'd experience if someone punched you in the arm. Most of the time you will feel nothing, but either way it's nothing to worry about and you'll just get used to it. Eventually, you won't feel anything at all! In rare instances, you could be having a reaction to the ester that involves a greater amount of pain and swelling.

Q: Do you recommend the usage of a 5/16 gauge or 1-inch insulin syringe to inject testosterone intramuscularly (thereby potentially reducing scar tissue formation)? What is your take on this?

A: This is a good question, and it bears an intelligent response. The use of an insulin syringe (27-31 gauge) to inject testosterone, both intramuscularly and subcutaneously, is strongly recommended (even though few physicians provide these options to their patients). These syringes are usually less than 0.5 inches long and have a very narrow needle barrel. Injecting with such a small needle drastically minimizes the chances of injection scarring, especially over a lifetime of injections.

One major consideration you should keep in mind during injections is your body fat levels. After all, you are taking a needle that is less than a half inch long and trying to reach into your muscle with it. If you have a high percentage of body fat, you may not be able to get through the fat into the target area. It is also extremely difficult to push the testosterone solution through the syringe when injecting because of the thinness of the needle, so take your time and become skllled at it. Many men are now using insulin syringes to inject their TOT subcutaneously. As already said in Chapter 8, feel free to give this option a try.

Q: I'm 32 and obese at 5'7" and 285 lbs. I'm seeing an endo-crinologist in a few days and I'd like to know what my options are?

A: Being FAT (i.e. obese) will limit your ability to experience optimal results while using TOT. Too many men think that they can live a FAT lifestyle and use TOT as a magic bullet to get good results - WRONG! Testosterone is not a panacea or a magic pill. It's one part of living an optimized lifestyle. Using TOT when you are obese can lead to issues with the aromatase enzyme, ultimately leading to high E2 readings (estradiol) that will likely cause negative estrogenic side effects. These effects include increased estrogenic fat deposition, moodiness, water retention, and feeling 'off' due to a lack of balance between testosterone and estrogen. More research is coming out by the day, indicating that being obese (with a testosterone deficiency) dramatically increases your risk of death[694].

Q: Does TOT make me sterile and unable to have children?

A: This is a myth. If you want to have children, make sure you include either **hCG, clomid**, and/or **hMG** therapy as part of your TOT protocol. As previously stated, you should also visit your urologist to get a **measured sperm count** in order to understand your baseline values before starting TOT. It also wouldn't hurt to freeze your sperm in the event of a worst-case scenario. Usually, TOT will not permanently damage your ability to get a woman pregnant. In the worst cases, we have seen a rigorous course of **hCG, clomid**, and/or **hMG** restore fertility within six months, and sometimes sooner than that. These 'worst cases' include men who were on TOT for more than 10 years and were totally inhibited via low luteinizing hormone (LH) and follicle stimulating hormone (FSH) levels. Even these men restored their fertility completely!

Q: With the sensationalist claims from 2014 through 2016 about testosterone increasing the possibility of CV (cardio-vascular) events like heart attacks, strokes, etc...and your

---

[694] Double Trouble: co-occurrence of testosterone deficiency and body fatness associated with all-cause mortality in US men. Clin Endocrinol (Oxf). 2017 Oct 25. doi: 10.1111/cen.13501. [Epub ahead of print]

THE TESTOSTERONE OPTIMIZATION THERAPY BIBLE

book clearly dispelling them as poorly interpreted data from older men in higher risk population groups, what is the prudent course of action knowing that there are NO CONCLUSIVE long-term studies proving the safety of TOT?

A: This a great question. We have already listed and discussed the myriad of studies documenting the safety and benefit of TOT in relation to the risk of cardiovascular disease. In fact, we've already proven that there are NO conclusive studies showing a definitive association between statistically significant ADVERSE cardiovascular events and TOT in otherwise normal men. The benefits of testosterone, as opposed to being wholly biochemical in nature, may be a function of the hormone's effect on fatigue. Secondly, it increases one's tendency to exercise and pursue a more physical lifestyle. This, by virtue, provides protection AGAINST coronary disease. No one questions the health-improving effects of exercise in aging individuals, right?

But let's play devil's advocate and assume the worst. From this standpoint, all you can say is that the data is somewhat mixed with respect to an overall consensus. However, considering that the "risk" associated with TOT is likely a function of flawed study design, we say HELL YES - it is WORTH the risk! At 46 years of age, aging backwards with respect to our appearance and measurement of our metabolic health, we are living proof that the reward crushes the perceived risk. And if you accept that TOT provides you the key to a real life of vigor and increased energy, is the tradeoff of having neither really worth it to you? If you answer YES, you should ask for a refund for your purchase. This book is not for you.

Q: I have had trouble finding a good TOT doctor in Denver without spending upward of $3,000 just to get started. I paid for my own lab work, used the bloodwork video you

536

have posted online and put myself on TOT using black market testosterone. So far, everything has been great.

Do you know of a doctor who would work with me on this, without forcing me to go on a hormonal/emotional roller-coaster just to "prove" that my natural levels are crap, and therefore qualify for a legitimate TOT prescription?

A: This is also a great question, and the folks at CHEKD[695] have provided me with the best answer. You would not need to stop your hormone supplementation. On your initial panel, they will detect you are taking an androgen. They will encourage you and all men in similar situations to be honest and transparent. If they know you are using testosterone, they will continue your TOT without disruption but will modify the protocol (i.e. your dosage) to get all of your numbers within an accepted and healthy range.

CHEKD's Expert Health Providers will want to know what you were using, for how long, and so on. If you are young (less than 35 years old) and are only using underground AAS, then the doctors will have you stop using AAS and do an HPTA stimulation protocol.

Q: What level do you attempt to keep your total testosterone, free testosterone and estradiol numbers at? I know it's all dependent upon an individual's biochemistry and needs, but just curious at where your levels remain on a week to week basis?

A: This question cannot be answered universally. We can paint a broad picture by saying that numbers should typically be within normal lab ranges (along with the absence of symptoms).

---

[695]   www.checkmybloodwork.com

Jay has been very open about his total testosterone lab readings that come from 150 mg of injectable testosterone per week (normally spread out over 2-3 injections, depending on lifestyle convenience). His peak (highest levels) to trough (lowest levels) over a 7-day moving average are normally about 1450 to 720 ng/dL, respectively. What's most important, however, is how one feels in the absence of side effects. We consistently hear from patients about their doctors trying to keep their total testosterone numbers in a 'mystical' but measurable range between X and Y. This is silly. As long as your physician understands the half life of the testosterone delivery system being used, only a super high level (likely over 2200 ng/dL) that is not measured within 24 hours post-injection would be any reason to lower your dosage and measure again.

Q: Can you define the optimal weekly dosage, and also discuss the upper range limit of weekly injectable testosterone dosages to stay within 'therapeutic levels'?

A: There is no such thing. What's optimal for you might not be optimal for me. Again, this is why it's imperative to work with a physician who is skilled at "dialing you in" while you are on TOT. "Normal" injectable dosage ranges are between 80-200 mg per week. The highest dose we have seen progressive physicians use to help a patient stay within accepted total testosterone levels is 250 mg per week. Therapeutic total testosterone levels are somewhere between 650-1500 ng/dL, and that number coincides with the elimination of negative side effects.

Q: Hi Jay and Jim! I'm an emergency room doctor transitioning into Integrative and Functional Medicine (i.e. leaving 'Sick Care'). I see so many well-known doctors who mention starting patients on hCG and an Aromatase Inhibitor when

starting TOT. Can most men receiving TOT do fine in the long term without hCG and Arimidex? To me, extra injections with hCG, on top of taking extra meds, makes compliance and biomarker evaluation more complicated.

A: Thank you for your question! You certainly raise some great points. Most of the progressive physicians in the optimization space will start patients on testosterone first, and then take bloods in 4-6 weeks to get a better idea of what type of estrogen response is taking place before treating it (if necessary). Of course, if the patient comes in with estrogen levels that require immediate action via treatment (normally with an aromatase inhibitor (AI) as the standard front line therapy), a conservative dosing approach with regular blood work is advised.

With **hCG**, it depends entirely on the needs of the patient. This means that if the patient desires fertility, starting with **hCG** may be the best course. If fertility is not a desire, starting the patient on testosterone and getting a baseline for blood work could be advantageous to see if **hCG** adds real-life value to the patient's TOT or not. Also, in regards to AI medications, the newest research - cited throughout this book - shows that they can wreak havoc on bone mineral density (BMD). We believe these medications should be used on rare occasions as a last resort. If they must be used, the minimum effective dosage (MED) principle should be applied with the immediate goal of weaning the patient off the AI as soon as a therapeutic level of estrogen (E2) (in the absence of symptoms) is attained.

Q: I wonder if you guys can offer your input on the relationship between TOT and obstructive sleep apnea.

A: We already discussed this in Chapter 12, but it bears repeating. We think the connection between obstructive sleep apnea and testosterone has to do with the tendency to gain water weight on testosterone, especially when estradiol levels are not properly controlled. Normally, this affects a small number of people. It also occurs in men with too much body fat. As we've stated multiple times in the book, reducing body fat will always improve EVERYTHING in relation to health, fitness and extending your life.

Q: I wanted to get your take on an aspect of my TRT that my physician seems to lack knowledge in. For the past 2 years, I was on 160 mg of testosterone cypionate (80 mg on Sunday, 80 mg on Thursday). I was also prescribed 0.25 mg of Anastrozole for use alongside each shot, but we discontinued it because we found that it dropped my sensitive E2 levels too low.

Then, my hematocrit levels seemed to jump up into the 51-ish percent range, so I began donating blood every 56 days. That didn't seem to regulate my hematocrit levels in the long run, so my physician slowly dialed back my testosterone dose, where it is now at 50 mg on Sunday and 50 mg on Thursday. My hematocrit levels seem to still be creeping up every 2 months, and now I am barely under the limit for where the Red Cross will allow you to donate blood.

Do you have any suggestions on how to keep hematocrit levels under control without having to do blood donations every 9 weeks for someone like me that appears to be more susceptible to polycythemia? I really don't want to drop my testosterone dose any lower.

A: This is a great question! The answer is found in Chapter 12, with a thorough explanation provided by **Dr. Rob Kominiarek** on understanding the difference between polycythemia and erythrocytosis. However, your question is worthy of answering in relation to your specific points.

First of all, your doctor (like most on this issue) is confused. It is not polycythemia vera, but erythrocytosis that is causing your hematocrit levels to increase. This is actually a good thing because you are increasing the oxygenated blood supply available to your body.

There are 3 things you can do.

- Increase the FREQUENCY (not the dosage amount) of your injectable testosterone dose to daily or every-other-day shots (i.e. NOT your total weekly testosterone dosage, that stays the exact same). As a result, each individual dose will be smaller.

- Improve your cardiovascular efficiency and drop body fat. Do steady state cardio at a heart rate of 125-140 BPM (i.e. low to moderate intensity), 4-7 days a week and 30-45 minutes per session.

- Have your platelets measured. Elevated platelets would be a much greater indication that you need to be phlebotomized. If there is no platelet elevation, besides following the first two steps, DO NOTHING as your levels are well within normal ranges (i.e. safe and healthy) as already discussed by **Dr. Kominiarek** in Chapter 12.

We would also ask you about how you are feeling.

If you are tired, sluggish, and feel out of breath, then that *may* be a sign of your blood thickening and a good indication that you should consider donating blood.

We can't blame your doctor here, as very few physicians understand this situation because it involves science that is currently being developed. Much of the accepted practices regarding phlebotomy are based off incorrect interpretations of past misunderstandings.

Dr. Neil Rouzier has research data he collected from his patients, and based on that data, he does not phlebotomize patients with hematocrit values under 55% when there is no corresponding elevation in blood platelets. As stated in the book with **Dr. Rob Kominiarek's** explanation in Chapter 12, if you feel fine when your hemoglobin levels are under 22 and hematocrit levels are under 54%, there are no conclusive studies indicating the need for therapeutic phlebotomy (as long as your physician is also checking your platelets for a corresponding elevation).

Q: What is your take on SARMs (Selective Androgen Receptor Modulators)? Are any of them truly worth using instead of TOT? What about in combination?

A: While there are numerous 'Fit Bros' and 'Underground Bodybuilding Board Gurus' who claim otherwise, we have read all of the research pertaining to this question. In comparison to TOT, the answer is an unequivocal NO. Not a chance, actually.

The use of typical SARMs such as Ostarine (there are many others that will go unmentioned) will not fix declining testosterone levels. Talking to many users from the underground fitness scene, it's a split decision where some people 'might have gotten an effect', while others claim adverse reactions or none at all. However, most of these men are using SARMs in a cyclical fashion and have no idea what is happening to their estrogen and testosterone levels while using them. The majority of these users are also NOT drawing proper labs to evaluate their biomarkers, nor are they working with physicians. If you have suboptimal hormone levels and have attempted to maximize them with proper lifestyle habits, then the best way to get optimized is with TOT.

Q: Is there hope for 30+ year olds who want to reach and maintain optimal testosterone levels without TOT? I think it's really hard to keep +800 ng/dL naturally at this age. Do you think it's possible if all of your lifestyle factors are optimized, or is it really just a case of trying to fix something that inevitably goes down hill (and TOT is thereby the best option for lifelong testosterone optimization)?

A: There are genetic components, and certainly an onslaught of environmental factors involved in trying to speculate if you will have your testosterone levels within an acceptable range at 30 years old. As we've clearly explained in this book, due to living in large populated areas, most male endocrine systems are under siege on a daily basis from environmental contaminants. As you get older, the ultimate way to fight the natural decline of your hormonal systems is through TOT with a progressive doctor who has a broad experiential based practice. There are some men (few, we might add) who can stay above 700 ng/dL of total testosterone and maintain high levels of free testosterone into their 50's. However, most men will feel the inevitable decline by ages 40 and up. And some men will experience it even sooner.

We highly recommend you optimize all the lifestyle factors that you can, and don't focus so much on hard numbers. If you are not experiencing negative symptoms, you are probably in the generally accepted total testosterone ranges of **500-900 ng/dL.** With that said, we strongly recommend you track your testosterone levels every year and see if you can identify a linear decline over time.

At 30 years old, if you don't have any negative symptoms present, simply get your hormone levels checked once a year and keep track of them that way. Of course, if you have low numbers AND the negative symptoms, then some type of intervention is warranted. Whether it's lifestyle changes (such as reducing cortisol, lowering body fat and improving adherence to proper nutrition and resistance training, etc.), or some type of clinical intervention (such as hormone optimization), do it NOW!

Most men today will see a decline in hormone levels, and a great majority of them will have symptoms that justify some type of correction. For most of those men, TOT becomes a lifelong solution for maintaining optimal levels of health.

Q: Can you provide advice for folks in the UK, where this type of medicine is perceived as legally selling 'steroids' (versus a perspective of well-being and anti-aging)?

A: This manual arms you with the information needed to have those types of conversations with healthcare providers. We highly recommend you have them read this book! There is more and more evidence accumulating on a daily basis which shows that out-of-range hormone levels represent a REAL global health risk[696]. As always, I would approach this subject with the end goal of preventing various disease processes.

When meeting with a clinician (physician), it is always advisable to print out the studies that you will base your arguments on. That way, you can make a clear and concise case for using TOT. Remember that these people are extremely busy! Therefore, if you don't make a great case in front of them with your claims backed up and available at that exact moment, you greatly decrease your chances of opening their minds on this subject. It is our opinion that within 10 years, TOT will be a widely

---

[696] Hagai Levine, Niels Jørgensen, Anderson Martino-Andrade, Jaime Mendiola, Dan Weksler-Derri, Irina Mindlis, Rachel Pinotti, Shanna H Swan; Temporal trends in sperm count: a systematic review and meta-regression analysis, Human Reproduction Update, Volume 23, Issue 6, 1 November 2017, Pages 646–659.

accepted practice, even in areas where it's currently viewed as 'fringe' (most of Europe and Asia).

Q: What's your take on long term risks vs. benefits going into one's 40s/50s/60s?

A: If you have a clinical need for TOT, not being on it and suffering the inevitable decline of your testosterone levels is far worse than feeling optimized and 'being unaware' of the long-term risks (if any). Would you rather get old and suffer, due to the fear of the unknown? It's not a good way to live your life!

Q: Free testosterone vs total testosterone for assessment: my free testosterone levels have dropped (-65% due to SHBG doubling), much more than my total testosterone levels (-35%) over the last 4 years. Are there any specific lifestyle recommendations you'd make to help reverse this?

A: Lose body fat, improve diet and exercise (via resistance and cardiovascular training). Fix everything naturally first via optimizing your lifestyle factors, and then medicate with TOT once all lifestyle factors are accounted for.

Q: I know 200 mg/mL injectable testosterone weekly is pretty common, but I'm on 100 mg/mL a week. If I want to know what gauge I should use to determine the dosage, would it be just "how I feel'?

A: Essentially, yes. It comes down to regular blood work in combination with how you feel. Two primary goals of TOT are to balance the ratio between testosterone and estrogen, and improve one's happiness. Happiness is defined as "I feel great, full of energy ready to take on the world."

Q: Is there a natural way to produce extra testosterone? I'm in my 50's now and would like to increase my libido. I'm wondering if there is a safe way to raise my testosterone levels?

A: Not really. If all your lifestyle factors are dialed in and you are genetically blessed, you can likely stay in mid-range until 40. But after that it's a downhill road, especially if you're living in densely populated areas (due to the environmental siege brought on by endocrine-disrupting chemicals).

Q: How do I find a reputable TRT clinic/physician in my area? What should I be looking for?

A: Great question. Look for an experiential-based practice. The physician should have a documented record of working with multiple patients (ideally hundreds), both males and females. Asking them if they've read our book will help too. If you've read the first book and this updated version, you will be fully educated, and be able to ask them the necessary questions. Remember to use the 10 questions found in Chapter 8, under "Vetting Your TOT Doctor."

Q: I had a great follow up with Defy's Dr. Justin Saya yesterday. I'm going to be switching to daily intramuscular (IM) injections with a 29-gauge, 0.5 inch syringe. I'm looking for injection sites to rotate. Any suggestions on which sites I can rotate on a daily basis?

A: Another good question. When considering the possibility of undergoing injectable TOT for the remainder of your life, remember that you'll be poking a lot of holes in your body. As such, understanding how to inject yourself with small gauge needles is definitely a learned art form. It takes time and practice, and you definitely want to make sure you minimize injection scarring. You should consider the upper arms (tricep/delt area), the lateral (outside) side of the quads, the outer glute and the lower abs (for those who are able to effectively inject subcutaneously). We demonstrate all of these injection locations in TOT University[697].

Q: I'm an older gentleman (just turned 63) and have never used testosterone in my life. I've probably been suffering from a deficiency for 20 years or so. Is it going to take me longer at my age to get dialed in (i.e. achieve an optimal balance between testosterone and estrogen) than it would if I had started TOT sooner?

A: Thank you for your question. We're really glad you made the decision to become proactive. It's never too late to optimize your health. As long as you don't suffer from any other unknown or unusual health problems, and work with a progressive & experienced physician who is skilled at working with patients like you, it should not take longer than 3-4 months to get you fully dialed in. And quite honestly, if you're severely deficient in testosterone, you should see noticeable improvements within a couple of weeks in your cognition, mood, sex drive and energy.

Q: I was recently diagnosed with Klinefelter's syndrome at the age of 24. My doctor is recommending I start TOT, but I would like to try and preserve my fertility at the same time. What are my best options?

A: Klinefelter's syndrome is the most common form of primary hypogonadism (Class 1), where men are unable to produce

---

[697]   www.TRTUniversity.com

sperm or sufficient levels of testosterone. Normally, men diagnosed with your condition become infertile, as the extra X chromosome affects your ability to produce sperm. The good news is that most studies show TOT being effective in allowing for a normal and productive life (improved cognition, normal fertility, enhanced sense of well being)[698]. There are also studies supporting specialised fertility techniques, such as microsurgical testicular sperm extraction and intracytoplasmic sperm injection[699], that have helped some men with Klinefelter's syndrome to father children. Also, make sure you are working with a physician who is experienced in working with men who are diagnosed with Klinefelter's.

Q: Thank you for taking the time to read this. I have read your TOT Bible, The Metabolic Blowtorch Diet, listened to most of the TOT Revolution podcasts, and been on TOT for about two months.

Against your recommendation, I began TOT with a body fat percentage of about 24%. My blood work prior to beginning TOT showed signs of subclinical hypothyroidism with a 9 TSH but normal T3 & T4. Full list of what I am taking: testosterone, HCG, Anastrozole, multivitamin, DHEA, vitamin D, whey protein, and the IC-5. I am endomorphic.

As I look to incorporate the Blowtorch diet, would you suggest I stick with intermittent fasting on training days until I get around 20%, then begin feeding on training days? Or, should I

---

[698] Serum Testosterone and Cognitive Function in Ageing Male: Updating the Evidence. Recent Pat Endocr Metab Immune Drug Discov. 2016;10(1):22-30.

[699] Sperm recovery and ICSI outcomes in Klinefelter syndrome: a systematic review and meta-analysis. Corona G, Pizzocaro A, Lanfranco F, Garolla A, Pelliccione F, Vignozzi L, Ferlin A, Foresta C, Jannini EA, Maggi M, et al. Hum Reprod Update. 2017 May 1; 23(3):265-275.

begin with the max fat loss protocol and still feed on training days now?

A: Great question. If you are not a newbie to training, we would do the diet as normal but reduce carbs significantly by 3PM on training days. Obviously, because you are an endomorph, your carbs need to be greatly reduced anyways. Make sure you are doing your cardio 2x per day on fasting days. We would also recommend you fast at least 18 hours (or longer preferably) on your fasting days. Also, no heavy meals after 8PM on long fasting days. Try to make them mostly fat and protein. We love casein protein, almond butter, MCT oil and cinnamon blended together in a shake. We also recommend you ask your doctor to prescribe you Metformin and dessicated thyroid.

Q: Thanks for your book and podcasts! Just a quick question concerning your emphasis in some of the podcasts on the destruction that the toxins in our environment have on the endocrine system. If one was to optimize their hormonal levels synthetically, would they still have to worry about the various toxins in the environment (and in food), or not as much?

Should they still be avoided as much as possible if one is fully optimized? I just don't see how it is possible to avoid the bombardment of toxins without spending fortunes on grass fed meat, personal care products made from natural ingredients, filtered water, or going outside! Even then, who knows how much we are still exposed to? Do you still avoid the toxins as much as possible by eating organic foods, grass fed beef and whatever else, or is it not as big of a deal provided you combat the toxin-induced effects with medications/ supplements (i.e. being hormonally optimized)?

A: This is a great question and your insights are correct. In a world which is increasingly harmful, not only to human beings but all forms of life, hormonal optimization is the best course of action to protect yourself. Consider it a fail safe against the daily bombardment to our endocrine systems. Furthermore, if one has the means to afford it, we still recommend taking further precaution by eating organic and/or grass fed meat and wild caught fish where possible. Also, using the preferred supplements and ancillary medications found inside this book will only further improve your results. We believe as time goes on, we will have research to verify the diseases created by these environmental toxins. Therefore, consider hormonal optimization as one part of your overall strategy to limit your exposure to them.

TOT Resources

Even though it can be confusing to sift through the information found on the web about testosterone, allow us to point you in the right direction to excellent websites, books and podcasts providing helpful information and answers to commonly asked questions regarding TOT.

TOTRevolution.com/Testosterone-replacement -therapy-resources

PRIVATE CONSULTING

If you take a look at the most impressive physiques in the world, whether as a weekend warrior or an athlete competing at the highest level, they all have one thing in common:

A professional, qualified coach who helps them dial in their nutrition, training and competitive mindset.

They don't waste time or bang their heads against the wall trying to figure out everything all by themselves. They leave all the hard thinking and decision-making to somebody else, so they can do the one thing they're supposed to do: Consistently execute the plan that is known to WORK!

If you want someone to guide you through your fitness and hormonal optimization journey, you can personally work with

*http://www.trtrevolution.com/testosterone-replacement-therapy-resources/

us 1-on-1. We will provide you with EVERYTHING YOU NEED, completely customized to your body type and goals.

Visit www.TOTRevolution.com/coaching to find out more. It might be the best decision you will ever make for optimizing your lifelong health!

ABOUT THE AUTHORS
Jay Campbell and Jim Brown

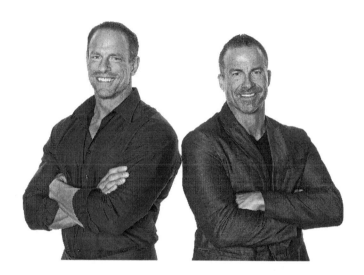

Jay Campbell is the Amazon best-selling author of *The Definitive Testosterone Replacement Therapy MANual: How to Optimize Your Testosterone for Lifelong Health and Happiness,* a 17-year TOT patient and a respected thought leader on hormonal optimization. Jay is the founder of TOTRevolution.com and the TOT Revolution Podcast, both of which are the definitive resources for all things testosterone, anti-aging, and life optimization. Jay is also a champion male physique competitor and the co-founder of FabFitOver40.com, the #1 site on the web for people who want high-quality and scientifically backed information on staying fit above 40.

Jim Brown is an elite athlete who began training as a bodybuilder at 13 years old. Over the course of 33 years, he has become knowledgeable in every aspect of body transformation, hormonal optimization and elite performance. Jim is the creator of the Forged Training System, a complete training program allowing for maximal muscle gain with minimal time spent on training[700].

Jay and Jim are the authors of *The Metabolic Blowtorch Diet: The Ultimate Guide for Optimizing Internet Fasting: Burn Fat, Preserve Muscle, Enhance Focus and Transform Your Health*[701]. Jay and Jim, in partnership with visionary entrepreneur Joshua Smith, are also the co-owners of OptimizedLifeNutrition. com (OLN), which produces the world's most powerful OTC nootropic supplement E-M-F (Energy Memory Focus). OLN offers a unique line of supplements that are essential for living a hormonally balanced and fully optimized life. They also offer *90 Days To Optimized*, a revolutionary lifestyle improvement program that's available online[702]. Jay and Jim also write for Iron Man Magazine as the Fitness Over 40 Experts.

---

[700] AdvancedForgedTraining.com

[701] http://www.metabolicblowtorchdiet.com/

[702] www.optimizedlifenutrition.com

The Science Team

Dr. Jim Meehan CEO of BodMd.com

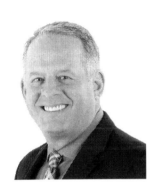 Dr. Meehan is not your typical doctor. Before his career in medicine, he was an award winning West Point cadet, medical sales executive, and entrepreneur. He's also a 5th degree black-belt in TaeKwonDo, NAGA World Jiu Jitsu Champion, and 2013 "Living Legend" inductee into the Martial Arts Masters Hall of Fame.

Dr. Meehan has advanced training in ophthalmology, medical informatics, functional medicine, interventional endocrinology, and nutrition. He is an expert in pain management, addiction medicine, diagnostic laboratory services, toxicology, pharmacogenetics, and the business of medicine. He created the Meehan Protocol™ for male hormone replacement and invented the MINDSET™ Wellness Operating System.

With these tools, he restores the health and lives of patients suffering from pain and addiction. His programs have helped thousands of patients optimize their health as well as reduce and eliminate their dependence on dangerous drugs.

Despite all of his accomplishments, he will tell you that his greatest joys come from his service to Christ, 26 years of devotion to his beautiful wife Cathy, raising five amazing children and watching them find their paths and purpose in the world, and enjoying every possible moment with his grandson Isaiah.

Dr. John Crisler

Founder of AllthingsMale.com and DrJohnCrisler.com

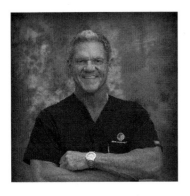

17 years ago, Dr. John Crisler pioneered the use of therapeutic testosterone to treat age related symptoms in men. Dr. Crisler is a world renowned expert on testosterone optimization therapy (TOT), having created several treatment protocols which have changed the way physicians everywhere care for their patients.

Today, physicians throughout the world rely on his expertise and training, and men and women accepted into his practice benefit from the most experienced care available. There are good reasons why men have travelled to be seen by him from every state, as well as dozens of foreign countries: "Dr. John" successfully treats the tough cases.

Realizing the need for a short yet comprehensive explanation to help his colleagues learn how to administer testosterone replacement therapy, he wrote the first version of "TRT: A Recipe for Success" in 2004. It showed how to provide, start to finish, optimum treatment for hypogonadism. It wasn't long before it became the most highly read paper in the history of the field of endocrinology.

Dr. Crisler can assist you and your doctor in fine tuning your prescriptions by offering advice via telephone consultation too. Call 1-517-485-4424 for more information.

Dr. Robert Kominiarek

Founder of RenueHealth.com, AmericasFitnessDoctor.com, AlphaMaleInstitute.com

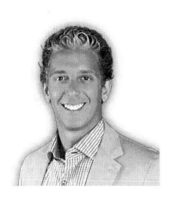

Dr. Rob Kominiarek D.O., FACOFP, is a board certified, Fellow of the American College of Osteopathic Family Physicians. Dr. Rob is a graduate of the Nova-Southeastern University, College of Osteopathic Medicine in Fort Lauderdale, Florida. He completed his residency training at Ohio University, Grandview Hospital and Medical Center in Dayton, Ohio. Dr. Rob is a medical advisor and director to emergency medical services, police departments and radio and television shows across the country. Dr. Rob is a veteran of the United States Army and is a best-selling author with a passion directed towards overall health of the mind and body through proper eating habits, regular exercise, appropriate supplementation, and the intelligent optimization of hormones when clinically indicated.

Dr. Rob Kominiarek D.O., FACOFP received his certification in Age Management Medicine with the nationally renowned Cenegenics Medical Institute. Cenegenics' certification in Age Management Medicine is jointly sponsored by Cenegenics Education and Research Foundation (CERF) and the Foundation for Care Management in Las Vegas, Nevada. CERF and the Foundation for Care Management are accredited with honors by seven sponsoring organizations, including the American

Medical Association and the American Board of Medical Specialties. Dr. Kominiarek is additionally certified in Advanced Bio Identical Hormone Replacement Therapy and regularly lectures for the Age Management Medical Group.

"Optimum health is no accident. It is the reward for taking a preventative and proactive approach towards your personal health. We at ReNue Health® have assembled some of the most advanced, comprehensive services available today and a responsive, dedicated staff who understand your goals and needs. You deserve nothing less. I have no financial conflicts of interest or ties to any pharmaceutical company. My only objective is determining the most effective, safest therapy for my patients. My mission is to engage my patients in the active pursuit of optimal health and to provide personalized superior care with an emphasis on preventive medicine, hormone optimization, and healthy aging."

Dr. Rob is an avid athlete who enjoys cycling, swimming, triathlons, soccer, tennis, soaring, skiing, Italian motorcycles, and automobile racing. He is a dedicated father who believes in practicing what he preaches, and as such lives a lifestyle dedicated towards healthy living and regular exercise.

Dr. H. Merrill Matschke

Board Certified Urologist. Fellowship trained expert in Andrology/Men's Sexual Health & Wellness, BetterLifeCarolinas.com

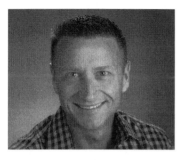

Dr. Matschke is a 15-year board-certified urologist in the Chicago area who recently left the "Sick Care Health Care" model to partner with Dr. Mickey Barber at BetterLifeCarolinas.com in the field of Preventative Medicine and Clinical Wellness.

He completed his medical degree and residency training in Urological Surgery from Northwestern University Feinberg School of Medicine. Dr. Matschke was then awarded a fellowship in Male Reproductive Medicine and Surgery with Dr. Larry Lipshultz at Baylor College of Medicine in Houston, TX. In practice for more than 15 years, Dr. Matschke has focused on the surgical and medical treatment of male sexual health and infertility, while serving to educate providers and patients on the benefits of optimal testosterone supplementation. He has lectured extensively on TOT throughout the country, speaking to both physicians and patients. Dr. Matschke received his certification in Age Management Medicine through the nationally renowned Cenegenics Medical Institute.

Dr. Matschke fully endorses the concept of optimized healthy living to avoid utilization of the "Sick Care" system. He strives to empower clients to invest in their health, with the ultimate goal of living a vigorous, healthy life at any age. He welcomes all clients interested in maximizing their healthspan to join him at BetterLifeCarolinas.com. He can be reached at the following:

@MatschkeMD on Twitter and DrMatschke@BetterLifeCarolinas. com. To schedule a consultation, call 843-737-2597.

Aaron Grossman

Founder of CHEKD

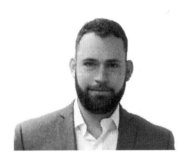

Aaron Grossman, MD is the Founder of CHEKD, America's #1 Optimization & Personalized Health company, helping top performers reach optimal levels of performance.

After graduating medical school at the prestigious University of Florida in 2014, Dr. Grossman jumped right into the entrepreneurial space, growing CHEKD nationally to help NFL & MLB athletes, top realtors, Inc. & Forbes Magazine-featured entrepreneurs, Fortune 500 CEO's, and other renowned physicians reach the top 3% of their fields.

Dr. Grossman has authored and published research in blood biomarkers, robotic surgery, cancer, kidney disease and male health, which has appeared in renowned publications such as the journal of urology.

CHEKD clients are having the best periods of performance in their entire careers after working with CHEKD. His pioneering approach in the fields of hormone, anti-inflammatory & metabolic optimization, incorporated with the latest technology, is setting the part for health optimization and adding actual years to the lives of CHEKD clients.

Shaun Noorian

Founder and CEO Empower Pharmacy

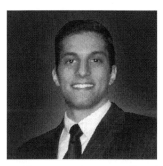

Shaun Noorian is the founder and CEO of Empower Pharmacy, a nationally licensed FDA-registered compounding pharmacy that specializes in compounded health and wellness medications. Shaun holds a degree in mechanical engineering from the University of Texas, and numerous certifications and accreditations in pharmaceutical compounding. He is considered an expert in the field of men's health medicines, medication compounding and pharmaceutical regulations, along with education tailored towards physicians and patients.

After being injured on the job and diagnosed with hypogonadism, Shaun gained his health and vitality back through compounded TOT medications. Not being satisfied with the quality of medications he was receiving through a local compounding pharmacy, Shaun knew he could add value to the industry and others diagnosed with the same condition. By using his background in engineering, manufacturing, and quality control, he now operates one of the nation's largest compounding pharmacies, serving hundreds of thousands of patients across the US.

Knowing all too well what it is like to go through TOT, Shaun finds his joy in helping fellow patients expand their access to quality, affordable medications. You can learn more about the most commonly prescribed men's health compounds at EmpowerPharmacy.com.

The Editing Team

Tom Zakharov

Fitness, Anti-Aging and Health Copywriter

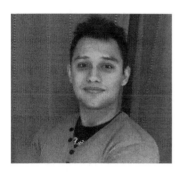 Tom Zakharov is an accomplished Canadian copywriter who has a strong passion for the written word. He has successfully worked with numerous clients across a diverse range of niches, having written virtually every type of copy under the sun.

When he isn't crafting persuasive copy for his clients, he's optimizing his latest high-performance writing strategies. His programs are for writers who want to consistently write more words at faster speeds while improving their overall production. He can be reached at

tom.zakharov@gmail.com or on **Twitter @TomZakharov**

Daniel Kelly,

Writer for TRTRevolution.com, Consultant for BalanceMyHormones.co.uk, Blogger for DanielKelly.eu

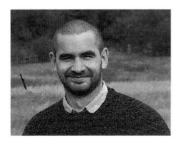

Daniel Kelly is a writer and entrepreneur. He's extremely passionate about men's health & fitness, and began blogging about it to share his passion with the world. What started out as a hobby evolved into a lifelong pursuit.

Daniel is a leading European authority for men under 35 on testosterone replacement therapy, training, mindset and men's health. He strongly believes that health should be your number one priority in life, because without it you are nothing. He also advocates taking responsibility for your own health, and not giving your power away by relying on someone else to look after it. Health is not something that's given to you - it's something you have to work at.

Daniel is a keen traveller and speaks several languages, including French, Spanish, German and Italian. His new companion book *Optimized Under 35: The Ultimate Hormonal Health Guide for Young Men* is due to be released in the middle of 2018. You can find him on his website **DanielKelly.eu** and on **Twitter @ danielkellytrt**

Austin Gunter Author,

Writer, Editor and Blogger
AustinGunter.com

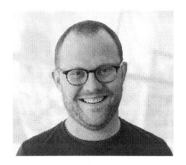

Austin Gunter is an eclectic and renowned San Francisco author who is focused on winning a 20-year battle with severe rheumatoid arthritis (by utilizing the strategies found in this book, of course). He is currently immersed in Taoist meditation, Qi Gong, and Tai Chi while self hacking his way to a fully optimized life.

You can find him on his site at AustinGunter.com, where he writes about hard questions worth asking, particularly when they're painful, require extreme honesty, explore weird parts of our lives, or require us to think dangerous thoughts.

He values connections, culture, and community. When he walks into a room, one of his primary goals is to catalyze the relationships everyone has with one another. This unique skill allowed him to become the master editor of this life changing book. You can also reach him on **Twitter @austingunter**

Alexander Juan Antonio Cortes,

Author and Blogger AlexanderJuanAntonioCortes.com

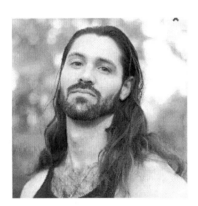

Alexander Juan Antonio Cortes has established a reputation for being an iconoclast in the fitness industry, and with a background as a trained dancer and choreographer, he brings a wholly unique perspective to the field of health and fitness.

Having been a personal trainer for close to a decade, his methods and perspectives on training, nutrition, and health optimization are based on real-world application and experimentation.

He has published hundreds of articles in print (and online) for major websites and publications, along with his own books that cover his training and dietary philosophies. He can be found on his website AT **alexanderjuanantoniocortes.com** or on **Twitter @AJA_Cortes**

A SINCERE REQUEST

The information found inside this book provides a real path to sustainable and fully optimized lifelong health. It can also prevents millions of men and women from suffering from hormone deficiencies.

In order for this book to reach as many people as possible, we're depending on you! Please do us a huge favor and write an honest (preferably 5 STAR)Amazon review. The more reviews it gets, the more this information will help others (just like you) escape from the condition of suboptimal hormonal levels and transform their lives. We are sincerely grateful for the time and effort you put into a writing a thoughtful review.

If you choose to leave us a 5 STAR AMAZON CERTIFIED REVIEW and send Jay an email (jay@trtrevolution.com) with a screenshot once it is uploaded and gets verified, we'll send you two surprise gifts.

BONUS GIFT #1: The EXACT answers doctors should provide when you use the "Questions To Ask Your Doctor" found in Chapter 8 in The TOT Bible.

BONUS GIFT #2: "A Day In The Life Of Jim & Jay" - This jam-packed PDF breaks down EVERYTHING we do on a daily basis. What supplements we take and when, our testosterone protocols, our morning and evening rituals, our training regimens, and more!

Thank you so much for reading *The TOT Bible: The Ultimate Guide to Living a Fully Optimized Life.* We hope you use this information to transform your own life.

To your ultimate health!

Jay and Jim

Made in the USA
Middletown, DE
18 April 2018